**A Contemporary Guide to Practice Management for Physicians, Managers, and Administrators**

Edited by:

Brian K. Iriye

Anthony C. Sciscione

Daniel F. O'Keeffe

© 2018 Brian K. Iriye, Anthony C. Sciscione, and Daniel F. O'Keeffe
All rights reserved.

ISBN: 0692994432
ISBN-13: 9780692994436

# Table of Contents

Introduction: Practice Management for the Maternal-Fetal Medicine (MFM) Subspecialist ... v

Chapter 1: The New System of Women's Health Care—2020 ... 1

Chapter 2: Management Structure for Successful Hospital-, Private-, and University-Owned Practices ... 21

Chapter 3: The Role of the MFM Subspecialist as a Medical Neighbor ... 25

Chapter 4: How Physicians Can Become Involved in Health-Care Changes ... 37

Chapter 5: The New Story of MFM Practice Leadership ... 49

Chapter 6: Physician Recruitment, Engagement, and Retention ... 65

Chapter 7: How to Set Up a New Associate in Your Practice ... 71

Chapter 8: Common Personnel Issues That Require Expertise in HR Management ... 77

Chapter 9: The Importance of Evidence-Based Medicine, Value, and Protocols in the MFM Practice ... 85

Chapter 10: How to Operate an Efficient Outpatient Ultrasound Practice ... 93

Chapter 11: Utilization of Advanced Practitioners in MFM—Nurse Practitioners, Nurse Midwives, and Genetic Counselors ... 103

Chapter 12: Physician Assistants in the MFM Practice ... 111

Chapter 13: Improving Clinical Process Efficiency within Your MFM Practice ... 117

Chapter 14: Performance Indicators for MFM Practices ... 139

Chapter 15: A Guide to Marketing Your MFM Business ... 163

Chapter 16: Contract Negotiations for MFM Subspecialists 101 ... 181

Chapter 17: Accounts Receivable Management / Accounts Collections ... 195

Chapter 18: Coding and Auditing Your Practice — 205

Chapter 19: Benchmarking Provider Work and Coding — 215

Chapter 20: Planning Your Office Space — 233

Chapter 21: Electronic Health Records / Practice Management Selection—A Guide to Making the Right Choice for Your Practice — 247

Chapter 22: Information Technology for Your Practice — 253

Chapter 23: Phone Systems and Service — 267

Appendix 1: Miscellaneous Employee Forms and Employee Manual — 273

Appendix 2: Common Employee Description Forms for the Medical Office — 301

Appendix 3: Patient Office Forms — 337

List of Contributors — 347

# Introduction

## Practice Management for the Maternal-Fetal Medicine (MFM) Subspecialist

Brian K. Iriye, MD

Practice management is the frequently ignored domain related to the improvement of clinical medical care. Often not discussed until problems arise and frequently overlooked until adversity affects the office, a poorly managed practice will have a negative impact on medical care. In contrast, a well-run and efficient practice will increase the likelihood of providing superior outcomes and better medical care. Our hope is that you have obtained this book to increase your knowledge of practice management principles prior to the onset of problems within your practice rather than after problems have occurred. Nonetheless, education in the field of practice management is sorely needed, as this knowledge is not imparted by the vast majority of training programs; graduates from maternal-fetal medicine (MFM) fellowships will almost universally agree that they are taught very little about practice management over the seven years of their residency and fellowship[1].

Unfortunately, a financially distressed practice, an office lacking in leadership, and a workplace with deficits in emotional intelligence will all handicap providers' ability to give their patients superior care. Members of the Society for Maternal-Fetal Medicine (SMFM) and of other medical societies often rely on the advice of other physicians to improve their management decisions but find few places to obtain that knowledge from their past training institutions. A mentor for clinical or research advice often simply does not possess training, experience, or education in practice management, so many MFM subspecialists are left without an adviser to depend on.

In constructing this book, the editors and authors hope to provide the reader with an educational and instructional path in running a practice—preferring you to enjoy initial success rather than have to learn primarily from your mistakes. Regardless of the practice type, the major principles are the same in almost every environment, whether university or hospital-based, company-owned, or private practice. Additionally, although this book is written by experts in MFM, the advice provided applies to many practice types in other medical fields. To think that the major principles are different dismisses the actual realities present in the modern health-care system, thus stifling the promotion of change and causing unnecessary delay in action.

The first *Maternal-Fetal Medicine Practice Handbook*, published by the SMFM in 2004, provided a wealth of information for the MFM subspecialist. At that time, practice management was discussed in general, but most providers did not fully appreciate the business aspect of a practice. Prior to 2004, health-maintenance organizations (HMOs) created an initial upheaval in

---

[1] Porter B, Iriye B, Ghamsary M. Maternal-fetal medicine physician and fellow perceptions of business in medicine. Am J Perinatol 2018 Jan; 35(1): 90-94.

payment and practice management. During the '80s and early '90s, private insurer premiums rose between 15 and 20 percent per year. The concept of managed care was a response to these increasing costs. The initial formation of HMOs and managed care temporarily reduced the healthcare spending curve by means of physician fee cuts, utilization controls via authorization, and the management of hospital stays and admissions. But the instruments of realizing these cost reductions created ill will among patients and physicians alike. Providers began to look at practice management as a means of keeping wages stable via governing their practices with some improvements in efficiency and business management. Whether the influence of HMOs eventually decreased because of political and media backlash or due to the tight labor market of the late '90s that claimed the initial life of managed care, the idea that practices should be managed became part of traditional practice philosophy.

Although practice environments differ, management philosophies in the medical field are relatively stable and universal. You may be joining a practice straight out of your fellowship or leading a university department as chair or department head. Alternatively, you may join an established hospital-owned practice or form a hospital-based practice where services previously did not exist. You may be contemplating starting your own practice or joining a corporate-owned entity. In all the above circumstances, it is imperative that you understand the practice conditions and ramifications of each decision. It is our goal that you will gain the knowledge to succeed in these seemingly diverse environments; although they may seem quite different, their management principles are abundantly similar.

Overall, the guiding rule in all medicine is "best care wins"—for the physician, the practice, and, most important, the patient—but the corollary should be that "superior practice management helps provide the best care." The management of the financial segment of a practice has a major effect on the level of patient care the practice provides through their ability to make equipment purchases, to maintain provider happiness through a reasonable workload and vacation times, to fund the performance of research, and to acquire and maintain a happy and exemplary ancillary staff.

The Medical Group Management Association (MGMA) annually looks at the traits of practices that are "better performers." Practices categorized as better performers are more likely to have spent money on equipment purchases and information technology in the previous twelve months, utilized advanced practitioners, performed practice surveys, and possessed incentivized compensation plans. An examination of ultrasound equipment alone provides evidence of care and an MFM practice's financial health.

Moore's law is the theory that computer processor speeds will double every eighteen months. Ultrasounds function as highly specialized computers. If processor speed doubles every eighteen months, then an upgraded ultrasound can theoretically double in frame rate or dramatically increase pixel density every eighteen months. Faster frame rates smooth real-time picture quality, while pixel density increases picture quality as well making a normal picture high definition (HD) or closer to "retina" quality. Moore's law tells us that six-year-old equipment can possibly be sixteen times slower, thus resulting in lower-quality images and reduced diagnostic capability. The average high-end ultrasound machine costs approximately $100,000 as of 2018, and service agreements cost $15,000–$20,000 per year. Clearly, having financial stability can improve your practice diagnostics.

The US Patient Protection and Affordable Care Act (PPACA) of 2010 has been the most recent impetus to cause large modifications in American health-care delivery. Although the two-thousand-page PPACA has many provisions, a major influence has been a push toward value care. Briefly, value care is defined as cost-efficient care that yields improved outcomes and patient experience. Wherever you stand on the law and its potential positive or negative effects, it is undoubtedly forcing changes toward increasing provider efficiency while trying to maintain or improve patient outcomes. This upheaval in the US health-care system is rewarding those who are trying to work with the new system. Providers and practices who resist the change run the risk of being bypassed while system changes are put in place. It is important that all providers have a working understanding of a few practice management principles to help them provide a group atmosphere that will promote optimal patient outcomes with reduced cost.

Within this book we have attempted to involve authors with expertise in many areas of practice management. No matter what level of knowledge you have in practice management, you should find much useful information throughout these pages and should learn new strategies that will help improve your practice. Reading through a chapter and realizing that you are already implementing much of what the author advises will lead to reassurance and confidence that you are doing many things well, which is also a bonus. Continually updating your knowledge of practice management principles and implementing change within your practice will both offer you not only tools for survival in a changing time, but also hope for further practice success while simultaneously providing an optimal environment for superior patient care.

# 1

## The New System of Women's Health Care—2020

### David C. Lagrew Jr., MD

One of the most appealing and challenging aspects of modern medicine is the presence of constant transformation, including provocative new discoveries, changing methods for practice and payment, and evolving roles of the practicing physician. Few physicians would say that practicing medicine today resembles how it was practiced at the time they started. In general, humans are averse to change; fortunately, most people who choose medical careers possess an underlying curiosity, an interest in learning new techniques, and a desire to improve the care they render. Unfortunately, the current (as of 2018) changes in health-care reform involve the relatively mundane parts of practice (such as payment methods, documentation tools, or quality measures) that even the most adventuresome struggle to find interesting. Regardless of our feelings, changes in the health-care sector will continue in an exponentially rapid fashion; to remain successful we must understand, accept, and adapt to this new world of health care.

We can draw from the experience of other industries that have gone through large-scale changes. Andrew Grove, former CEO of Intel, has described how nearly all businesses that enjoy long-term success must learn how to go through "inflection points."[1] Grove describes how executives must begin to see that "what worked before doesn't work now." This realization often occurs after a long period of unbroken success. During downward spirals, companies often experience periods marked by unhappy and unengaged workers, runaway costs, inefficient production, high rates of production defects, safety issues for workers, and poor customer satisfaction. Innovative and ultimately successful businesses adapt to these new environments and view these "strategic inflection points" as opportunities for reinvention and reorganization that will lead to further success.[2] Using Grove's definition, it is easy to say that health care has reached a strategic inflection point.

The medical advances of the last several decades have produced medications, treatments, and procedures that have led to amazing miracles for patients, professional and financial success for providers, and more productive workers for businesses. We have truly enjoyed a long period of unbroken success. But these successes are now tainted by skyrocketing costs, increasing rates of chronic diseases, and inconsistent and disparate outcomes based on location, race, and financial status. Our workforce (physicians and other clinicians) are unhappy and unengaged. One group

---

[1] Andrew Grove, *Only the Paranoid Survive* (New York: Doubleday, 1996), 34.
[2] Ibid., 46–48.

has found that 60 percent of physicians wished they had chosen a different profession.[3] We ourselves appear to have reached our inflection point.

To gain this understanding for jumping the inflection point to achieve further success, it is important that we appreciate (1) the reasons that health care is changing and why change is required, (2) the guiding principles that should be utilized for the changes to achieve desired outcomes in health care, (3) an understanding of the types of transitional forces that will be needed, and (4) an acceptance of what we as clinicians will need to do to make these changes and be successful in the new world of medicine. In the field of obstetrics and gynecology, it will be necessary to embrace these changes to improve the health of the women we serve.[4]

## The Reasons for Change

Why is all this change necessary? Most often we seem to have things working pretty well in our office or clinic. We may believe small adjustments and changes are necessary, but on the whole our patients seem to be satisfied and doing well clinically. The pressure for changes seems to be coming from external sources such as the government, third-party payers, medical groups, or hospitals. In many practices, though, subtle but real signs are visible that pressures are coming from within. Stable or decreasing income against rising costs and red tape, difficulty in finding new partners to join and to work reasonable schedules, and narrowing networks from payers that exclude traditional sources of payment are all becoming more common.

What external factors are leading to change? These include a trio of factors that create an almost perfect storm: (1) rapidly rising health-care costs, (2) changing patient demographics, and (3) provider changes.[5] Examining these in some detail will explain much of the reason for the need for change.

### First and Foremost—Cost

Most experts agree that the cost of our current system is not sustainable and often unaffordable for patients, providers, and payers. According to the US Centers for Medicare and Medicaid Services (CMS) National Health Expenditure Projections from 2012–2022, "health spending is projected to grow at an average rate of 5.8 percent," which is 1 percent faster "than expected average growth in the Gross Domestic Product (GDP)." Recently we have seen some slowing, with the sluggish economic recovery from the recession holding this increase to 4 percent; however, "improving economic conditions, Affordable Care Act (ACA) coverage expansions, and the aging of the population" drove an increase in the 2014 rate to over 6 percent.[6] At this current

---

[3] Mark William Friedberg et al., "Factors Affecting Physician Professional Satisfaction and Their Implications for Patient Care, Health Systems, and Health Policy." Rand Corporation / American Medical Association, 2013.

[4] David C. Lagrew Jr. and Todd R. Jenkins, "The Future of Obstetrics/Gynecology in 2020: A Clearer Vision. Why Is Change Needed?" *American Journal of Obstetrics and Gynecology* 211, no. 5 (2014): 470–74.

[5] Ibid., 470–74.

[6] Jason Hockenberry and Kenneth Thorpe, "Slow Health Care Spending Growth Moderates GDP Growth in the Short Term and Policy Targets Should Reflect This." *Health Affairs*. Accessed January 20,2018. http://healthaffairs.org/blog/2014/10/16/health-care-spending-growth-moderates-gdp-growth-in-the-short-term-and-policy-targets-should-reflect-this/.

pace, by 2020, the cost of US health care will reach over 20 percent of GDP despite the changes in the Affordable Care Act, although some evidence shows that the exchanges have held down the double-digit increases in premiums, as evidenced by the California experience.[7] Since some 40 percent of Americans are covered by government-paid insurance (16 percent via Medicaid, 14 percent via Medicare, and 8 percent via government employment[8]), this rising burden of health-care costs is a significant contributor to unsustainable federal deficits[9] and has seized the attention of lawmakers. The Harvard economist and health-care policy specialist David Cutler has posited that "the United States does not have a deficit problem—it has a health care problem."[10] The Congressional Budget Office projects that between 2015 and 2024, the annual budget shortfalls will rise substantially from a low of $469 billion (2015) to around $1 trillion (2022 through 2024), based mainly on the aging population, rising health-care costs, the expansion of federal subsidies for health insurance, and growing interest payments on federal debt.[11]

In the private sector, US businesses, which are already struggling to remain competitive in a global economy, are further challenged by continued inflation in their health-care costs and have recently begun to control their portion by giving employees high-deductible plans. According to the Kaiser Family Foundation, the average annual premium for family coverage rose from $5,845 in 1999 to $18,764 in 2017. While the rate of increase has slowed somewhat since then, the costs have still risen 55 percent since 2007. In addition, the percentage of covered workers with an annual deductible of at least $1000 dollars has increased from 34% in 2012 to 51% in 2017. The cost of high-deductible plans are around $1,100-$2,300 less for a family plan, but the average worker still paid $1,020 for single coverage and $4,599 for a family plan in 2017[12] All these rises lead to the government, businesses, and individuals straining to be able to pay for rising health-care costs.

When compared to other countries, Americans pay far more for coverage without many measurable improvements in clinical outcomes. For businesses, this competitive disadvantage is magnified by the fact that other developed countries either have contained their costs to levels less than 50 percent of American standards or have transferred the cost of health coverage to government-run systems. According to the Organization for Economic Cooperation and Development (OECD), in 2012 the United States spent 2.5 times the amount the average OECD

---

[7] CoveredCA.com, "Health Insurance Companies and Plan Rates for 2016: Keeping the Individual Market in California Affordable." Accessed January 20, 2018. http://www.coveredca.com/PDFs/7-27-CoveredCA-2016PlanRates-prelim.pdf.

[8] US Bureau of Labor Statistics, "The Employment Situation—October 2017." News release. http://www.bls.gov/news.release/pdf/empsit.pdf; Kaiser Family Foundation, "Health Insurance Coverage of the Total Population." Accessed January 20, 2018. http://kff.org/other/state-indicator/total-population/.

[9] Congressional Budget Office, "The Updated Budget Projection: 2014–2024." Accessed January 20, 2018. http://www.cbo.gov/publication/45229.

[10] John Ydstie, "Reining in Health Care Costs Key to Trimming Deficit." National Public Radio. Accessed January 20, 2018. www.npr.org/2014/02/06/272349662/reining-in-health-care-costs-key-to-trimming-deficits.

[11] Congressional Budget Office, "The Updated Budget Projection: 2014–2024."

[12] Kaiser Family Foundation, "Employer Health Benefits 2017 Annual Survey." Accessed January 20, 2918.. http://files.kff.org/attachment/Report-Employer-Health-Benefits-Annual-Survey-2017.

country spent on health care. This translates to the United States spending $8,233 per person, compared to an average of $3,268 per person in the OECD countries.[13]

As expected, market forces may have already begun the process of reducing the steady rise of health-care costs with alterations such as the increase of high-deductible plans, increased transparency in quality and costs, and the presence of health-care exchanges (as mentioned above). This situation has led CMS to proceed away from traditional fee-for-service (FFS) payment models to 80 percent being risk-sharing models by 2018.[14] Consumers are also responding because the great recession of 2008 reduced family income and thereby the funds for elective procedures/care, which resulted in a dropping off of these types of care. Companies and insurers responded to the increased costs by introducing more high-deductible plans, which transfer a greater proportion of costs to patients and have prolonged this reduced utilization.[15] Exposed to the out-of-pocket costs, the public is demanding increased transparency, and patients want to be empowered with improved cost data when making their health-care decisions. The health-care exchanges, as provided by the ACA, have also adopted the high-deductible approach in most cases; this change is thought to be a factor in containing insurance costs by disincentivizing utilization and shifting cost to the patient.[16]

It is not clear that the increased cost of health care has led to better outcomes for Americans. In support, some point to us leading the world in health-care research and in cancer care and survival. The United States has the highest survival rates for colorectal and breast cancer.[17] The latter claim is disputable, as discussed by Gilbert Welch, MD, in his book *Overdiagnosed: Making People Sick in the Pursuit of Health*. Dr. Welch points out that overscreening for cancers such as thyroid and breast cancer has led to these claims of better survival, since more cases that would have spontaneously regressed or not led to a cancer death are counted as "survivors." He supports his claims by pointing out that death rates from these cancers have not dropped.[18] Despite these successes, the US health-care system consistently scores poorly on measures of "quality, efficiency, access to care, equity, and the ability to lead long, healthy and productive lives."[19] The Commonwealth Fund ranks the US health-care system last among seven industrialized countries for these measures.[20]

---

[13] OECD, "OECD Health Data 2012: US Health Care System from an International Perspective." Accessed January 20, 2018. http://www.oecd.org/unitedstates/HealthSpendingInUSA_HealthData2012.pdf.
[14] US Department of Health and Human Services, "Federal Register: Medicare and Medicaid Programs; CY 2016 Home Health Prospective Payment System Rate Update; Home Health Value-Based Purchasing." Accessed January 20, 2018. http://www.gpo.gov/fdsys/pkg/FR-2015-07-10/pdf/2015-16790.pdf.
[15] Kaiser Family Foundation, "Health Insurance Coverage of the Total Population."
[16] CoveredCA.com, "Health Insurance Companies and Plan Rates for 2016."
[17] Kaiser Family Foundation, "Health Insurance Coverage of the Total Population."
[18] H. Gilbert Welch, *Less Medicine, More Health: 7 Assumptions That Drive Too Much Medical Care*, 1st ed. (Boston: Beacon Press, 2015), 58–64.
[19] The Commonwealth Fund, "US Ranks Last among Seven Countries on Health System Performance Based on Measures of Quality, Efficiency, Access, Equity, and Healthy Lives." Accessed June 25, 2010. http://www.commonwealthfund.org/Newsletters/The-Commonwealth-Fund-Connection/2010/June-25-2010.aspx.
[20] Ibid.

Given these discussions, many experts, patients, and politicians believe we are not getting a good value for our investment in health care. As a result of these rising costs and questionable value, both government and business leaders are demanding changes to the health-care delivery system and the removal of an estimated $750 billion in medical-care waste.[21] Prominent speakers such as Atul Gawande have suggested that we "shift focus from delivering stuff to delivering outcomes" (to quote the title of one of his keynote speeches) to reduce wasteful and unnecessary care.[22]

## Different Patient Demographics

Several patient demographic factors will influence the volume and type of care provided; these factors include aging, obesity, prior surgeries, and increased population diversity (i.e., race or ethnicity). The most significant demographic change to affect health care is the aging of the US population. An increase in the population of older Americans is occurring because of increased life expectancy and the maturing of the baby-boomer population.[23] In 1970, the United States had 20,065,502 people (9.8 percent) older than sixty-five years of age; this number had increased to 40,228,712 (16.1 percent of the US population) by 2010, and by 2020 it is projected to have grown to 54,804,470. This change will increase the rates of gynecologic conditions such as menopausal issues, pelvic organ prolapse, urinary and fecal incontinence, and cancer.[24] We know from actuarial data that these patients require several times the amount of health-care resources as their younger counterparts.[25] By age eighty, they require nearly twelve times the inpatient charges per capita as compared to forty-year-old patients. This situation will lead to expensive increases in inpatient utilization at an increasing rate until 2020–2022, when the yearly increase will plateau at 0.89 percent, and outpatient increases will similarly occur.[26] In gynecologic care, and all medicine, our own success at preventing and treating infections, cancers, and long-term medical disorders in women of younger ages has increased the life expectancy for US women from 75.6 in 1970 to 80.8 in 2007.

The aging of the population is not just occurring in patients over the age of sixty-five. Societal norms are leading to an increasing number of obstetrical patients with advanced maternal age as women delay childbearing. The average age of first birth in the United States increased from 21.4 in 1970 to 25.0 in 2006. Statistics show that although women in their twenties continue to

---

[21] D. M. Berwick and A. D. Hackbarth, "Eliminating Waste in US Health Care," *Journal of the American Medical Association* 307, no. 14 (2012): 1513–16; Bradley C. Strunk, Paul B. Ginsburg, and Michelle I. Banker, "The Effect of Population Aging on Future Hospital Demand," *Health Affairs* 25, no. 3 (2006): w141–w149.

[22] Atul Gawande, "Atul Gawande: Shift Focus from Delivering Stuff to Delivering Outcomes." American Hospital Association Health Forum, uploaded July 24, 2015. http://www.hhnmag.com/Daily/2015/July/atul-gawande-deliver-outcomes-video-summit-weinstock.

[23] US Census Bureau, Population Division, "Projections of the Population by Age and Sex for the United States: 2010 to 2050 (NP2008-T12)." Accessed August 14, 2008. https://www.acl.gov/sites/default/files/Aging%20and%20Disability%20in%20America/2010profile.xls.

[24] B. C. Strunk, P. B. Ginsburg, and M. I. Banker, "The Effect of Population Aging on Future Hospital Demand," *Health Affairs* 25 (2006): W141–49.

[25] Ibid., W142.

[26] Ibid., W147.

make up the largest number of deliveries, the birth rate is falling in this age group. Over the same time period, deliveries among women older than thirty-five years of age have increased eightfold, making them the most rapidly increasing proportion of delivering mothers by age group.[27] These factors, coupled with the overall aging of the population, have led experts to declare this to be "the age of chronic conditions" such as congestive heart failure, diabetes, hypertension, and hyperlipidemia.[28]

Other factors besides age are leading to complex health-care situations. Dietary and activity changes have led to skyrocketing rates of obesity, which affects rates of women's medical issues such as abnormal uterine bleeding, stress urinary incontinence, or complications arising from more difficult operative procedures.[29] In addition, current practices will change the types of patients we will be seeing in the near future. The effects of the increased cesarean rate of the past few decades have led to a tremendous increase in placental complications and more difficult gynecologic surgeries.[30]

On the positive side, we may see less cervical dysplasia from beneficial therapies such as the HPV vaccination[31] and other new treatments that have led to better control of chronic conditions. Unfortunately, the net effect will still be an increasingly higher risk and a more complex population. This is occurring at a time when those financially responsible are demanding cost containment, so the net effect will be more complex care for reduced reimbursement. In addition, we cannot expect relief from medical legal pressures or patient demand for services. Based on the concept of "overdiagnosis," Dr. Welch also predicts that patients in the future will be more likely to question the need for routine screening and will demand better counseling and education about the risks and benefits.[32]

Another factor is the increasing patient diversity over the last three decades, and this trend has shown no evidence of slowing. The United States of 2050 will be a demographically changed nation from that of today: for example, whites will no longer be in the majority. The US minority population, currently 30 percent of the total population, is expected to exceed 50 percent sometime before 2050. This increased diversity of the population will result in changes in the prevalence of certain diseases in various geographic regions and will challenge providers to learn cultural differences and languages; therefore, the need to understand the unique needs of this

---

[27] J. A. Martin et al., "Births: Final Data for 2010," *National Vital Statistics Reports* 61, no. 1 (2012): 1–71; T. J. Mathews and B. E. Hamilton, "Delayed Childbearing: More Women Are Having Their First Child Later in Life," *National Center for Health Statistics (NCHS) Data Brief* 21 (2009): 1. http://www.cdc.gov/nchs/data/databriefs/db21.pdf.
[28] US Department of Health and Human Services, Health Resources and Services Administration, "Women's Health USA 2010: Life Expectancy." Women's Health USA 2011. Rockville, MD: US Department of Health and Human Services, 2011. http://mchb.hrsa.gov/whusa10/hstat/hi/pages/207le.html.
[29] C. L. Ogden et al., "Prevalence of Childhood and Adult Obesity in the United States, 2011–2012," *Journal of the American Medical Association* 311, no. 8 (2014): 806–14.
[30] E. A. Clark and R. M. Silver, "Long-Term Maternal Morbidity Associated with Repeat Cesarean Delivery," *American Journal of Obstetrics and Gynecology* 205, no. 6 (supplement, 2011): S2–10.
[31] J. Cuzick et al., "Overview of the European and North American Studies on HPV Testing in Primary Cervical Cancer Screening," *International Journal of Cancer* 119, no. 5 (2006): 1095–1101.
[32] Welch, *Less Medicine, More Health*; H. Gilbert Welch, *Overdiagnosed: Making People Sick in the Pursuit of Health*, 1st ed. (Boston: Beacon Press, 2012), 81–83.

patient base—to converse with them and be educated in their language/cultural systems and susceptibilities—will increase.[33]

## New Types of Caregivers / Practice Pattern Changes

Experts also predict a coming doctor shortage in primary care and targeted specialties. The Association of American Medical Colleges (AAMC) has suggested that, despite increased training, "the United States faces a shortage of more than 91,500 physicians by 2020—a number that is expected to grow to more than 130,600 by 2025."[34] This physician shortage is due to the increasing number of patients and the retirement of baby-boomer physicians. One 2015 report has stated that half the physician workforce at that time was over the age of fifty-five, with approximately 250,000 physicians likely to retire by 2020.[35] These potential physician shortages are exacerbated by generational, gender, and regulatory factors. Baby-boomer obstetrician-gynecologists (ob-gyns) trained in an environment that included long work hours, sleep deprivation, and an emphasis on independent practice. This training environment resulted in ob-gyns who practiced in a similar fashion during their career and who were more likely to prioritize work-related activities over home life. They are being rapidly replaced by the millennial generation, who were trained in an environment more focused on adherence to guidelines, a team approach to medicine, and the risks of sleep deprivation. They expect more from their jobs, are more focused on family life, and are more likely to switch jobs frequently.[36]

Women now represent 80 percent of all residents in obstetrics and gynecology and approximately 50 percent of all active ob-gyns,[37] and most women remain the primary caregiver for their children; this has resulted in surveys consistently suggesting that women expect more work-life balance than their male predecessors.[38] The net effect of these generational and gender changes is a workforce who works fewer hours per week and will require greater numbers of workers and/or improved efficiency. This effect is being augmented by the changes to residency training in 2003 and 2011 that have placed significant restriction on work hours.[39] While studies are still forthcoming on their full impact, these changes to residency training, which are meant to reduce errors due to fatigue, have possibly led to other complications, with residents graduating with

---

[33] J. Kotkin, "The Changing Demographics of America: The United States Population Will Expand by 100 Million over the Next 40 Years. Is This Reason to Worry?" *Smithsonian*. August 2010, http://www.smithsonianmag.com/40th-anniversary/the-changing-demographics-of-america-538284/#0RV3oYTWHTJyrTmS.99.

[34] American Association of Medical Colleges, "GME Funding: How to Fix the Doctor Shortage." https://www.aamc.org/newsroom/keyissues/physician_workforce/.

[35] IHS Inc., *The Complexities of Physician Supply and Demand: Projections from 2013 to 2025*. Prepared for the Association of American Medical Colleges (Washington, DC: Association of American Medical Colleges, 2015), 3; Physicians Foundation Inc., *Physicians and Their Practices under Health Care Reform* (2009).

[36] E. Jovic, J. E. Wallace, and J. Lemaire, "The Generation and Gender Shifts in Medicine: An Exploratory Survey of Internal Medicine Physicians," *British Journal of Sociology* 58: 297–316.

[37] W. F. Rayburn, "The Obstetrician Gynecologist Workforce in the United States: Facts, Figures, and Implications 2011," American College of Obstetrician Gynecologists, 2011.

[38] Richard A. Cooper et al., "Economic and Demographic Trends Signal an Impending Physician Shortage," *Health Affairs* 21, no. 1 (2002): 140–54.

[39] R. M. Antiel et al., "Effects of Duty Hour Restrictions on Core Competencies, Education, Quality of Life, and Burnout among General Surgery Interns," *Journal of the American Medical Association Surgery* 148, no. 5 (2013): 448–55.

fewer hours of valuable surgical/clinical experience and increasing errors caused by more frequent patient handoffs.[40]

In addition, nonclinical physician leader roles in medical staff functions, administrative duties, and quality-improvement efforts will be needed to implement and participate in a redesigned system. In a study from Jonathan Lomas and fellow researchers in 1991, the authors showed that workers demonstrated improvement in their case-lowering cesarean rates when educated by strong physician opinion leaders to successfully augment education and protocol changes,[41] and others have outlined the critical role of medical leadership and the need for effective interventions to improve quality of care and to control costs.[42]

## Getting Going in the Right Direction; Finding True North

Focusing on the problems and challenges can be daunting. Fortunately, thought leaders have come up with an excellent guidepost to lead us in the right direction. Dr. Donald Berwick and his colleagues at the Institute for Healthcare Improvement (IHI) have developed a simple description of the primary outcomes desired for future changes. They defined a framework called the Triple Aim that seeks to (1) improve the health of the population, (2) obtain the best experience for the patient, and (3) control costs.[43] By balancing any change or choice against these principles, an innovator or health-care system can improve patient care, satisfy society's goals, and ensure success. Any successful solutions to health-care reform must incorporate all three goals.

Recent history has shown a classic example of care redesign failing because the Triple Aim was not balanced. Health-maintenance organizations (HMOs) flourished during the early 1990s. According to the National Bureau of Economic Research, by 1998, 75 percent of Americans were insured in some form of managed-care plan, and 48 percent were covered by HMOs. These organizations succeeded in reducing health-care spending, with the report suggesting that for every 10 percent of growth in managed care, the country saw a 0.5 percent drop in health-care spending.[44] The strict practices and harsh restrictions of patient choice, however, did not satisfy the second aim of "obtaining the best experience for the patient."[45] Indeed, many argued at the time that cost controlling led to the underutilization of necessary care for patients. These practices led to a severe public backlash and the passage of patient's rights laws that curbed many of these practices, which in turn led to changes that diminished HMOs' abilities to control costs. In

---

[40] S. Sen et al., "Effects of the 2011 Duty Hour Reforms on Interns and Their Patients: A Prospective Longitudinal Cohort Study," *Journal of the American Medical Association Internal Medicine*, 173, no. 8 (2013): 657–62.
[41] J. Lomas et al., "Opinion Leaders vs. Audit and Feedback to Implement Practice Guidelines: Delivery after Previous Cesarean Section," *Journal of the American Medical Association* 265, no. 17 (1991): 2202–27.
[42] Ibid.; D. Blumenthal and A. M. Epstein, "Quality of Health Care, Part 6: The Role of Physicians in the Future of Quality Management," *New England Journal of Medicine* 335, no. 17 (1996): 1328–31.
[43] D. M. Berwick, T. W. Nolan, and J. Whittington, "The Triple Aim: Care, Health, and Cost," *Health Affairs* (Millwood) 27, no. 3 (2008): 759–69.
[44] National Commission on Physician Payment Reform, "Report of the National Commission on Physician Payment Reform," March 2013. http://physicianpaymentcommission.org/wp-content/uploads/2013/03/physician_payment_report.pdf.
[45] Berwick, Nolan, and Whittington, "The Triple Aim," W142.

contrast, research has shown that in certain situations, the medical home model can satisfy all three goals of the Triple Aim by improving the health of the population, improving the patient experience, and containing costs, thus providing a sustainable model of care.[46]

## Transformational Forces: Changes Necessary to Achieve the Triple Aim

What kind of changes are needed to achieve the Triple Aim? What types of innovations, care models to reduce costs, changes that improve a population's health, or methods that maximize the patient/provider experience will help to do this? In an effort to categorize these changes, Todd R. Jenkins and I divided them into four major groupings of transformational forces,[47] which include: (1) payment reform, (2) care system reform, (3) digital conversion of clinical data and health information technology, and (4) disruptive clinical innovations.[48] These forces are additive and complementary to one another in improving health care. Each of the transformational forces contains certain "disruptive ideas" that, particularly if enacted simultaneously, should improve care and accelerate improvement.[49] (See figure 1.1[49])

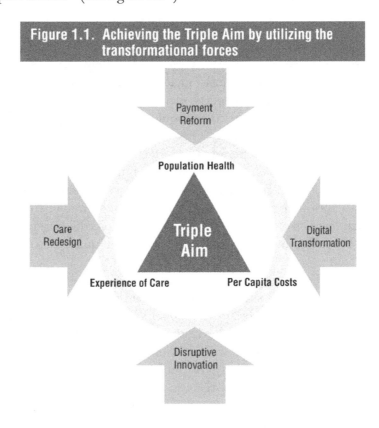

Figure 1.1. Achieving the Triple Aim by utilizing the transformational forces

---

[46] M. E. Domino et al., "Enhancing the Medical Homes Model for Children with Asthma," *Medical Care* 47, no. 11 (2009): 1113–20.
[47] D. C. Lagrew Jr. and T. R. Jenkins, "The Future of Obstetrics/Gynecology in 2020: A Clearer Vision; Finding True North and the Forces of Change," *American Journal of Obstetrics and Gynecology* 211, no. 6 (2014): 617–22.
[48] Ibid.
[49] Ibid.

## Force 1—Payment Reform: Transitioning Away from Fee-for-Service Medicine to Value-Based Care

Changing away from a FFS model ensures that providers will be incentivized and aligned with the goals of the Triple Aim. As discussed above with the quote from Dr. Gawande, we need to "shift focus from delivering stuff to delivering outcomes."[50] Estimates have noted that physician salaries and related costs only make up 20 percent of health-care expenses, but the decisions and treatments that health-care providers recommend influence up to 60 percent of overall spending. The 2012 National Commission on Physician Payment Reform recommended a five-year plan to move from FFS payments to do away with inherent incentives for both public and private payment systems.[51] The current FFS model incentivizes overutilization. This model increases the quantity of care provided but does not incentivize improvements to the health of the population, improvements to the patient experience, or reductions in costs.

There is almost uniform agreement in Congress that movement away from FFS medicine is needed; the process is being baked into the 2015 "doc fix" Medicare reform bill, which passed in the Senate by a 92–8 vote.[52] In a value-based payment system, the payer shifts the risk of overutilization to the provider side and adjusts incentives to reward for quality and satisfaction rather than volume of care. While most experts seem to agree on moving in that direction, the precise type of payment system (or systems) that should be used remains unclear. Multiple models of rewarding outcomes have been proposed. These new models vary from rewarding based on performance standards, such as pay-for-performance (P4P) models, to "full-capitation" models in which a provider organization is given a lump-sum reimbursement to cover expenses at a per-member-per-month (PMPM) basis. In between these extremes are various partial models such as bundled payment for an episode of care or shared-savings programs where providers and payers split savings or potential losses from a projected model. To avoid the negative backlash seen from older HMO models, balancing measures of satisfaction and quality are necessary to prevent underutilization.[53]

As an example, envision how such models would influence obstetric and gynecologic care: imagine a model for a "mother-baby pregnancy episode" in which all providers must divide a single payment for all the services rendered for both mother and baby. Instantly we are financially at risk for delivering a baby prematurely or for the increased costs of an unnecessary cesarean section or ultrasound examination. Similarly, obstetricians are strongly incentivized to evaluate their care and identify confounding medical risks to the mother and infant.[54] A more traditional

---

[50] Gawande, "Shift Focus from Delivering Stuff to Delivering Outcomes."
[51] National Commission on Physician Payment Reform, "Report of the National Commission on Physician Payment Reform."
[52] Billy Wynne, "May the Era of Medicare's Doc Fix (1997–2015) Rest in Peace. Now What?" *Health Affairs*, April 14, 2015. http://healthaffairs.org/blog/2015/04/14/may-the-era-of-medicares-doc-fix-1997-2015-rest-in-peace-now-what/.
[53] Lagrew and Jenkins, "The Future of Obstetrics/Gynecology in 2020," 618–19.
[54] Ibid., 619.

model involves packaging the cost of surgical procedures, such as "bundling" a hysterectomy, and compensating all the involved providers (gynecologist, anesthesiologist, pathologist, and hospital staff) from a single bundled payment with bonus incentives for meeting quality and satisfaction measures. Therefore, in order to maximize profit, every member of the health-care team is responsible for the cost, patient satisfaction, postoperative disability and recovery time, and clinical quality. This strategy could lead to a comprehensive assessment of new modalities to include cost analysis and quality (such as robotics) and could result in the use of these modalities in the most cost-efficient manner.

In the office setting, a capitated form of payment for care rewards less direct patient contact and more utilization of cost-effective communication techniques such as phone and e-mail communication. One would expect dramatic changes in performance of certain tests where capitation for screening and preventative care—such as Pap screening, mammograms, and vaccination—would improve compliance with best-practice goals for outcomes. Payments based on patient-satisfaction ratings incentivize good staff-patient communication and prompt follow-up. When not incentivized by volume-based models, ob-gyns are more likely to participate in what is known as team medicine, which utilizes lower-cost ancillary providers / health coaches and makes more appropriate specialty referrals.[55]

## Force 2–Care Redesign: Team-Based Care to Take Advantage of Everyone's Strengths and Time Constraints

Team-based care is founded on the concept that each patient has an appropriately assembled group of providers to meet her individual needs who provide for "efficient care, an excellent patient experience, and good clinical outcomes," as Jenkins and I wrote in our 2014 article "The Future of Obstetrics/Gynecology in 2020."[56] Teams are multidisciplinary, they involve various types of providers, and they usually involve transferring work to ancillary providers, thus leading to cost/time savings for advanced providers so they can perform high-level tasks. Health coaches, nutritionists, and pharmacists also have knowledge bases that allow for special counseling. In this model, physicians, nurse practitioners, and midwives are often directing rather than performing much of the direct patient care. In many cases the patients themselves (and family caregivers) are empowered with the knowledge and tools to become caregivers themselves.

In primary care, the concept is exemplified in the patient-centered medical home model (PCMH), where team medicine focuses on the needs of specific populations and the needs of individual patients to ensure that they receive the necessary care and the appropriate preventative care.[57] This model appears to be widely applicable to multiple populations, has resulted in

---

[55] Ibid., 620.
[56] Ibid., 620.
[57] Domino et al., "Enhancing the Medical Homes Model"; National Commission on Physician Payment Reform, "Report of the National Commission"; M. L. Paustian et al., "Partial and Incremental PCMH Practice Transformation: Implications for Quality and Costs," *Health Services Research* 49, no. 1 (2014): 52–74; R. S. Nocon et al., "Association between Patient-Centered Medical Home Rating and Operating Cost at Federally Funded Health Centers," *Journal of the American Medical Association* 308, no. 1 (2012): 60–66.

significant savings and reduction in unnecessary care,[58] and has been shown to have good clinical outcomes and staff satisfaction. The model will be even more applicable in a value-based care model.[59] New legislation describes provider organizations that can assemble the providers, necessary tools, and facilities to provide care such as accountable-care organizations (ACOs), which can be thought of as PCMHs on steroids; they accept a diverse population of patients and distribute payments to providers in a shared savings model.[60] To date, the early results have been mixed in these organizations' ability to lower costs; a minority of the ACOs succeed in lowering costs or improving quality, which underlines the fact that different segments of the population will require different payment solutions.

The fields of obstetrics and gynecology have well-established protocols for preventative women's care, routine prenatal care, and follow-up, although we are just beginning to employ the advanced techniques of care coordination and home care that are used in most medical-home models. Newer innovative prenatal models include so-called group prenatal visits, which allow patients to partner with other patients to provide self-teaching and emotional support.[61] In addition, advanced team-based care involves all the providers for a patient's needs and is likely to incorporate the "mother-baby" team so that obstetricians and pediatricians are likely to be considered as a single team working toward cost containment, patient experience, and population health.

Another important concept is the adoption of evidence-based protocols, which include checklists with critically timed, standardized actions and responses based on scientific evidence. These are designed in the form of crew-management protocols, such as those used in aviation, which have reduced errors and improved outcomes. The AIM project (the Alliance for Innovation on Maternal Health) for improving patient safety is based on this concept of every organization adopting a minimal set of key changes to obtain improvements in specific areas.[62] These bundles are executed by adopting change concepts from performance improvement toolkits designed to improve care. A good example includes the obstetrical hemorrhage toolkit developed by the California Maternal Quality Care Collaborative, which has been implemented and shown to reduce transfusion rates and to improve maternal outcomes.[63] [64]

The widespread standardization of evidence-based medicine (EBM) with constant monitoring and improvement of processes will be dependent on organizations having electronic

---

[58] National Commission on Physician Payment Reform, "Report of the National Commission."
[59] Lagrew and Jenkins, "The Future of Obstetrics/Gynecology in 2020," 620.
[60] National Commission on Physician Payment Reform, "Report of the National Commission"; Lagrew and Jenkins, "The Future of Obstetrics/Gynecology in 2020," 620.
[61] S. D. Tandon et al., "Improved Adequacy of Prenatal Care and Healthcare Utilization among Low-Income Latinas Receiving Group Prenatal Care," *Journal of Women's Health* (Larchmont) 22, no. 12 (2013): 1056–61.
[62] E. K. Main et al., "National Partnership for Maternal Safety: Consensus Bundle on Obstetric Hemorrhage," *Obstetrics & Gynecology* 126, no. 1 (2015): 155–62.
[63] D. Bingham et al., "A State-Wide Obstetric Hemorrhage Quality Improvement Initiative," *MCN: The American Journal of Maternal/Child Nursing* 36, no. 5 (2011): 297–304.
[64] L. E. Shields et al., "Comprehensive Maternal Hemorrhage Protocols Improve Patient Safety and Reduce Utilization of Blood Products," *American Journal of Obstetrics and Gynecology* 205, no. 4 (2011): 368.e1–8.

records and clinical data.⁶⁵ The support staff and costs of redesign are likely to drive further provider and payer consolidation, so the expectation is for larger group practices and alignment with hospitals.⁶⁶ Doing so will reduce the number of small practices but would also be more in line with the desires of more recently trained physicians and other providers.⁶⁷

## Force 3—Digital Transformation: Vast Amounts of Clinical Electronic Data

At the current rate, by 2020 the transformation of clinical data into electronic records will likely be nearly complete. The past few years have seen an exponential rise in the number of offices and hospitals that have converted to electronic records. The landscape is still shifting, however, and consolidation has taken place from many vendors into a successful few. Many providers have chosen their vendors by whether they were the least expensive or easiest conversion for their clinic or office. Unfortunately, many vendors have not obtained enough market share to allow for continued development of the kind of robustly functioning electronic medical record system that would have capabilities for documentation, result retrieval, ordering, or decision support and interoperability (i.e., the ability of systems to exchange information) with outside systems. In the next few years, this failure to modernize their software, combined with medical group consolidation forcing practices to adopt to different electronic records systems, will lead to a large number of practices converting from one electronic record to another, rather than conversion from paper to electronic.

A similar situation, to a lesser degree, may be seen in hospitals, but clearly there will be a need to convert systems from a hospital's initial choices. Those physician practices and organizations that lack these robust IT solutions will be at a disadvantage and will be unable to function as part of an effective clinical team. Recent years have seen an increasing push to solve interoperability concerns, which will likely drive more consolidation and regulatory push. It will also be necessary to solve problems related to semantic interoperability, security issues, and data definition issues. The patient's record will then be a collection of information obtained locally and from other sources of care.⁶⁸

In addition to enhanced interoperability of systems, provider frustration with poorly designed interfaces and workflows has led to a big push in design enhancements, which will improve usability. This will lead to office visits being more efficient and effective, in turn resulting in a reduced number of physical office visits and potentially a reduced provider workload. The electronic format will also drive increased utilization of telemedicine. Patients will be able to obtain routine care for standard low-risk ailments via e-visits, which can be managed via electronic communication rather than through physical visits. This format for care meets the time needs of

---

[65] Lagrew and Jenkins, "The Future of Obstetrics/Gynecology in 2020," 621.
[66] National Commission on Physician Payment Reform, "Report of the National Commission."
[67] Lagrew and Jenkins, "The Future of Obstetrics/Gynecology in 2020," 462.
[68] D. C. Lagrew Jr. and T. R. Jenkins, "The Future of Obstetrics/Gynecology in 2020: A Clearer Vision; Transformational Forces and Thriving in the New System," *American Journal of Obstetrics and Gynecology* 212, no. 1 (2015): 28–33.

the patients and is markedly more efficient for providers.[69] E-visit patients are typically screened by physician extenders who utilize evidence-based protocols, which allows prompt replies and electronic prescriptions. Kaiser Permanente and the Veteran's Administration (VA) system have both demonstrated their ability to provide specialty care and to much more efficiently distribute expertise in this way.[70]

These opportunities for care will be augmented by telehealth (patient-only interactions) in which detailed clinical education and instructions regarding conservative, patient-directed treatment can be provided. Patients will be able to go to their primary-care physician's office in order to have a consultation with a remote subspecialist, thus saving time and increasing satisfaction for both parties. Under the current FFS payment system, telemedicine has been somewhat delayed (in terms of getting payers to see the benefit and in defining proper coding), but under value-based systems, telemedicine has begun to show clear benefits.

Keeping data in electronic form has many other benefits. The structured data can trigger point-of-care and embedded-decision support that will get much more powerful as more data becomes available. Feedback reporting to providers can be automated, and new analytic tools will let providers review and analyze their own practice patterns for personalized process improvements. In addition, trends from big data analysis may allow systems improvement and interventions to be ongoing. Comparative effectiveness research will be markedly enhanced with the ability to combine clinical and financial data in ways that were never before possible. Electronic formatting also allows clinicians to quickly sort and review the massive amounts of increased data from new imaging techniques, genomics, and other exploding sources of data that would have overwhelmed paper-based systems.[71]

## Force 4—Disruptive Clinical Innovations

The history of medicine has demonstrated that while improvements in care mostly happen in an incremental way, certain techniques and developments can radically change and improve medical care and therefore can be described as disruptive.[72] Indeed, many of these advances will actually change the essence of delivering health care by preventing or curing diseases and reducing complications, thus markedly improving patient outcomes and cost. Where and when these breakthroughs will occur is often difficult to predict, but in an age of exponential improvements and technological advances, we should expect an explosion of these advances. Where and when these discoveries will occur is beyond the scope of this chapter, since many promising ideas often are not feasible economically or to scale to large distribution. Health-care entities in the future will need dedicated individuals and facilities to help keep abreast of innovations and their particular impacts on their institutions. We can name some of the more promising potential innovations in

---

[69] L. J. Finney Rutten et al., "Patient Perceptions of Electronic Medical Records Use and Ratings of Care Quality," *Patient Related Outcome Measures* 5 (2014): 17–23.
[70] G. B. Raglan et al., "Electronic Health Record Adoption among Obstetrician/Gynecologists in the United States: Physician Practices and Satisfaction." *Journal for Healthcare Quality* 39 (2017): 144–52.
[71] Lagrew and Jenkins, "The Future of Obstetrics/Gynecology in 2020," 31–33.
[72] Ibid., 470–74.

obstetrics and gynecology that have the potential to be quite disruptive. For examples, table 1.1 lists some of the possible technologic advances that may disrupt our current practice; the following discussion highlights a number of possible disruptions.

| Table 1.1. Examples of transformational forces | | | |
|---|---|---|---|
| **Payment Reform** | **Care Redesign** | **Digital Transformation** | **Disruptive Clinical Innovations** |
| • High deductible policies<br>• Pay for performance by quality and utilization adjustments<br>• Bundled payments: low-risk mother-baby pair, high-risk diagnosis, procedural such as cesarean birth, total "ultrasound care" for pregnancy<br>• Capitated care<br>• Inclusion of nonmedical expenses to payer such as time from work, transportation costs | • Team-based care<br>• Patient-centered medical home<br>• Preventative care/health maintenance<br>• Accountable care organizations<br>• Evidence-based protocols/order sets<br>• Group prenatal visits | • Electronic medical records<br>• Transitions of care documents<br>• Health information exchange<br>• Patient portals<br>• Electronic visits<br>• Telemedicine<br>• Big data analytics/comparative effectiveness research (CER) | • Gene testing for risk analysis<br>• Gene therapy<br>• Genetic tumor analysis<br>• Personalized therapy based on genomic/epigenomic testing<br>• Computer-aided image analysis of ultrasounds, CT, MRI<br>• Computer-aided pathologic testing<br>• Minimally invasive therapy<br>• Stem-cell therapy<br>• Regenerative medicine |

*Genomics and Epigenomics*

By 2003, the Human Genome Project (HGP) had identified over 20,500 genes in human DNA, but the task of linking these genes to human diseases and conditions has only just started.[73] The technological advancements in equipment for analyzing genetic material has allowed for rapid analysis at lowered costs and reduced time of discovery. In 2013, scientists uncovered that the 90 percent of "dark matter DNA" that sits between known genes contains the switches for these genes, which explains how control could lead to expression or lead to problems such as cancerous growth.[74] The field of epigenetics, which the *Merriam-Webster Dictionary* describes as "the study of changes in organisms caused by modifications of gene expression rather than alteration of the genetic code," is just starting to be understood.[75] As we begin to appreciate the "on-off" switches of our genome, we will better understand how individuals can have the same genes and yet not the same phenotype and expressed disorders. The application of genomic/epigenomic knowledge will likely result in improved diagnoses and potential new therapies.

Genetic advancements can potentially allow diagnoses to be earlier, less invasive, and more accurate. The widespread application of noninvasive prenatal diagnostic techniques has become available to analyze free fetal DNA strands floating in maternal blood during early pregnancy.

---

[73] L. Hood and D. Galas, "The Digital Code of DNA," *Nature* 421 (2003): 444–48.
[74] I. Y. Choi et al., "Perspectives on Clinical Informatics: Integrating Large-Scale Clinical, Genomic, and Health Information for Clinical Care," *Genomics & Informatics* 11, no. 4 (2013): 186–90.
[75] *Merriam-Webster Dictionary*, s.v. "epigenetics," www.merriam-webster/com/definitions/epigenetics.

These appear superior to other noninvasive testing techniques among high-risk patients; if validated in low-risk populations, it is clear that these techniques will likely replace hormonal-based screening[76] by markedly reducing invasive sample testing and will result in lowering the number of procedure-related losses. The impact to costs will be augmented by lower numbers of follow-up ultrasounds. The effect should be a reduction in "decision points," at which patients are given equivocal information, and better cost control to meet the Triple Aim. Scientists demonstrated similar potential for improved noninvasive testing for single gene defects in 2012 when an analysis of maternal blood and paternal saliva yielded the entire fetal genome in an Italian cystic fibrosis (CF) study.[77] The success or failure of these techniques will require time as well as clinical studies with large numbers of participants.[78]

The applications will also potentially affect non-obstetrical women's health screening. Next-generation DNA testing of stool samples has been shown to correctly identify 85 percent of polyps and colorectal cancers.[79] While not considered a diagnostic test, such testing could replace costly, unpopular (less than 70 percent compliance), and invasive tests such as colonoscopy screenings. The net effect may improve population screening as increased numbers of patients become compliant with mailing in a stool specimen rather than scheduling a colonoscopy. An additional gynecologic application of such DNA screening is in the improved detection of gynecologic malignancies. DNA probe testing has been performed on routine Pap specimens and has been shown to detect 100 percent of endometrial cancers and 41 percent of ovarian cancers.[80] Once again, success will depend on these tests being more accurate and leading to fewer false diagnoses, at an acceptable cost.

Genomic/epigenomic testing will also lead to the ability to design tailored, patient-specific therapy. An explosion of identified genes such as BRCA1/2 will help identify those patients who should receive more timely interventions that are specifically designed for their unique genome.[81] Choosing the most effective drug based on the presence of certain genotypes (such as which type of statin to use for hypercholesterolemia) can result in improved responses to medications.[82] With

---

[76] E. R. Norwitz and B. Levy, "Noninvasive Prenatal Testing: The Future Is Now," *Reviews in Obstetrics & Gynecology* 6, no. 2 (2013): 48–62.

[77] A. Bustamante-Aragonés et al., "Non-Invasive Prenatal Diagnosis of Single-Gene Disorders from Maternal Blood," *Gene* 504, no. 1 (2012): 144–49. doi: 10.1016/j.gene.2012.04.045.

[78] "Cell-Free DNA Screening for Fetal Aneuploidy," Committee Opinion #640, American Congress of Obstetricians and Gynecologists, September 2015. http://www.acog.org/Resources-And-Publications/Committee-Opinions/Committee-on-Genetics/Cell-free-DNA-Screening-for-Fetal-Aneuploidy.

[79] I. Lansdorp-Vogelaar et al., "Stool DNA Testing to Screen for Colorectal Cancer in the Medicare Population: A Cost-Effectiveness Analysis," *Annals of Internal Medicine* 153, no. 6 (2010): 368–77.

[80] I. Kinde et al., "Evaluation of DNA from the Papanicolaou Test to Detect Ovarian and Endometrial Cancers," *Science Translational Medicines* 5, no. 167 (2013): 167ra4.

[81] P. M. Campeau, W. D. Foulkes, and M. D. Tischkowitz, "Hereditary Breast Cancer: New Genetic Developments, New Therapeutic Avenues," *Human Genetics* 124, no. 1 (2008): 31–42.

[82] E. Link et al., "SEARCH Collaborative Group. SLCO1B1 Variants and Statin Induced Myopathy: A Genomewide Study," *New England Journal of Medicine* 359, no. 8 (2008): 789–99; T. K. Ma et al., "Variability in Response to Clopidogrel: How Important Are Pharmacogenetics and Drug Interactions?" *British Journal of Clinical Pharmacology* 72, no. 4 (2011): 697–706.

the advent of multiarray genomic testing, a patient could be screened for hundreds of such genes in the future, and precise medications could be prescribed to be most effective in that patient.

Finally, the identification of specific tumor-producing genes will lead to more accurate diagnoses, drugs targeted toward these cancerous tissues to "switch off" their anaplastic growth, and the development of specific drugs for use with specific tumor-gene abnormalities rather than the use of organ site–based therapy.[83]

*Computer-Aided Diagnosis*

Computer-aided diagnosis will also expand with the digitization of clinical information. In 2012, Microsoft research labs in Great Britain demonstrated algorithms for reading CT and MRI images.[84] Such advances will lead to ultrasound machines where algorithms can be run on digitized volumes to obtain biometrics and screen fetal anatomy and abnormalities. This capability should improve accuracy and, coupled with remote reading—which will allow experts to read ultrasounds to review images much more rapidly and accurately—reduce the human workforce needed for ultrasound screening. This has already been demonstrated in mammography readings, which have been improved with the addition of computer-aided reading.[85] Coupled with traditional telehealth communication videoconferencing, detailed imaging will be more widely available to patients in remote settings and should reduce imaging times. The net effect of the increased use of artificial intelligence should be a lowering of undiagnosed anomalies and reduced costs per scan.

*Minimally Invasive Therapies*

Surgery will likely continue the trend toward minimally invasive techniques and care redesign. The current controversies related to robotic surgery highlight those seen in all new technology,[86] but surgeons will continue to feel the pressure on how to perform the least invasive techniques to provide maximal surgical outcomes with minimal disruption of a patient's life. This trend will be driven by patient satisfaction and payment reform that incorporates disability time under total cost of care, as shorter recoveries allow the resumption of productivity sooner. Advances in equipment and market pressures should make the technology more cost effective than current equipment. Operative techniques will be augmented by better preoperative imaging and intraoperative use of dyes and markers to highlight tumors and lymph nodes.[87] These techniques should reduce operative times and costs.

---

[83] National Cancer Institute, "NCI-Molecular Analysis for Therapy Choice Program (NCI-MATCH)." Updated June 6, 2017. http://www.cancer.gov/about-cancer/treatment/clinical-trials/nci-supported/nci-match.
[84] D. Zikic et al., "Decision Forests for Tissue-Specific Segmentation of High-Grade Gliomas in Multi-Channel MR," *Medical Image Computing and Computer-Assisted Intervention* 15, part 3 (2012): 369–76.
[85] C. S. Park et al., "Detection of Breast Cancer in Asymptomatic and Symptomatic Groups Using Computer-Aided Detection with Full-Field Digital Mammography," *Journal of Breast Cancer*, 16, no. 3 (2013): 322–28.
[86] Lagrew and Jenkins, "The Future of Obstetrics/Gynecology in 2020," 29.
[87] E. C. Rossi, A. Ivanova, and J. F. Boggess, "Robotically Assisted Fluorescence-Guided Lymph Node Mapping with ICG for Gynecologic Malignancies: A Feasibility Study," *Gynecologic Oncology* 124, no. 1 (2012): 78–82.

Teleconferencing should allow for routine intraoperative consultations with remote experts. In addition to surgical techniques, invasive radiological intervention and less invasive techniques such as in-utero surgeries, hysteroscopic procedures, and ablative techniques will allow for lower costs and quicker patient recovery.

*Stem-Cell Therapy and Regenerative Therapy*

In addition to these advances, various discoveries in basic science have suggested that advanced genetic therapies that replace defective genes or turn off tumor-promoter genes or turn on suppressor genes offer hope that genetic abnormalities or translational errors can be corrected and cure diseases altogether. Stem-cell therapies for diseases such as sickle cell anemia and other hemoglobinopathies can be given to fetuses and newborns and may correct defects before the children are affected. In-utero surgical corrections may prevent long-term damage and chronic health problems, thus reducing patient suffering and health-care costs related to these problems. In urogynecology, the science of building stem cell–regenerated organs, such as urinary bladders, offers great hope for replacement organs.[88]

# Conclusion

Regardless of their promise, the innovations that will ultimately be used will be determined by their efficacy and benefit, as measured by the Triple Aim goals. The four types of transformational forces are all linked together and must occur in an orchestrated fashion.[89] For example, payment reform must reward better usage of efficient digital medicine and new technology, which provides cost-effective care with better outcomes for patients, as determined by comparative effectiveness research (CER). Care redesign must incorporate the new technology for maximum efficiency, as is being done in the manufacturing and service sectors. When used together, the benefits will multiply and accelerate the process of health-care improvement. Ultimately, the care providers and organizations that succeed in the new world will have to be comfortable with implementing change in an organized and rapid fashion.

In "The Future of Obstetrics/Gynecology in 2020," our paper on this subject we mentioned earlier, we described the "winners" in this process as having the following qualities:

- They will be individuals who study the new technology and understand its benefits and limitations.
- They will adopt the concept of "best designed medicine" and give careful empathetic thought to how they deliver care to their patients.
- They will be team players who are experts in documenting their thoughts and plans.
- These providers will carefully transition their patients from various care settings and seamlessly pass appropriate information to the next provider.
- Successful MFM subspecialists in the new system will understand that these are not "their patients" but rather "I am their doctor."

---

[88] A. K. Sharma, "An Examination of Regenerative Medicine-Based Strategies for the Urinary Bladder," *Regenerative Medicine* 6, no. 5 (2011): 583–98.
[89] Lagrew and Jenkins, "The Future of Obstetrics/Gynecology in 2020," 28.

- They will assume responsibility for their patients, know their own limitations and freely ask for assistance.
- They will preserve their personal touch with patients but be team players who treat all members of the team with respect and professionalism.
- They will be those with expertise in team medicine and special knowledge of new technologies.[90]

Successful leaders will be skillful in quality improvement and transparent about sharing their performance metrics. The focus will be on the quality of their care, not the volume of care, and they will understand how important patient experience is as a part of quality care. They will focus on the needs of their patients and empower patients by (1) educating them or the family caregiver in understanding their diagnoses and choices, (2) helping them to actively participate in the care plan, and (3) accepting the patient's desires in a nonjudgmental fashion.[91] Everyone's goal will be to see the patient return to a full state of health.

Understanding these principles will be easier when providers practice empathy: by seeing care from the patients' view and respecting their concerns. Obviously, adopting the technological and institutional changes we have discussed will be important, but success will ultimately rely on the human factor. For motivation it is helpful to remember that, regardless of our current health status, we are highly likely, except in extreme cases, to be patients ourselves. Perhaps the best providers will be those who understand how it feels to be a patient.[92]

To summarize this chapter:

- Women's health care will continue to change rapidly because of various factors, including cost pressures, changes in characteristics of providers and patients, and technological developments.

- Providers can adapt to the changing world by using the Triple Aim concepts to choose the best path forward.

- Transformational forces of payment reform, care redesign, digital transformation, and disruptive technologies, if used correctly, should improve patient care and provider satisfaction.

- The most successful providers will be those who learn to adapt to change and lead the transformation.

---

[90] Lagrew and Jenkins, "The Future of Obstetrics/Gynecology in 2020," 33.
[91] Welch, *Less Medicine, More Health*, 193.
[92] Lagrew and Jenkins, "The Future of Obstetrics/Gynecology in 2020," 33.

# Management Structure for Successful Hospital-, Private-, and University-Owned Practices

Daniel F. O'Keeffe, MD

Medicine is now a business. When we went through our training to become physicians, not many of us learned how to run a business. Medicine has been changing quickly since the passage of the US Patient Protection and Affordable Care Act (PPACA). Our relationship with payers, hospitals, patients, and referring physicians is now drastically different. Entering this new world, many providers have found themselves ill prepared to succeed in this time of rapid change.

More physicians who are coming out of residency are now choosing to be employees rather than independent practitioners. Established practices are selling to large groups or hospitals, under the impression that they will gain freedom from the burden of the business of medicine. Unfortunately, this is a misconception. The lack of providers who are taking part and leading in these changing situations has transformed our role into simply being a commodity in the healthcare machine. We will lose standing, influence, and the power to make meaningful changes in our practices and lives. So what can we do to continue to have a say in what we do and where we go? How can we make sure our practice will be successful? Whatever type of practice you are in, be it private, hospital, or university, there are basic guidelines and tenets that you as a physician should enact to be successful. Without having a map for a difficult journey, it is highly likely that you will not find your destination. Even if you do have a map, you will need people who have the skills to use it to ensure success in reaching your destination.

A strategic plan is the map that will help us navigate on our journey. This is a *must* for a practice. It provides direction, solidifies purpose, and ensures consistency for all participants to move forward while going in the same direction to achieve their goal. Practices often benefit from a professional facilitator to help them develop a strategic plan. A practice needs the commitment and buy-in of all physicians and staff in this plan to accomplish true success. The goals of the practice should be written out and approved. Generally, a strategic plan contains between four to six goals, with objectives under each goal. These objectives are very specific tasks that define the methods and timing by which the goals will be achieved. Following this, you should have:

- A timeline—be specific, since you cannot let this be free floating;
- Required resources—these must be categorized and funded;
- Accountability—list who is accountable (this must be one person);
- Measurements—describe what constitutes success.

When you create a strategic plan, choose an offsite location for development meetings; this will aid in avoiding distractions. Your physicians and key staff will need at least one day and possibly two to develop the plan.

All practices should have a medical director. This person should demonstrate interest and be willing to take time (and also be provided the time) from clinical practice, education, and research to perform these valuable tasks. The performance of these tasks should not negatively affect this person's compensation and possibly should enhance it due to the after-hours work, worry, and planning this role takes. The compensation of roles does indeed show the importance of a duty to the practice. A medical director should possess training in transformational leadership and the skills required to be in this position. (If needed, the medical director can take courses at the Academy for Leadership and Development from the Society for Maternal-Fetal Medicine or at the American Association for Physician Leadership.) The physicians of the group and administration of the hospital or university should:

- Respect and support the person in this position;
- Allow the medical director equal pay;
- Provide protected time to perform business functions (away from clinical time);
- Provide support to learn the necessary business skills.

The medical director's responsibilities should include:

- Assisting with business contracting—interacting with the medical director of the particular health plan to show the value of the practice;
- Communicating in a timely fashion with all partners from both the clinical and business side of the practice;
- Modeling conflict resolution within the practice;
- Setting up a quality/performance-review process for the practice;
- Selecting and mentoring emerging leaders from the practice;
- Providing vision for the practice, which includes keeping the practice moving in a positive direction and following the strategic plan as well as knowing where medicine is heading and prepare for it (e.g., the PPACA and all its ramifications);
- Setting up a structure to measure, benchmark, and ensure quality care;
- Creating a system to ensure timely and accurate communication with referring physicians;
- Being part of technological initiatives (i.e., electronic medical records, website, social media);
- Providing strong medical leadership. Obtaining a seat at the table with the various players in the health-care puzzle will help keep the physicians in a stronger position. The most successful practices/divisions all have great medical leadership.

Having a professional administrator in addition to the medical director can lead to a more powerful team to ensure practice success. All practices consisting of three or more physicians should have a professional administrator. The emphasis is on the word *professional*—a person who has had training and experience in doing this. The biggest mistake many medical practices make is to promote outstanding staff (nursing, billers, and coders, for example) into positions they have insufficient training or skills to perform. If you are going to do this, make sure that they get the

# 3

## The Role of the MFM Subspecialist as a Medical Neighbor

James Keller, MD, MHSA

In 1971 a little-known musician named Barry Manilow sung in a new ad campaign for a Midwest-based insurance company. That jingle, "Like a Good Neighbor, State Farm Is There," is still the foundation for State Farm, a company now so large that as of 2017 it is number thirty-three on the Fortune 500. State Farm's website describes being a good neighbor as being there for their customers. The modern-day maternal-fetal medicine practice and maternal-fetal medicine subspecialist (MFMS) not only need to practice quality medicine—for this is presumed for all practices and physicians—but they also need to be there for their customers.

For the MFMS, the customer comes in many forms: the patient, the patient's family, the referring physician, the payer, and possibly the employer of the MFM provider. Throughout this book, we have discussed the changing paradigm of health-care delivery. No matter what model is proposed, the overarching theme is that the health-care system must deliver better care to more patients for less money. For the obstetric community to meet this challenge, the MFMS will have to play an integral role. In a system where a favored model of care is referred to as the patient-centered medical home (PCMH), the role of the subspecialist is that of a supporting neighbor, much like the theme of State Farm. Practices that support patient-centered care in PCMHs are referred to as patient-centered specialty practices (PCSPs). The purpose of this chapter is to describe the role of the MFMS as a medical neighbor. At the end of the chapter, we will discuss the pathway to formal recognition by the National Committee for Quality Assurance (NCQA). Regardless of a practice's decision to pursue such official recognition, their success as an MFMS will depend on following the principles of being a good medical neighbor.

## Rationale

With the paradigm shift occurring with value-based care, although it may be irrelevant to assign the responsibility of the role of the subspecialist from a provider an isolated provider instead to a part of a team, two main drivers are involved: price and quality. It is no accident that the intersection of price and quality is often referred to as "value."

Value = Quality ÷ Price

Let's look at a scenario where the MFMS practices in an isolated manner. A patient is referred to an MFMS at thirty-three weeks because the referring obstetrician has a concern about fetal growth. The patient herself makes the call, which is taken by an untrained front-desk attendant. The patient is scheduled two days from the call for an ultrasound, umbilical artery Doppler, nonstress test (NST), and a consultation. The patient arrives and spends thirty minutes reviewing her history with the nurse and undergoes her NST. This is followed by an ultrasound that shows the fetus is actually in the 44th percentile, but Dopplers are performed anyway, and the MFMS reviews all this with the patient during a brief consultation. The patient returns to the obstetrician, who may or may not have received a report from the MFMS, and finishes the remainder of her pregnancy having weekly NSTs and amniotic fluid evaluations.

A few years ago, this scenario may not have been a concern. In reality, the referring physicians were happy, as their patients received comprehensive evaluations. The MFMSs were happy, as their offices were kept busy, with a significant generation of revenue. Even a typical patient—who, most likely, by virtue of her being pregnant and in light of her subsequent hospitalization, would be unconcerned about copays and deductibles—would also be happy, as her doctor had obviously cared enough to send her to a specialist, and she may have even walked away with a keepsake photo. Assuming these interventions did not lead to an untoward outcome, one could rationalize that there was no problem with the care. But remember that quality at any price does not translate into a good value.

Let's now look at why the above example would not work in today's world. Remember, nobody is questioning the intent of the MFMS or the quality of care the patient receives. The reality is that back when volume was considered the mark of success, MFMSs such as this were practicing in a successful manner. But as the marker of success transitions from volume to value, an MFMS's care of a particular patient such as this would not be considered successful, even if there was a healthy mom and baby at the end.

So what would this patient's care look like in a value-based paradigm? Most likely the cost of care would be a consideration for everyone involved. The patient would most likely have a higher copay and deductible, which would cause her concern and hardship if she were referred for unneeded intervention. At a minimum, even if the referral were necessary, she would expect that only the required testing would be performed. The obstetrician may be the de facto primary-care physician for this patient during her pregnancy.

One of the methods for payers who are assuming responsibility for controlling costs may be evaluating the performance of the obstetrician. What about the MFMS? A poor neighbor wouldn't care about the referring physician's and patient's financial concerns. Previously, and in some communities, the patient and referring physician would have no choice but to acquiesce to low-value care, as long as the quality was decent. But the successful MFMS of today and tomorrow would care. The referring obstetrician (or his or her partners) would no longer utilize a low-value MFMS; in the future, as a primary-care physician, the referring obstetrician may control the flow of dollars with the flow of patients. By illustrating how a good neighbor MFMS would handle the above case, we will highlight several elements of a successful patient-centered specialty practice. Several elements of the efficiencies required are described elsewhere in this book.

The call from the patient would have been screened and the patient's history and records obtained prior to her being seen, if possible, thus eliminating a significant portion of the burden on the nursing staff as well as on the patient. A flow would have been developed so that, had the ultrasound revealed normal growth, neither a Doppler study nor an NST would have been performed. A midlevel provider could easily have explained to the patient why no further testing had been performed, and most important, the findings would have been communicated to the referring obstetrician, thus obviating the need for the weekly NSTs.

Assuming the quality is the same and remembering that value is quality divided by price, a simple mathematical calculation shows that the second scenario has created twice the value as the first. So how does one become a good medical neighbor, and how does one succeed financially in such a model?

Two things must be realized before we continue. The first is that the reader is strongly advised to read the chapters by Brian K. Iriye and Elizabeth Williams (10 and 11), Thomas Lee (13), and Arnold W. Cohen (16), which describe strategies for running an efficient practice and workforce as well as contracting in a way in which value is rewarded. The second is to ask this question: Is it unrealistic to think that the MFMS will generate the same type of salary in a value-driven world? The good news is that if one wants to and is willing to take financial risk, then large rewards might be obtainable. The other good news is that the opportunity to drive value as a good medical neighbor is so inherent in the practice of maternal-fetal medicine that value-based compensation should continue to provide the MFMS with a favorable salary.

## Patient-Centered Medical Homes

Before examining the elements of a successful subspecialty practice, one must first grasp the basic elements of a patient-centered medical home (PCMH) as a model of practice. The term "medical home" was first used by the American Academy of Pediatrics in 1967 as a way to provide care to children with special needs. The current model of the PCMH is one with broad goals: to improve outcomes, safety, and efficiency while increasing both patient and provider satisfaction. This is no small feat, as many feel that any move to increase efficiency means increasing work output per associate, while increasing value means restricting access to care for the patient. Neither would be true for a well-functioning and successful PCMH. The data to date are unclear on many of the financial aspects of the PCMH, but a systematic review from 2013 confirmed that the effect on patient and associate satisfaction has been positive.[93] Although there is no universal agreement on the components necessary for a practice model to be called a PCMH, the above-mentioned systematic review identified the following components to be most common:

- Patient-centered orientation to the whole person
- Care that is coordinated across the health-care system and community
- Enhanced access to care that uses alternative methods of communication
- A systems approach to quality and safety

The question remains: What is the relevance of the PCMH to obstetric care? Because this chapter focuses on the role of the MFMS—and thus the patient-centered specialty practice (PCSP) and the role of the specialist in serving the PCMH—one needs to understand what maternity care

---

[93] G. L. Jackson et al., "The Patient-Centered Medical Home: A Systematic Review," *Annals of Internal Medicine* 158, no. 3 (2013): 169–78.

in a PCMH may look like. Even those who question whether obstetricians or systems will embrace the PCMH model for maternity care certainly cannot ignore the core values listed in table 3.1 as being key elements to a successful practice. Thus, for MFMSs to be successful neighbors or parts of successful PCSPs, they must envision what the obstetric PCMH would look like and need. To do this, let's expand the above components to include possible examples. Remember, this is a generalist model; the role of the MFMS will be added in later.

Before we take a deeper dive into how the MFMS serves this model, it is important to remember that by the virtue of many MFMS practices providing primary obstetric care, the core values of a PCMH may need to be instituted into a specialty practice. While we transition into a discussion of the role of the medical neighbor, remember to refer back to the core components and values of the PCMH. This will serve as a commonsense template as to what services you can provide your referring physicians and their patients in order to be considered a good neighbor. In addition, it highlights which services will bring value not only to the care you provide but also to the care they provide.

### Table 3.1. A model obstetric PCMH

| PCMH Component | General Obstetric Example |
|---|---|
| Wide-ranging team-based care | Expanded service on-site Ultrasound, labs, pharmacy |
| Patient-centered orientation to the whole person | Behavioral health, dentistry |
| Care that is coordinated across the health-care system and community | Seamless access to referrals for services not contained in PCMH |
| Enhanced access to care that uses alternative methods of communication | Easy access to professionals in asynchronous manner (e-mail, Skype) |
| Systems approach to quality and safety | Transparent outcome reporting Use of evidence-based care protocols |

## The Medical Neighborhood

As health care becomes more and more complex, most people think of the health-care system as a mass of people and places with very little coordination or communication between them. Most patients feel that the responsibility to coordinated care falls on them, thus leading to poor satisfaction and a system that hardly supports superior outcomes. In other words, most patients would not describe their care as being patient centered. The patient-centered medical home goes a long way toward treating the whole patient and placing an emphasis on patient-centered care, but the reality of modern medicine is that complex disease processes require specialty care. It is the relationship between primary providers and specialists that defines the transition from home to neighborhood. At this point we hope to describe the essential components of a patient-centered medical neighborhood, followed by a brief review of how the concept is functioning. Finally, we will describe the process of accreditation as a patient-centered specialty practice, which is a key component of the neighborhood.

The US Agency for Healthcare Research and Quality (AHRQ), in its white paper "Coordinating Care in the Medical Neighborhood: Critical Components and Available

Mechanisms,"[94] describes the medical neighborhood as the patient-centered medical home and the constellation of other clinicians who provide health-care services to patients within it, along with various community and social-service organizations and state and local public-health agencies. This long definition purposely defines the neighborhood as being important for the care of the individual as well as carving out the neighborhood's place as a foundation for population health.

One of the more interesting concepts to consider is that the hub (i.e., the PCMH) and spoke (specialist) relationship may be reversed based on the disease state and the community the patient resides in. A patient with a severe chronic autoimmune disorder may have his rheumatologist as the spoke. This is particularly important if a patient with a significant obstetric issue accesses her primary obstetric care from a maternal-fetal medicine practice but also may need to access community resources or other specialties, perhaps even her primary-care provider—thus inverting the typical hub-and-spoke relationship that a specialist practice generally falls into (see figures 3.1 and 3.2).

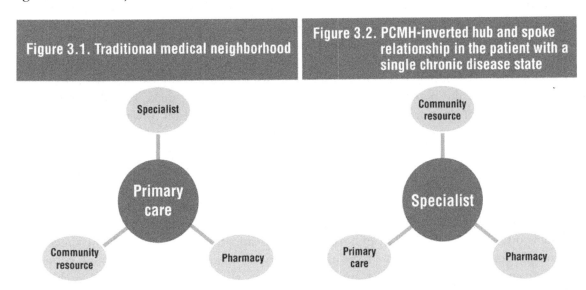

Several highly functioning integrated health systems or health plans have the components of a functional neighborhood, just as many specialty practices have all the characteristics and components of an accredited patient-centered specialty practice. While the components for accreditation will change over time, a medical neighborhood has certain key elements: (1) sharing of clinical information through a strong information technology (IT) platform; (2) care teams built around the needs of an individual patient; (3) clear methods of transition between settings of care; (4) community relationships; (5) clear understanding of components' roles; and (6) patient engagement and participation.

---

[94] E. F. Taylor et al., "Coordinating Care in the Medical Neighborhood: Critical Components and Available Mechanisms," Agency for Healthcare Research and Quality, US Department of Health and Human Services, 2011.

# The Finances of the Medical Neighborhood

While the above six elements form the medical foundation of the neighborhood, the concept falls apart on many levels when attention is not paid to the payment models. Within this book the reader will be made aware of the transition from fee-for-service (FFS) to payment models, which range from providing a value component to an FFS model to one where organizations take on the full risk for the health-care costs of a population. While the transition is happening rapidly, the necessity for the better coordinated care that a medical neighborhood will bring is a reality today.

In their review of the patient-centered medical neighborhood in the *New England Journal of Medicine*, Xiaoyan Huang and Meredith Rosenthal emphasized the importance of the economic model.[95] Relevant to the MFMS is the fact that except for those in systems such as Kaiser Permanente, most MFMS have little experience with anything else other than FFS models. Primary-care physicians have had much more experience in managing the cost of health care and managing complex chronic conditions across continuums. The medical home will not function with the two entities living with different payment models. Because the foundation of the medical home is the coordination of care across the continuum, some of the dollars that would have been spent on procedures in older models would now be put toward reimbursing professionals for coordination of care. The person coordinating the care, however, must do just that and not act as a gatekeeper. The role of the person or practice acting as the hub is to make sure that the patient follows along the line of the correct spoke and that care and information flows in both directions in an efficient manner.

The restriction of care rather than the coordination of care will be too reminiscent of restrictive health-maintenance organizations (HMOs) and will cause the concept of the medical neighborhood to lose credibility. Financial models in the medical neighborhood will need to be aligned around shared risk and reward for the primary-care physician and the specialist alike. One of the models often seen in medical neighborhoods is subcapitation. In this model, the specialist is paid a monthly fee for each patient in the neighborhood, regardless of the amount of service provided. The subcapitation of specialists and subspecialists, while attractive on many levels, is not without risk. On the one hand, once the volume aspect of any compensation model is removed, the volume of procedures performed tends to decrease as well. While this generally results in cost savings, it is not always in the best interest of the patient. Two factors can negatively affect the patient. A specialist may withhold treatments that are expensive or time consuming but advantageous. The counterbalance to this would be both objective and subjective. From an objective point of view, one would hope that specialists who withhold or decrease the intensity of appropriate therapies would fall out in quality or satisfaction metrics, which would make them less desirable to formal neighborhoods. Subjectively, primary-care physicians would likely recognize this behavior and steer consultations away. While many specialists still will derive a portion of their income from productivity, the loss of business should have a greater impact than the savings achieved by withholding care.

---

[95] Xiaoyan Huang and Meredith B. Rosenthal, "Transforming Specialty Practice—The Patient-Centered Medical Neighborhood," *New England Journal of Medicine* 370 (2014): 1376–79.

Specialists are at risk themselves. If primary-care physicians are not at risk for the cost of specialty care, then they may refer patients whose problems are appropriately handled at the level of primary care, thus utilizing resources that the specialist may be responsible for. When joining a medical neighborhood as a specialist, it is important to remember that the personality, skills, and work ethic of your primary-care physicians may be just as important as any structural or financial model.

**The Why and How of the Medical Neighborhood**

While successes and failure have been reported for the patient-centered medical home, most feel that the rationale for the system of care is so strong that the homes will stay in one form or another as a model of coordinating care. Huang and Rosenthal describe the PCMH as necessary yet not sufficient for managing the two major concerns of health care in the United States: cost and fragmentation of care. As previously mentioned, solely placing primary-care physicians in control of costs raises the failed specter of the gatekeeper of the '80s and '90s.

The other issue that points to the need for specialist participation in the neighborhood is that specialists account for the overwhelming majority of health-care costs, even in a well-designed, waste-free system. It was this realization that led the American College of Physicians (ACP) to produce a position paper in 2010 titled "The Patient-Centered Medical Home Neighbor: The Interface of the Patient-Centered Medical Home with Specialty/Subspecialty Practices."[96] This paper acknowledged that improved care integration and coordination requires specialists and subspecialists; the value of this acknowledgment cannot be underestimated, especially with respect to the role of the MFMS.

The ACP described the following processes that a specialty practice must engage in to be an effective PCMH neighbor (PCMH-N):
- Ensures the bidirectional nature of integration of care
- Ensures that consultations complement the aims of the PCMH
- Clearly guides the determination of responsibility in co-management situations
- Engages in patient-centered care (quality, safety, access)
- Supports the PCMH as having overall responsibility for the coordination and integration of care

The interaction between the PCMH and the PCMH-N occurs in the following manner. An obstetric/MFM interaction is included at each step to illustrate the role of the MFMS as a PCMH-N.

---

[96] American College of Physicians, *The Patient-Centered Medical Home Neighbor: The Interface of the Patient-Centered Medical Home with Specialty/Subspecialty Practices* (Philadelphia: American College of Physicians, 2010); policy paper. (Available from American College of Physicians, 190 N. Independence Mall West, Philadelphia, PA 19106.)

1. *Preconsultation exchange to clarify the need for referral.* For the MFMS practice, this would mean a process for the referring physician to set up consultations—making sure the patient presents at the correct gestational age and is seen in an appropriate amount of time, given the acuity of the disorder. A mechanism for transmission and review of previously obtained data (e.g., ultrasounds, labs, prenatal records) is necessary.

2. *Execution of the formal consultation.* For the MFMS practice, this could include the ultrasound, or interactions with nonphysician providers such as diabetic educators and genetic counselors.

3. *Establishment of a co-management process.* In this process, the PCMH, the PCMH-N (i.e., the MFMS), and the patient are clear about the level of participation and role of each.
   - *Co-management with shared management or principal management for the disease.* For the MFMS, the "disease" may be as general as a high-risk pregnancy—say a patient with a previous history of a preterm delivery—where the MFMS may be involved in the initial evaluation and surveillance, but the general obstetrician would continue with regular prenatal care and delivery.
   - *Co-management with principal care of the patient with a consuming illness for a limited period.* For the MFMS, this may be assuming care of a hospitalized gravida during pyelonephritis. If any follow-up is necessary, then this must be communicated to the PCMH.

4. *Transfer of the patient for totality of care.* This may be a higher-order multiple gestation or a twin-twin transfusion syndrome, where the obstetrician may not have the skill to undertake (or be comfortable participating in) the care of the patient or whose care may be solely the delivery of the patient. It is critical for the success of the PCMH-N that the relationship between the primary-care physician and specialist is not considered hierarchical but a partnership. Tasks should be performed by the home or the neighbor based on the efficiency of the system. If a patient needs a quantitative VDRL (venereal disease research laboratory) test repeated in a serial manner, then that might be the responsibility of the home. Follow-up on a fetal fibronectin may best be accomplished by the neighbor. Again, the relationship best works with robust communication and respect.

When the MFMS decides to become a PCMH-N, it is important that the relationship, although guided by the principles of patient-centered care and common sense, should be spelled out in as much detail as is reasonable. The agreement should be reviewed annually, but ongoing dialogue between members of the MFMS office (PCMH-N) and the PCMH is critical to the success of the relationship.

Patient-centered medical homes already receive financial incentives for coordinating care in many models, in the form of coordination fees or increased reimbursement per interaction. The ACP recommends involving the PCMH-N in incentive structures that support the specialist role in care coordination. Given the perceived excess of health-care dollars going to specialists, this may not happen. The advantages of participating as a PCMH-N would be having access to a larger patient pool for the MFMS. In addition, an improved coordinated-care process could make the work of the MFMS more efficient, which would result in financial advantages in the absence of specific financial incentives.

The last key aspect is the description of the role of the MFMS in the PCMH-N. As the MFMS becomes more involved in at-risk contracts such as subcapitation, the ability to provide care in unique and more efficient ways will be critical. Two processes that are components of the successful home, and thus should translate to the specialist neighbor, are telemedicine and asynchronous communication and consultation.

Especially in a subcapitated environment, MFMSs will benefit by providing services to a larger population than they may have in an unstructured fee-for-service (FFS) environment. If every patient needed to be seen in person and if all communication was unstructured, the MFMS-N would be overwhelmed. Enhanced telemedicine capabilities for ultrasound and consultations would be necessary to support a functional MFMS practice.

Evaluation and communication need to be possible in an asynchronous nature as well. The ability of the MFMS to batch studies from multiple sites and review them in a central location at her convenience is much more consistent with the methods used by other imaging specialists. Payers would need to recognize that on-site presence is not necessary to deliver optimal care. MFMSs must also develop systems of efficient communication with both patients and the PCMH. Physicians from the PCMH will be less likely to request that an MFMS be interrupted if they become used to receiving an answer to an electronic query in a timely manner. The same could be true with patient questions. In a subcapitated environment, answering an e-mail query, perhaps to discuss a simple lab result, could obviate a visit that would not bring further value to the patient, the specialist, or the PCMH.

## Are the PCMH and PCMH-N Effective?

In a formal sense, the value of the PCMH and neighborhood has yet to be proven. In a 2014 study commissioned by the Rand Corporation, two large groups of patients from a single state—over one hundred thousand people in all—were compared. Those who were cared for within a formal medical home fared only slightly better in one of the multiple measures that were evaluated: management of kidney disease among diabetic patients.[97] Analysis of data from the state of Minnesota, however, report their own experience, which showed improvement in both outcome and cost.[98] It is not surprising that value will be difficult to show at first. With all new processes, clinician administrators as well as patients will face a learning curve. In addition, value is always difficult to measure, especially in health care, when the cost of care is still rising in all spheres. Regardless, health care will need to address novel approaches in order to better coordinate care for patients through an ever-complex system.

---

[97] M. W. Friedberg et al., "Association between Participation in a Multipayer Medical Home Intervention and Changes in Quality, Utilization, and Costs of Care," *Journal of the American Medical Association* 311, no. 8 (2014): 815–25.
[98] D.R. Wholey et al., "Evaluation of the State of Minnesota's Healt Care Homes Initiative Evaluation Report for Years 2010-2014." Accessed February 11, 2018.

**Formal Certification**

Less clear is the need for formal certification. Certainly, highly functioning accountable-care organizations and integrated health-care systems are practicing the components of the PCMH-N system of care without formal certification. Formal certification serves two purposes. First, there may come a time when the financial structure—things like incentive payments for outcome or stipends for care coordination—may require formal accreditation. Second, smaller groups may need the guidance of a formal accreditation process as a roadmap to creating their own PCMH-N systems.

The National Council for Quality Assurance (NCQA), a nonprofit organization that was formed in 1990, measures quality and credentials over many in-patient and outpatient domains. Step-by-step processes for obtaining accreditation can be found on their website, and the reader is urged to access this information prior to any such accreditation process, as standards my change. To be recognized as an NCQA-specialty practice, a practice must demonstrate competence along these six standards:
1. Track and coordinate referrals;
2. Provide access and communication;
3. Identify and coordinate patient populations;
4. Plan and manage care;
5. Track and coordinate care;
6. Measure and improve performance.[99]

These six standards serve as a template for care for all specialty and subspecialty groups. Regardless of your intent to obtain certification, paying attention to these facets will make your practice a much more effective referral partner, thus bringing value to patients, referring practices, and the health-care system as a whole.

## Summary

- The patient-centered medical home (PCMH) is a model that is being used more often in the delivery of health care in the United States.

- Several experts have recognized that the PCMH alone, excluding specialists, will not be able to effectively coordinate care or control health-care costs.

- A specialist, through certification or practice modification, can become an effective specialty practice; doing so will augment the PCMH in becoming a PCMH-Neighborhood.

---

[99] National Committee for Quality Assurance (NCQA), "Introduction to Patient-Centered Specialty Practice (PCSP) 2016 Recognition Program." 2016.
http://www.ncqa.org/Portals/0/Programs/Recognition/PCSP%202016%20Standards%20Training%20Slides%2009.06.2016.pdf?ver=2016-09-06-230710-457. Accessed December 26, 2017.

- Exercising communication, coordination, respect of culture, and a clear understanding of the role of the home and the specialist (or neighbor) in the care of each patient is the only way to achieve an effective neighborhood.

# 4

## How Physicians Can Become Involved in Health-Care Changes

### Donna D. Johnson, MD

The US Affordable Care Act (ACA) was passed on March 23, 2010. The ACA has ushered in the most extensive changes in health-care delivery in the United States since the introduction of Medicare and Medicaid in the 1960s. Health-care reform under the ACA is by no means complete and will continue into the near future. Physicians may choose to sit back and watch the changes occur and then comply; alternatively, they may become more educated about health-care strategies and economics and become more involved in the reformation process. To become engaged is simple, but it does take time. The trade-off is that you will be able to help control health-care delivery to your patients, improve quality of care, and save health-care dollars. Physicians can become involved on three levels: at the national, state, and local-hospital levels.

Although the scope of this chapter is not to discuss national politics, national politics cannot be ignored. Among the 115th US Congress, three physicians were elected into the Senate and ten into the House of Representatives. Two of the physicians were obstetrician/gynecologists.[100] When important health-care legislation comes before Congress, ideally physicians will contact their own representatives to discuss their professional views and educate the representatives on the issue. Representatives do listen to their constituents. If physicians do not want to be personally involved, then they can contribute money to political action committees that represent the interests of the physicians.

For example, the American Congress of Obstetricians and Gynecologists (ACOG) has a political action committee to lobby for or against bills that affect women's health care. The Society for Maternal Fetal Medicine's Health Policy and Advocacy Committee and chief advocacy officer promote causes at the federal level and educate policymakers about the impact that specific health-care rules and regulations have on women with high-risk pregnancies. The amount of legislation debated at the national level that affects women's health is not trivial. The 112th Congress voted fifty-five times on legislation that targeted women's health and potentially how we treat patients.[101] The legislation ranged from contraception coverage and preventative care to nutritional support for at-risk women.

Other legislation, such as the Medicare Sustainable Growth Rate (SGR), can have a significant impact on physicians. This bill, enacted in 1997, was a method to ensure that the yearly

---

[100] AMA Patients + Action Network, "Physicians of the 115th Congress." Accessed December 27, 2017. https://www.patientsactionnetwork.com/physicians-115th-congress.
[101] Henry Waxman, "New Report on the Anti-Women Voting Record of the 112th Congress Identifies 55 Anti-Women Votes by House Republicans." *Vote Smart*. September 5, 2012. https://votesmart.org/public-statement/739853/new-report-on-the-anti-women-voting-record-of-the-112th-congress-identifies-55-anti-women-votes-by-house-republicans#.WkXrUSOZOgQ.

increase in Medicare expense per beneficiary did not exceed the country's growth in GDP. Each year the payments for physician services would change based on the previous year's total expenditures. If the prior year's total expenditures exceeded the target set by Congress, then payments to physicians decreased. The SGR was replaced in 2015 with the Medicare Access and CHIP (Children's Health Insurance Program) Reauthorization Act. This new policy rewards the health-care system by quality of care over volume of care and will, we hope, create a health-care system that prioritizes the health and well-being of patients. Under the Medicare Access and CHIP Reauthorization Act, physicians should benefit from more stable reimbursement from Medicare, and patients should benefit from the quality initiatives.

State politics cannot be ignored, either. Medicaid is administered through the Centers for Medicare and Medicaid Services (CMS), a federal program, but Medicaid rules and regulations differ from state to state. Medicaid expansion is an excellent example. As of 2017, only thirty-three states and the District of Columbia have agreed to participate in this program.[102]

On many issues, physicians can have a significant impact and should become involved. Prior to becoming engaged, a physician should understand his or her state's basic Medicaid system. Your state may have one Medicaid service, or it may have several Medicaid health-maintenance organizations (HMOs). Usually if the state has multiple HMOs, then it sets basic coverage guidelines for each insurance company. Below are a few examples of how being active may be beneficial to you.

## Three Examples from South Carolina

In the first example, South Carolina changed from using a single fee-for-service (FFS) entity to using seven different Medicaid HMOs. Each organization had a different drug formulary, and each had its own preauthorization process to obtain 17-hydroxyprogesterone for the prevention of preterm birth. The process itself often prevented patients from getting the appropriate treatment in a timely manner. One physician constructed a simple form for the preapproval process. He then met with each medical director to explain how onerous the preapproval process for 17-hydroxyprogesterone was for obstetricians. He proposed a unified process to each medical director and explained the potential benefits for the insurance company. Access to the medication would be better, so more preterm labor would be prevented, thus lowering their cost for premature infants. As a result of his efforts, a unified preapproval process was adopted by all the insurers. The physician then obtained a small community grant to educate physicians throughout the state of South Carolina about the benefits of 17-hydroxyprogesterone and the uniform process for obtaining preapproval.

In the next example, the passage of the Balanced Budget Act of 1997 and the Telemedicine Communications Act of 1996 enabled payment for professional telemedicine consultation in 1999. Under Medicaid, each state had the authority to develop its own mechanisms to pay for

---

[102] Kaiser Family Foundation, "Status of State Action on Medicaid Expansion. Timeframe: As of November 8, 2017." https://www.kff.org/health-reform/state-indicator/state-activity-around-expanding-medicaid-under-the-affordable-care-act/?currentTimeframe=0&sortModel=%7B%22colId%22:%22Location%22,%22sort%22:%22asc%22%7D.

telemedicine services. Some states, such as Arkansas, were early adopters of telemedicine for obstetrical triage and care.[103] In 2006 South Carolina Medicaid had no coverage for telemedicine service. To improve access to high-risk obstetrical care in rural communities, one medical school in the state established a telemedicine network between rural obstetrical offices and federally qualified clinics. One physician then met with leaders in the South Carolina Department of Health and Human Services (SCDHHS) to solicit coverage for telemedicine services. The physician presented the problem of increased perinatal morbidity and mortality in rural areas and proposed telemedicine as a solution to improve access to risk-appropriate care. After the presentation, the physician asked if the SCDHHS would cover telemedicine consults. If the answer was no, then the physician asked the group to identify any barriers that might prevent Medicaid coverage. A follow-up meeting was then scheduled to address any lingering issues. In fewer than three months, Medicaid agreed to pay for telemedicine obstetrical services. In subsequent years once telemedicine became more acceptable, this physician served on the state telemedicine committee that established the requirements and indications for telemedicine services in the state. Other insurance companies then adopted the guidelines established by Medicaid.

In the final example, South Carolina formed a Birth Outcomes Initiative. This group has over one hundred stakeholders, including the SCDHHS, BlueCross BlueShield of South Carolina, the South Carolina Hospital Association, the March of Dimes, and many large industries in the state. The goal of the Birth Outcomes Initiative is to improve health outcomes for newborns throughout the state's population. To improve breastfeeding rates in the South Carolina population, the Birth Outcomes Initiative rewarded hospitals that obtained Baby Friendly Certification, which can only be achieved through a joint effort of the physicians, nurses, and hospital leadership working together. Grants were given to hospitals to assist in the education process for the team.[104]

## Other Options

A key goal of the Affordable Care Act is to improve the quality and lower the cost of health care. Hospitals cannot do this alone and must partner with physicians to do so. The approach the medical community takes to build accountability into their health-care organization depends on the structure of the local health-care system. For example, Kaiser Permanente's approach of directly employing physicians may alter their quality improvement efforts from those of a private hospital. The purpose of implementing accountability is to develop and organize processes necessary to improve the quality of health care while controlling costs.

The most stringent arrangement is accountable-care organizations (ACOs), which provide high-quality care to Medicare patients across providers (such as primary-care physicians and specialists) and settings (inpatient, outpatient, and long-term care facilities) over time. The goal of

---

[103] Rural Health Information Hub, "ANGELS: Antenatal & Neonatal Guidelines, Education and Learning System." December 28, 2010. https://www.ruralhealthinfo.org/community-health/project-examples/681.

[104] South Carolina Health Connections Medicaid, "South Carolina Birth Outcomes Initiative Dramatically Improves Infant Health, Saves Millions of Dollars." November 7, 2013. www.scdhhs.gov/press-release/south-carolina-birth-outcomes-initiative-dramatically-improves-infant-health-saves.

coordinated care is to ensure that patients, especially the chronically ill, get the right care at the right time while avoiding unnecessary duplication of services and preventing costly hospitalizations. When an ACO succeeds in delivering high-quality care and spending health-care dollars more wisely, the ACO shares in the savings it achieves for the Medicare program.[105] Obstetricians and gynecologists can play a pivotal role in ACOs by providing health-care maintenance for women and education about disease prevention.

CMS has other programs that reward quality as well. One of the most-discussed initiatives is the bundled payment initiative. In the current system, Medicare pays hospitals and other service providers separately. In contrast, fee-for-service (FFS) payment systems reward the quantity of service and not the quality. As a result, patient care is often fragmented and not coordinated well between facilities such as the hospital and rehabilitation services. With bundled payments, one payment will be received for an episode of care. Actual expenditures are reconciled against a target price set by CMS for an episode of care. If the total expenditures are below the bundled payment amount, then CMS shares those savings. But if the total expenditures are above the bundled payment amount, then CMS recoups part of the payment. The payment is made to the hospital, and then the hospital pays physicians and other practitioners.

By focusing on quality of care and outcomes for a single episode of care, CMS is incentivizing hospitals, doctors, and other providers to work together to provide high-quality coordinated care for their patients. Physicians who provide a high quality of care at a lower cost are likely to be compensated more via sharing of cost savings than physicians who provide a high quality of care at a higher cost. Physicians can be proactive and assist hospitals in implementing evidence-based practice plans for patients.[106]

## The Case of Hospital-Acquired Infections

An excellent example of how physicians and hospitals can work together to improve quality of care and to reduce cost is hospital-acquired infections (HAIs). HAIs increase patient morbidity and mortality as well as hospital expenses. The cost of the five most common HAIs contributes $10 billion annually to the US health-care budget. The two most common HAIs found in obstetrical services are surgical site infections (SSIs) and catheter-associated urinary tract infections (CAUTIs). Of the two, SSIs are the most common health care–associated infections and account for 31 percent of all HAIs among hospitalized patients.

Hospitals alone cannot reduce SSIs. In fact, the reduction of SSIs starts in the maternal-fetal medicine physician's practice. High-risk obstetrical patients often have predisposing factors to SSIs, such as diabetes and obesity. Physicians should encourage their patients to control their blood sugar tightly prior to surgery. Once the patient is admitted for surgery, the physician and

---

[105] US Centers for Medicare & Medicaid Services, "Accountable Care Organizations (ACO)." May 12, 2017. https://www.cms.gov/Medicare/Medicare-Fee-for-Service-Payment/ACO/.
[106] Centers for Medicare and Medicaid Services, "Better Care, Smarter Spending, Healthier People: Improving our Health Care Delivery System." January 26, 2015. www.cms.gov/Newsroom/MediaReleaseDatabase/Fact-sheets/2015-Fact-sheets-items/2015-01-26.html.

staff take additional steps to prevent an SSI: the physician can ensure that appropriate antibiotics are administered prior to the surgical incision, the patient's pubic hair should be clipped and not shaven, and at the time of surgery, physicians can scrub their hands appropriately and wear clean surgical attire. During the postoperative period, all health-care providers should wash their hands prior to examining the patient. If the patient develops an SSI within thirty days of the procedure, the hospital is required to report the case. SSI rates are reported and published by the Centers for Disease Control. These data are available for patients to examine so they can then make decisions on where to receive their care.

A team approach is essential to attain the lowest possible number of HAIs. Physician engagement and leadership are essential for success. Physician and nursing leadership must work as a team to establish a protocol that incorporates best practices. Physician leaders can then encourage their colleagues to follow the best-practice guidelines. Once a HAI is identified, the physician and infectious disease nurse can review the case to ensure that the HAI is correctly diagnosed and reported. Together they can review the case to determine if all components of best practices were followed. We assume that procedures are hardwired, but we often find surprises when we review cases. Recently in our hospital, a surgeon had an increase in his rate of SSIs; upon review of his cases, we found that patients were not getting the appropriate antibiotics they needed in a timely fashion.

Everyone benefits from lower HAIs. Patients are happier when they don't have complications. Potential patients can review HAI rates by hospital. Thus, patients may shop for hospitals with lower HAIs. Physicians who work at these hospitals can attract more patients to their practice. The hospital and the health-care system save money by avoiding complications. Therefore, reducing HAIs is a win for everyone.[107]

## Reducing Elective Deliveries

Another example of how a hospital administration and physicians can work as a team to improve quality and decrease cost is by reducing elective deliveries less than thirty-nine weeks of gestation. Infants born after an elective delivery between 37 0/7 and 38 6/7 weeks have higher complications than infants born at or beyond 39 0/7 weeks. Multiple studies have shown that early-term infants have a higher risk of respiratory complications as well as nonrespiratory complications such as jaundice. More than 15 percent of early-term deliveries may require admission to the neonatal intensive care unit (NICU). In addition to infant morbidity and mortality, the risk of a cesarean delivery is higher when a mother is induced with an unfavorable cervix.

Although elective deliveries prior to thirty-nine weeks have not been recommended, the rate has continued to increase nationwide. Patients prefer to have a planned day to go to the hospital, since they could then make plans for other children and have time for out-of-town relatives to be present. Often the patient could also choose to be induced by the physician with

---

[107] D. Sharp, T. Palmore, and C. Grady, "The Ethics of Empowering Patients as Partners in Healthcare-Associated Infection Prevention," *Infection Control and Hospital Epidemiology* 35, no. 3 (2014): 307–09. doi:10.1086/675288.

whom she had the closest relationship within a group. Physicians liked the practice because they could have more control over when the patient labored and could reduce the disruption to the office practice. But the cost to the health-care system continued to increase until a national campaign was launched to stop the practice.[108] Advocacy groups such as the Leapfrog Group began to report elective deliveries less than thirty-nine weeks as a quality measure that was publically displayed.[109]

Employers, who often bear a significant cost of health care, also began to take note. In at least one state, Medicaid stopped paying hospitals for an elective induction at less than thirty-nine weeks. Thus, most hospitals implemented programs to significantly reduce elective inductions at less than thirty-nine weeks. A physician "champion" usually joined forces with the hospital to implement a program to greatly decrease these elective deliveries. Some of the methods that were used successfully included "hard stops," "soft stops," and education for patients and physicians. With hard stops, the hospital simply would not admit a patient for an induction of labor less than thirty-nine weeks until a physician champion had reviewed the patient's history. With soft stops, the physicians who admitted patients to the hospital agreed to stop this practice, usually after education about the hazards of this practice and the underlying costs. Once elective early-term deliveries have been significantly decreased or entirely stopped, the hospital as well as the physicians can use this quality and cost-saving measure to negotiate with insurance companies.

## Lean Principles and Waste

Until recently, hospitals catered to individual physicians' desires without consideration of waste in the system. With the introduction of value-based care, hospitals have attempted to make their systems more cost efficient. One method some hospitals have used is lean principles. Lean principles originally began in the automobile industry but have since spread to other industries. *Lean* used in this sense is a customer-centric methodology used to continuously improve any process through the elimination of waste in the system. The ultimate goal is to provide a perfect product to the customer at the best value through a process that has zero waste.[110]

One of the main components of waste in the medical system is individual physician variation. The operating room is one place with wide variation that is very costly to the hospital. Standardization of surgical procedures allows team members to become more experienced and efficient. If a surgical procedure is performed in the same way every time, then all components of the system will become better organized. Uniformity also allows the amount of supplies to be greatly reduced. Supplies are less likely to become outdated and need to be discarded. By using more of the same supplies, hospitals can take advantage of the larger discount companies often offer when they order more supplies. With less variation, surgical trays, for example, are less likely

---

[108] American College of Obstetricians and Gynecologists, "Nonmedically Indicated Early Term Deliveries," Committee Opinion no. 561, *Obstetrics & Gynecology* 121 (2013): 911–15.
[109] The Leapfrog Group, "Early Elective Delivery Rate." Accessed October 31, 2017. http://www.leapfroggroup.org/ratings-reports/early-elective-delivery-rate.
[110] N. J. Sayer and B. Williams, *Lean for Dummies*, 2nd ed. (Hoboken, NJ: John Wiley & Sons, 2012).

to be defective and require resterilization. Setup in the OR is simpler and perfected more easily. The scrub nurse can anticipate the needs of the surgeon, and operating times can be reduced.

Physicians must buy into lean principles to implement changes. First, information must be gathered to determine all the steps to a procedure from the beginning to the end. Next, the literature should be reviewed to determine the best evidence-based way to perform the procedure. Next, each step of the operation must then be standardized. Physician leaders must then encourage their peers to adopt a universal means to perform a surgical procedure. Physicians who adopt the lean principles save health-care dollars and are more valuable hospital staff members than physicians who do not.

Since the Institute of Medicine (IOM) report *To Err Is Human* was published in 1999, health-care systems have focused on eliminating medical errors.[111] Medical errors are defined as the failure to execute an appropriate plan of care, or the use of an incorrect plan of care to treat a problem. An example of failure to execute an appropriate plan of care is performing surgery on the incorrect site. Failure to execute a plan of care is often a symptom of our fragmented health-care system and demonstrates that the system lacks adequate checks and balances. An example of an incorrect plan of care is the removal of a pregnant patient's gallbladder to treat right upper quadrant pain in a patient with preeclampsia with severe features: new onset hypertension, proteinuria, and right upper quadrant pain. Errors can occur in all stages of treatment, from diagnosis to treatment to preventative care.

A medical error that results in an injury is defined as a preventable adverse event. At the time of the IOM's report, adverse events occurred in 2.9 to 3.7 percent of patients; the risk of death from an adverse event is estimated to be 6.6 to 13.6 percent. From this data, between forty-four thousand and ninety-eight thousand patients are thought to die each year due to medical errors. This means that the number of patients who die from medical errors is greater than mortality from traffic accidents, breast cancer, or AIDS combined. Errors are also very costly. The estimated annual cost of errors is between $17 billion and $29 billion, half of which is for the extra medical care required to treat the patient; the other half is the cost to society in lost wages, long-term care, and other items. Both patients and health-care providers suffer from errors. Besides the medical problems caused by the error, patients lose trust in the health-care system. Health-care providers are embarrassed and often lose morale.

The IOM recommended a four-pronged approach to improve safety: (1) develop tools and perform research to help us better understand issues regarding patient safety, (2) develop a nationwide reporting system, (3) raise expectations for patient safety throughout health-care organizations, and (4) implement a safety system to ensure that patients are safer.[112] Hospitals felt pressure to promptly create a culture of safety. To gain more physician buy-in, many institutions

---

[111] K. T. Kohn, J. M. Corrigan, and M. S. Donaldson, *To Err Is Human: Building a Safer Health System* (Washington, DC: National Academy Press, 1999).
[112] Institute for Healthcare Improvement, "Patient Safety Leadership WalkRounds." May 10, 2017. http://www.ihi.org/resources/Pages/Tools/PatientSafetyLeadershipWalkRounds.aspx.

have recruited physician leaders to direct the change in hospital culture. Physician leaders examine safety as well as quality.

Safety and quality go hand in hand and have many similarities. Quality of care is defined as health-care services that increase the likelihood of desired health outcomes and that are consistent with current medical knowledge. Quality also improves efficiency in the health-care system. Systems with high quality of care are often safer. In smaller hospitals, one physician serves both roles, but in larger hospitals the roles are often divided.

# Effective Leadership

Physician administration and nursing leadership are essential to achieving and sustaining a culture of safety. Effective leadership is the most critical component. In 2006 the Joint Commission (formerly the Joint Commission on Accreditation of Healthcare Organizations, or JCAHO) identified ineffective leadership as a significant contributing factor in 50 percent of sentinel events—any unanticipated event in health-care settings that results in death or serious physical or psychological injury to a patient that is not related to the natural course of the patient's illness.

To change culture, leaders must convince everyone in the organization of the importance of patient safety. One very effective tool to show everyone the significance of safety is to conduct safety rounds as a team. At a minimum, physician and nurse leaders must conduct the safety rounds, but others, such as environmental services, social work, and pharmacy leaders, may join. The leadership meets with the group and asks open-ended, nonjudgmental questions. The questions are aimed at identifying any system deficiencies that may cause patients harm. Issues are recorded and addressed, and then appropriate feedback is given to the frontline people. The leadership's visibility and involvement demonstrates to the group the importance of patient safety to the organization. Safety walk rounds do not need to be confined to inpatient units; safety rounds can be conducted in outpatient clinics as well. As others buy into patient safety, five minutes at the beginning of the shift or clinic can be dedicated to discussing issues that may affect patient safety, such as short staffing and how to reach the physician on call for the day.[113] These huddles form an important setting of the culture of safety, efficiency, and value for all patient settings.

The leadership of all medical teams should embrace a methodology to capture all adverse events and near misses. Using more than one method appears to be the most effective strategy to do this. One popular system to report an adverse event or safety concern is the utilization of a computerized safety network.[114] Through this network a report is generated and sent to designated staff members. The reports are then examined for systematic and personnel issues. Another method is to use patient surveys. A patient's perception of the environment is valuable and can offer an additional perspective to the team. Patients observe health-care professionals making

---

[113] Ibid.
[114] C. E. Milch et al., "Voluntary Electronic Reporting of Medical Errors and Adverse Events: An Analysis of 92,547 Reports from 26 Acute Care Hospitals," *Journal of General Internal Medicine* 21, no. 2 (2006): 165–70.

rounds, answering the call system, and administering medication. If patients have significant problems, they often report problematic areas on their patient satisfaction surveys.

An additional approach that is often employed is an automatic trigger system to alert leadership that a case should be reviewed. Specific criteria are chosen by the hospital's quality and safety program. Two examples are a patient returning to the operating room for a surgical complication, or surgeons performing an unexpected procedure at the time of surgery, such as a hysterectomy at the time of a cesarean section. In obstetrics, a secondary reviewer should review adverse events because adverse events can occur irrespective of the quality of patient care. For example, a diabetic patient may have an intrauterine fetal demise despite having the best obstetrical care.

## Teamwork, Simulation Training, and Communication

Teamwork is essential to deliver safe care for a patient. The benefits of teamwork are obvious in "highly reliable" organizations such as those found in aviation and disaster response, as well as in sporting events, where teamwork almost always triumphs over individual talent. As Andrew Carnegie said, "Teamwork is the ability to work together toward a common vision. It is the fuel that allows common people to attain uncommon results." The best and most effective teams practice.

Simulation has been introduced into medicine to allow groups of people to practice clinical scenarios without any concern for patient risk.[115] Simulation is important in obstetrics, because some catastrophic events are rare. Multidisciplinary groups such as anesthesiologists, nurses, and obstetricians can practice together. Their performance can be critiqued, and immediate feedback can be given. Simulation events can be repeated to reinforce specific team behaviors.

A rare obstetrical scenario where simulation works exceptionally well is a maternal cardiac arrest. The hospital code team usually practices together, but codes rarely involve obstetrical patients and obstetrical providers. Simulation brings the hospital code team and the obstetrical team together to practice without the intense pressure of a true emergency. Clinical roles can be clearly delineated. For example, the obstetrical team should concentrate on the fetus, while the medical team should concentrate on maternal resuscitation. While the medical team concentrates on running the code, the obstetrical team must displace the uterus to help improve cardiopulmonary resuscitation and must prepare for a cesarean delivery if necessary. The medical team must regularly update the obstetrical team. Once the simulated code is complete, the teams can debrief. The simulation can be repeated again if necessary to work out the details of teamwork. As health-care organizations have become more aware that teamwork is as important to patient care and safety as medical treatments and sophisticated technology, simulation training for the physicians, nurses, and supporting staff has become an integral part of patient quality and safety.

---

[115] AHRQ Patient Safety Network, "Simulation Training." June 2017.
https://psnet.ahrq.gov/primers/primer/25/simulation-training?q=simulation+138.

Communication is an essential component of teamwork for improving safety in health care. For example, JCAHO has found that communication problems are the most common root cause of perinatal injury and death. Poor communication or miscommunication has been found to be involved in 72 percent of obstetrical cases with adverse outcomes[116]. Health-care systems are now working on more effective communication strategies. Good communication is essential every day for every patient.

## SBAR

Kaiser has developed SBAR (a tool adapted from the US Navy), which refers to *situation, background, assessment*, and *recommendation*.[117] For example, a nurse reports to a physician that a patient has been having back discomfort for most of the evening. She informs the physician that this patient is a primigravida who has been hospitalized for five days with premature ruptured membranes at twenty-six weeks of gestation. She has monitored the patient for the past hour and has not picked up any contractions. The patient's BMI is 35. The nurse's assessment may center on the concern that the patient is in labor, and the nurse may recommend that the provider check the patient.

In contrast, the physician's reaction would be much different if the nurse had believed the scenario might be consistent with musculoskeletal pain and recommended administering a muscle relaxant. SBAR offers a simple way to standardize communication and allows both the nurse and doctor to have a common expectation. SBAR should not be limited to interactions with nurses and physicians but should be used between any two members of the health-care team.

## TeamSTEPPS

The US Department of Defense and the Agency for Healthcare Research and Quality have developed another effective way to improve communication in clinical service. Team Strategies and Tools to Enhance Performance and Patient Safety (TeamSTEPPS) is based on twenty-five years of research on teamwork, team training, and culture change. While SBAR aims to improve communication between individual people, TeamSTEPPS introduces tools and strategies to improve team performance in health care. Although teamwork is essential for patient care, and it results in fewer errors, team members are rarely trained together, and teams often do not have consistent members from shift to shift and patient to patient. To further complicate matters, team members come from separate disciplines and possess diverse educational backgrounds. For example, obstetricians, anesthesiologists, nurses, pharmacists, scrub technicians, lab technicians, and blood-bank employees must work as a team at the time of a catastrophic postpartum hemorrhage. Simply installing a team structure does not ensure that the team will operate effectively. Teamwork is dependent on the willingness of the group to cooperate, to coordinate

---

[116] Preventing infant death and injury during delivery. Sentinel Event Alert #30. Oakbrook Terrace, Illinois: The Joint Commission on Accreditation of Healthcare Organizations. July 21, 2004.

[117] Institute for Healthcare Improvement, "SBAR Toolkit." December 11, 2017. http://www.ihi.org/resources/Pages/Tools/sbartoolkit.aspx.

care interventions, and to communicate while remaining focused on the optimal outcome for all patients. TeamSTEPPS equips health-care providers with a common set of knowledge, skills, and attitudes to effectively work together and communicate. TeamSTEPPS builds the framework that carries over from day to day and between teams; in this way, excellent teamwork does not require team members to practice and work together on a permanent basis.

TeamSTEPPS can be implemented in three phases. The first phase is a site assessment, which entails determining the readiness of the institution, identifying opportunities for improvement, and identifying barriers to implementing change. To be successful, the site must have the appropriate resources, such as leaders who are willing to work to change the culture. Having one or more physician leaders is key. The next phase is planning, training, and implementing TeamSTEPPS. TeamSTEPPS is not one program with a single method to improve communications. Instead, TeamSTEPPS is extremely adaptable and is tailored to each organization. An implementation plan is developed in this initial phase, and training is executed. Leaders must be committed to the plan and must communicate the plan to others. The final phase is sustainment. In this phase leaders provide opportunities to practice and celebrate wins. Outcomes are measured so that feedback can be given; processes are fine-tuned or modified as needed.[118] Without the commitment of cultural change, the program will not be successful.

An example of how a team can work well together is during an emergency cesarean delivery. In our institution, we used to have a paging system to summon the necessary team to perform the delivery, but its fragmented nature sometimes meant that a key person for the procedure was not notified promptly. Thus, our physician and nursing leaders engaged the entire team to come up with a solution. A group page was then sent to the anesthesiologist, obstetrical attending physician, neonatal attending physician, and charge nurse as well as the appropriate residents on each service. The unit secretary can easily activate the group with a single page. This second system worked well until the patient was taken to a different operating room than usual. The team ultimately found the room, but the surgery was delayed by several minutes. Hence, our leadership reconvened and changed the information contained within the page. Each shift the team is different, but the process remains the same. When team members enter the operating room, their roles are now clearly defined.

## Conclusion

In summary, the Affordable Care Act has stimulated significant health-care changes and reform. Never before have physicians been required to partner with hospitals to improve quality, safety, and clinical outcomes at a lower cost. Physician leaders must partner with university and hospital leadership if both groups plan to be financially viable in the new paradigm. The partnership oversees many aspects of care, from eliminating waste to improving patient satisfaction and care quality. In the meantime, two aspects of health care are certain: health care will continue to change,

---

[118] Agency for Healthcare Research and Quality, "TeamSTEPPS." Accessed January 18, 2018. www.ahrq.gov/professionals/education/curriculum-tools/teamstepps/.

and our physician and practice leaders must maintain constant vigilance to bring increased safety and value to patients and the system.

# 5

## The New Story of MFM Practice Leadership

Daniel F. O'Keeffe (MD), Michael R. Foley (MD), and Idahlynn Karre (PhD)

Maternal-fetal medicine (MFM) practice leaders face immense challenges. In a time of change and demands for greater accountability, MFM practice leaders must step forward with a clear understanding of themselves and why they want to lead change in health care. When workforce issues require MFM practice leaders to be excellent managers of talent as well as premier subspecialty physicians, the personal and professional requirements are great. Medicine and leadership become integrated into every element of daily practice. Leaders must know why and where they want to lead their colleagues, staff, team, organization, and profession. Most important, MFM practice leaders need to know and be able to use a critical set of leadership knowledge, skills, and best practices to help them as they manage talent, time, relationships, change, and influence. This chapter will discuss six elements of leadership during times of change:

1. Lead yourself exceptionally well
2. Lead with "why" and core values
3. Lead with strengths
4. Lead through relationships
5. Lead by engaging in conversations that matter
6. Lead with influence

## Lead Yourself Exceptionally Well

Before leading others, you must lead yourself exceptionally well. You must understand your values, motivations, and purpose. If you don't know why you are doing something, then you can't be passionate about it. People who follow you want to know what you stand for, what you value, and what motivates your behavior.

The Gallup organization has a low-cost, high-impact tool called Motivation Cards for helping you (and those around you) talk about what motivates one's best work. Figure 5.1 shows a few motivators from the Gallup Motivation Cards.[119] Consider your top three motivators from this list. What are the inherent values in each motivator? How do you behave when that motivator is at the center of your life and work? What primary purpose do your top three motivators give you?

---

[119] Gallup, "Motivation Cards" (2015). www.store.gallup.com.

### Figure 5.1. Gallup motivation cards

**Gallup's Personal and Professional Motivations**
1. Being recognized as an expert in your field
2. A day when you get all your work done
3. Getting credit for your accomplishments from your colleagues
4. Making an outstanding contribution to your community
5. One of your direct reports, or someone you trained, is promoted
6. Being named best developer of new medical talent in your specialty
7. A letter of appreciation from a patient
8. Being elected by your peers to represent or lead your organization
9. Authority to make your own decisions about your work
10. Responsibility for developing a new department or division
11. Your child nominating you for mother/father of the year
12. The flexibility to arrange your work schedule to accommodate work/life integration
13. Learning a new skill or subject that is interesting to you
14. A simple "thank you" from your colleagues, staff, or team members
15. Increased responsibility or workload

—Gallup Motivation Cards

After considering your personal motivations, connect them to your career in medicine and leadership. Why did you go into medicine? What are your motivations for being a physician? Why do you want to lead? What is driving you to want to lead change in MFM? Before you can lead others, you need to know the answers to these questions.

### Figure 5.2. Personal and professional mission statements

*"I will be a lifelong learner focused on creating harmony in my life to truly provide great care for my patients. I must first lead myself before I can lead others."*

*"I am committed to building long lasting relationships, leading with my strengths and taking great care of my health and well-being. In this way, I can give attentive and compassionate care to my patients. This is my 'Why' for effective leadership in the medical arena. I can and will make a difference in the lives of others."*

—Personal and Professional Mission Statements from
SMFM Leadership Academy

You must be able to integrate your passion for medicine and your passion for leadership into a personal and professional mission statement that you can communicate clearly and succinctly to others. Figure 5.2 includes sample mission statements from members of the SMFM Leadership Academy course.[120]

As you craft your mission statement, know that you make a difference; this is the most fundamental truth in leadership. Before you can lead, you have to believe that you can have a positive impact on others. You have to believe in yourself. That's where all leadership begins. Figure 5.3 shows what Jim Kouzes and Barry Posner have written in *The Truth about Leadership*.[121]

**Figure 5.3. The truth about leadership**

*"Everything you will ever do as a leader is based on one audacious assumption. It's the assumption that you matter. Before you can lead others, you have to lead yourself and believe that you can have a positive impact on others. You have to believe that your words can inspire and your actions can move others. You have to believe that what you do counts for something. Leadership begins with you."*

—Jim Kouzes and Barry Posner, *The Truth about Leadership*

You know what motivates you. You can articulate it clearly in a personal/professional mission statement. You understand your passions for medicine and leadership. You have purpose and drive. Does it ever feel like you are running on empty and need to refuel? Leading an MFM team is important and courageous work. It takes a lot of energy. Your focus is on serving patients, helping others learn and grow, and building practices and offices of excellence. Do you feel as though you don't have the time or means to look after yourself—to refresh and renew?

As "servant leaders", we long for the mental and emotional equivalents of a stimulating breath of fresh air and a reviving splash of cool water. Do some days feel as if you can barely muster the personal resources to get through the day, let alone lead? We may be having more days when our personal energy and productivity are waning. We wish for abundant energy, contagious passion, and a truly fulfilling, integrated, and harmonious life.

We believe one of the best contemporary resources on personal wellness is Tom Rath's book *Are You Fully Charged? The 3 Keys to Energize Your Work and Life*.[122] Using the metaphor of a fully charged battery for personal and professional wellness, Rath reminds us that we are at our best at work, with our family and friends, and in our communities when we are fully charged. The good news is that being fully charged does not require taking lengthy retreats for finding the meaning in life, making new friends at cocktail parties, preparing to run a marathon, or completing

---

[120] SMFM Leadership Academy (2012–2018), *SMFM Academy for Leadership and Development*. www.SMFM/Leadership: https://www.smfm.org/events/37-academy-for-leadership-and-development.
[121] Jim M. Kouzes and Barry Z. Posner, *The Truth about Leadership: No-Fads, Heart-of-the-Matter Facts You Need to Know* (San Francisco: Jossey-Bass, 2011), 74.
[122] Tom Rath, *Are You Fully Charged? The 3 Keys to Energizing Your Work and Life* (New York: Missionday, 2015).

a fad diet. Rath shares generous data, scientific research, and practical, simple suggestions related to the three keys for being fully charged, as shown in figure 5.4.[123]

### Figure 5.4. The three keys to energizing your work and life

**Meaning: Doing something that benefits another person**
Meaningful work is driven by deep internal motivation
Your work should improve your overall wellbeing
You create meaning when your strengths and interests meet another person's needs
Instead of responding to every ringing bell, focus on less to do more
Work in bursts, take frequent breaks, and keep the mission in mind

**Interactions: Creating far more positive than negative moments in our daily lives and work**
Our wellness depends on interactions, no matter how brief, with people around us
Focus most of your time and attention on what IS working
Practical goals and good questions create speed and productivity
Social networks that we often take for granted profoundly shape our lives
Spending time and resources on people and experiences yields the greatest return for wellness
We do better work when we collaborate and have shared incentives
The more you focus on another person's strengths, the faster they grow

**Energy: Making choices that improve mental and physical health**
When you eat, move, and sleep well, you can do more for yourself and others
Eating well starts with healthier defaults and decisions, making every bite count
Being active throughout the day matters for your health and wellbeing
The more you move, the better your mood
Every hour of sleep is an investment in your future, not an expense
Your daily actions can keep chronic stress from accumulating
Your reaction to a potential stressor is more important than the stressor itself

—Tom Rath, *Are You Fully Charged?*

## Summary: Lead Yourself.

To summarize this first element, people who follow you want to know your motivations, strengths, vision, and purpose. Most of all, they need to know your passions for medicine and transformational leadership. They need to know that you want to help them as individuals, as a team, and as an organization deliver excellence in service to one another and to those you serve.

---

[123] Rath, *Are You Fully Charged?*

They need to see you managing your energy and working toward work/life integration and harmony. As an MFM practice leader, you must model the way.

## Lead with "Why"

To lead others, start with "why." If you don't know why you do what you do, how can you expect anyone else to know the basic essence of your work? For others to know why you exist as an MFM practice leader, you must first have clarity about your own core values, vision, and mission. Inspire others and enlist them in a shared vision.

You, your colleagues, and your team must have a shared understanding of the kind of team, office, and organization you want to be. For clarity on this essential leadership behavior, we offer the Golden Circle, a valuable tool for understanding excellence in leadership, from Simon Sinek's book *Start with Why: How Great Leaders Inspire Everyone to Take Action*.[124] Sinek's TED Talk of the same title is available on YouTube and TED.com. Figure 5.5 shows a graphic of the Golden Circle, which differentiates "why" you do what you do from "how" you do it and "what" the outcomes will be. The best leaders and most successful organizations start with "why."

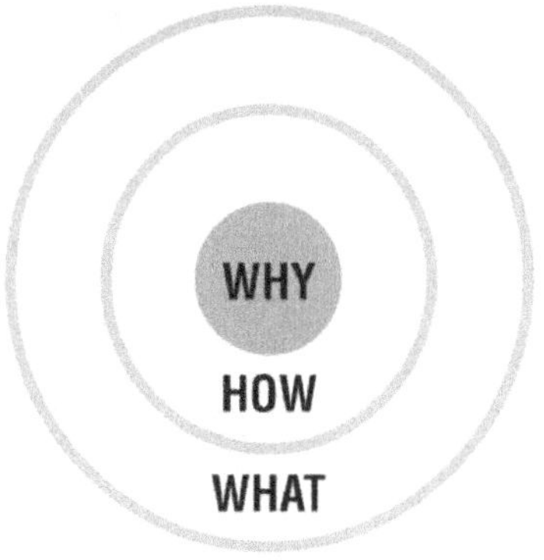

The Golden Circle works most effectively when MFM practice leaders have clarity of *why*, discipline of *how*, and consistency of *what*. No one section of the Golden Circle is more important than any other. The most important leadership behaviors are to start with *why* and create a balance across all three circles.

**Figure 5.5: The Golden Circle from *Start with Why***

**Why**: Very few organizations know *why* they do what they do. *Why* is not a matter of making money. *Why* is a purpose, cause, and belief. It's the very reason your organization exists. This is the first conversation you need to have with your colleagues and team.

**How**: Some organizations know *how* they do what they do. These are the things that make them special or set them apart from their competition. These are the actions that you and your team take to bring your work to life. They must be aligned with your values, guiding principles, strengths, and beliefs.

**What**: Every organization knows *what* they do. These are the products they sell or the services they offer. When *what* you do is derived from your core values (*why*) and balanced

---

[124] Simon Sinek, *Start with Why: How Great Leaders Inspire Everyone to Take Action* (New York: Penguin Group, 2011). See also Simon Sinek, "Start with Why: How Great Leaders Inspire Action," TED Video, 18:04, filmed September 2009. https://www.ted.com/talks/simon_sinek_how_great_leaders_inspire_action.

with the actions you and your teams take (*how*), you create systems, processes, and open and honest behaviors. As an MFM practice leader, you create a culture of safety and excellence. *What* you do becomes extraordinary.

In addition to the Golden Circle, MFM practice leaders must know and be able to use the "five practices of exemplary leadership" from *The Leadership Challenge*.[125] Jim Kouzes and Barry Posner have conducted intensive research on leadership since 1982. Their book *The Leadership Challenge* is widely considered the seminal text of leadership.

Kouzes and Posner have consistently chosen not to focus their research on famous people in positions of power who make the headlines. Instead, they have always wanted to know what the vast majority of good leaders do, focusing on ordinary people who get extraordinary things done for their teams, offices, and organizations. They have concentrated their research on people who lead project teams, manage departments, lead medical staffs, administer schools, organize community groups, and volunteer for civic organizations. Their research found five practices and ten commitments of exemplary leadership (see table 5.1).[126]

| Table 5.1. The Leadership Challenge | |
|---|---|
| **Leadership practices** | **Leadership commitments** |
| Challenging the process | 1. Search out challenging opportunities to change, grow, innovate, and improve<br>2. Experiment, learn, ask good questions |
| Inspiring a shared vision | 3. Envision an uplifting and ennobling future<br>4. Enlist others in a common vision by appealing to their values, interests, hopes, and dreams |
| Enabling others to act | 5. Foster collaboration by promoting cooperative goals and building trust<br>6. Strengthen people by giving them the opportunity to do what they do best, developing competence, offering visible support |
| Modeling the way | 7. Set the example by behaving in ways that are consistent with shared values<br>8. Achieve small wins that promote consistent progress and build commitment |
| Encouraging the heart | 9. Recognize individual contributions to the success of every project<br>10. Celebrate team accomplishments regularly |

Leaders need to use the research on exemplary leadership to help lead with *why*. When leading change, *challenge the typical process* of starting with 150 rational reasons, strategies, "hows," and "whats" that could be used in your MFM practice. Begin instead with core values—why. Make sure core values are shared by your entire team. Inspire a shared vision. Put that vision (why) at the center of all you do.

*Challenge the process* by agreeing to talk respectfully and openly about all issues related to work, collegiality, team, and office. Create systems, better thought processes, and best practices in

---

[125] Jim M. Kouzes and Barry Z. Posner, *The Leadership Challenge: How to Make Extraordinary Things Happen in Organizations*, 5th ed. (San Francisco: Jossey-Bass, 2012).
[126] Ibid.

communication to achieve the *how* of the Golden Circle. Make sure that the *what* of every day creates a culture of discipline, engagement, honesty, and trust.

*Enable others to act* by fostering collaboration. Make collaboration the default method of *how* and *what* you do. Develop norms of how all members of the team are going to communicate. Make them nonnegotiable. Create a culture of accountability where every person is a part of the solution, not the problem. Create safety. Develop an open, honest culture where all members of your practice are encouraged to speak up. Encourage and model respectful honesty without repercussions. Make it safe for colleagues and staff to bring up difficult issues, and assure them that they will not be intimidated or reprimanded for doing so. Figure 5.6 illustrates what Margaret Wheatley has written in *Finding Our Way*.[127]

> **Figure 5.6. Finding our way**
>
> "All of us can reach entirely new levels of possibilities together. To achieve these, we need to begin conversations about purpose and shared significance and commit to staying in them. As we stay in the conversation, people start to work together rather than convince each other of who has more of the truth. We are capable of creating wonderful and vibrant communities when we discover what dreams of possibility we share. And always, those dreams become much greater than anything that was ever available when we were isolated from each other."
>
> —Margaret Wheatley, *Finding Our Way*

In summary, MFM leaders need to know why they are doing what they are doing. So do their teams. Create a shared vision anchored in the very core of all you do—your values. Create highly functional behavior, communication, and a culture of engagement and discipline. Whatever you do comes from why you do it. Your *why* carries transformative power because it comes from you. When shared by your team, it inspires and enables others to be in service of one another and of your patients.

## Lead with Strengths

Be a talent scout; focus on and lead with strengths. In 1969, a group of Gallup scientists led by Dr. Donald O. Clifton began to investigate a series of questions that could differentiate the various ways of naturally thinking, feeling, and behaving that make someone uniquely successful. Gallup brought its research to bear in 2001 with the publication of the Clifton StrengthsFinder (CSF) online assessment tool. Since 2001 the CSF has been administered to millions of people worldwide. This forty-five-year research endeavor by Clifton and the highly respected Gallup organization provides a way of assessing innate talents organized around thirty-four signature themes of strength, as shown in figure 5.7.[128]

---

[127] Margaret Wheatley, *Finding Our Way: Leadership for an Uncertain Time* (San Francisco: Berret-Koehler, 2007), 21.
[128] Thomas Rath, *StrengthsFinder 2.0* (New York: Gallup Press, 2007). See also www.shop.gallup.com.

### Figure 5.7. Thirty-four themes of talent and strength

| | | |
|---|---|---|
| Achiever | Context | Intellection |
| Activator | Deliberative | Learner |
| Adaptability | Developer | Maximizer |
| Analytical | Discipline | Positivity |
| Arranger | Empathy | Relator |
| Belief | Focus | Responsibility |
| Command | Futuristic | Restorative |
| Communication | Harmony | Self-Assurance |
| Competition | Ideation | Significance |
| Connectedness | Includer | Strategic |
| Consistency | Individualization | Woo |
| | Input | |

Surround yourself with others who have complementary and different strengths. If you like to get things done, then make sure someone on your team has the strength to analyze details and see patterns in data. If you like to generate ideas, then look for the person on your team who thinks strategically. If you prefer to have a few close personal relationships, then have someone on your team who can win others over and welcome people to your practice and good work.

Cast your staff in roles that will give them an opportunity to use their strengths every day. Visit YouTube and watch Marcus Buckingham—speaker, author, and champion of the strengths movement—talk about the importance of strengths for personal, professional, team, and organizational excellence.[129] Figure 5.8 illustrates what Buckingham has written in *Go Put Your Strengths to Work*.[130]

### Figure 5.8. Go put your strengths to work

*"The strongest teams are not made up of perfectly well-rounded people, they are strong because they are made up of strong people who bring their strengths to a well-rounded team."*

—Marcus Buckingham, *Go Put Your Strengths to Work*

We each possess a unique combination of strengths and lesser talents. Our greatest potential for growth lies in our areas of strengths. The most up-to-date research by Gallup has

---

[129] Marcus Buckingham, "The Business Case for Strengths," YouTube video. https://www.youtube.com/watch?v=1KeNfhw7bK0&t=21s, 12:39, 2013.
[130] Marcus Buckingham, *Go Put Your Strengths to Work: 6 Powerful Steps to Achieve Outstanding Performance* (New York: Free Press, 2007). See also www.TMBC.com ("The Business Case for Strengths") and YouTube: "Trombone Player Wanted." https://www.youtube.com/watch?v=QfQdiVpcnGI. 15:37, 2015.

found two reasons for this—one biological, and one emotional. The biological answer is that we will learn, grow, and be most engaged and energized in our areas of strengths. Genetic differences are wired into each of us—a unique network of synaptic connections creates distinct patterns of thought, feeling, or behavior. These become our strengths. The emotional answer is that we will feel most energized and challenged when we are working in our strengths. We are more likely to be resilient, persistent, self-confident, and effective in those areas where we have developed some mastery. We will transfer these powerful thoughts, feelings, and behaviors to new challenges. As leaders, we can find the answers to growth and development by focusing on strengths.

In summary, exceptional performance occurs when leaders nurture talent and strengths. The most successful leaders build on their own strengths by knowing what gives them energy, motivation, and excellence in their life and work. Great leaders nurture the talents and strengths of their colleagues and teams by giving others opportunities to apply their talents in roles that suit, stretch, and build on strengths.

## Lead through Relationships

Leadership is a relationship. Relationships are at the center of all we do and hope to do as leaders. Leadership is about working with and guiding people. It's about achieving positive interactions and outcomes. If there is one thing we have learned over decades of studying and teaching leadership, and in working with numerous outstanding leaders, it's this: leadership is a relationship.

Maintaining meaningful relationships with your colleagues, teams, organizations, and those you serve is complex and cannot be reduced to a simple set of skills. Every relationship is unique and special, with its own set of possibilities. Relationships take time, energy, and commitment. We can't take them for granted. Leaders must be mindful of monitoring and mentoring relationships on a daily basis if they are to meet the challenges in today's MFM practice management and healthcare leadership.

When it comes to nurturing leadership relationships, everything begins with the ability to think about people other than ourselves. This is the most basic principle of building and maintaining strong interpersonal relationships. A favorite *Peanuts* comic strip by Charles Schulz shows Lucy swinging on the playground as Charlie Brown reads to her, "It says here that the world revolves around the sun once a year." Lucy stops abruptly and responds, "The world revolves around the sun? Are you sure? I thought it revolved around me." *Peanuts* reminds us to check our egos at the door and focus on building and nurturing relationships to help others grow and develop, to create high-performing teams, and to achieve excellence for those we serve.

Great leaders nurture communication channels by communicating all the time. In fact, they overcommunicate. Leaders create a shared vision and reaffirm it clearly and often. They communicate both verbally and nonverbally—in words and deeds. They "walk the talk." Research indicates that about 93 percent of the meaning that is communicated in any transaction is communicated nonverbally.[131] As MFM leaders, *what* you do may be far more important that *what* you *say*. We leaders must be mindful of the nonverbal messages we are communicating. Studies on interpersonal communication have confirmed that words such as *we*, *our*, and *let's* are part of the language of integrated empowered relationships and teams: "We have a good thing going" or "Let's work on this together." Use phrases like "our team" and "our department."

The language we choose to use is not the only strategy for building relationships at work. The ultimate empowerment tool for MFM practice leaders is to lead with questions— nonjudgmental questions. The better we become at asking effective questions and listening to the answers, the more consistently we and the people with whom we work can accomplish mutually satisfying outcomes, be empowered, reduce resistance, and create a willingness to pursue innovative change.

When we ask questions of others and invite them to search for answers with us, we are not just sharing information; we are sharing responsibility and helping everyone on the team be a part of things. Asking questions rather than telling people the answers engages the team in discussions and dialogue that matter and will strengthen the team as a whole. A nonjudgmental questioning culture is a culture in which responsibility is shared. Research on organizational excellence has found that outstanding leaders increase their ratio of question to answers by five to one.[132]

In summary, building strong relationships provides the foundation for open and honest communication. A culture of speaking one's truth and speaking truth to power will be the outcome of relationship building. When times get tough, or work expectations fail to meet their mark, having a foundation for talking when the stakes are high is critical.

## Lead by Engaging in Conversations That Matter

It all comes down to the number twelve. Ten million interviews spanning 114 countries and conducted in forty-one languages explain what every leader needs to know and be able to do about having conversations that matter. Rodd Wagner and James Harter's 2006 book *12: The Elements of Great Managing*[133] published decades-long research by the Gallup organization on talent management. The research found the twelve questions that will produce team engagement, increased productivity, retention, customer/patient satisfaction, safety, and excellence. In the book, Wagner and Harter share discoveries in the fields of neuroscience, game theory, psychology, sociology, and economics that provide a compelling story and convincing evidence about what we must do each day to create excellence and sustained individual success through talent management and leadership of teams.

The answers to the following questions—and the subsequent conversations and professional development that transform negative responses into positive responses—are at the

---

[131] Mehrabian, A. (1972). *Nonverbal Communication*. New Brunswick: Aldine Transaction.
[132] Jim Collins, *Good to Great* (New York: HarperCollins, 2001).
[133] Rodd Wagner and James Harter, *12: The Elements of Great Managing* (New York: Gallup Press, 2006).

core of leading and managing others through conversations that matter. The 12 Questions (Q12) are found in Figure 5.9.[134]

> **Figure 5.9. The 12 questions**
>
> 1. I know what is expected of me at work?
> 2. I have the materials and equipment I need to do my work, right?
> 3. I have the opportunity to do what I do best every day?
> 4. In the last 7 days, have I received recognition or praise for doing good work?
> 5. My supervisor, or someone at work, seems to care about me as a person?
> 6. There is someone at work who encourages my development?
> 7. At work, my opinions seem to count?
> 8. The mission/purpose of my organization makes me feel my job is important?
> 9. My coworkers are committed to doing quality work?
> 10. I have a best friend at work?
> 11. In the last 6 months, someone at work talked to me about my progress?
> 12. This last year, I had opportunities at work to learn and grow?

The Q12 work in concert to help us understand the unwritten social contract between leaders and teams. With the Q12, we can work to achieve engagement for individual and team success. Starting with clear expectations and the right materials and equipment, understanding and maximizing strengths, building a culture of recognition and praise, caring about one another, nurturing growth and development through timely and strength-based feedback on performance outcomes while fostering opportunities to learn and grow—these are the 12 Questions that will help MFM practice leaders engage in conversations that matter with colleagues and staff. Figure 5-10 shows what Wagner and Harter state in the same book.[135]

> **Figure 5.10. The elements of great managing**
>
> *"The leaders who are the best at getting the most from people are those who give the most to them."*
>
> —Rodd Wagner and James Harter, *12: The Elements of Great Managing*

Research findings from the corporate-consultant company VitalSmarts are also essential for MFM practice leaders; in particular, the VitalSmarts-affiliated books *Crucial Conversations: Tools for Talking When the Stakes Are High* and *Crucial Accountability: Tools for Resolving Violated Expectations, Broken Commitments, and Bad Behavior* are must-reads.[136] Crucial conversations are conversations that

---

[134] Adapted from Wagner and Harter, *12: The Elements of Great Managing*.
[135] Ibid.
[136] Kerry Patterson, Joseph Grenny, Ron McMillan, and Al Switzler, *Crucial Conversations: Tools for Talking When Stakes Are High*, 2nd ed. (New York: McGraw-Hill, 2011); Kerry Patterson, Joseph Grenny, David Maxfield, Ron McMillan, and Al Switzler, *Crucial Accountability: Tools for Resolving Violated Expectations, Broken Commitments, and Bad Behavior*, 2nd ed. (New York: VitalSmarts, 2013).

matter. A crucial conversation is a conversation where stakes are high, emotions are strong, and opinions vary. The VitalSmarts newsletter, as well as monthly leadership videos by Joseph Grenny and David Maxfield, are free and easily accessible resources for MFM practice leaders.[137] These tools all provide essential reading and skills development for anyone who needs tools for starting a difficult conversation or trying to hold someone accountable for work achievements.

While space and the focus for this chapter do not provide the opportunity to delve deeply into all the crucial conversation tools available to leaders from VitalSmarts or through the SMFM Leadership Academy, one basic concept is essential here. As individuals and members of teams, we each enter conversations with a reservoir of past experiences, opinions, feelings, theories, expectations, thoughts about others involved in the conversation, and the topic at hand. As Patterson and his VitalSmarts coauthors state in *Crucial Conversations*, "This unique combination of thoughts and feelings makes up our personal pool of meaning."[138] This pool of meaning informs and propels every action. The authors of *Crucial Conversations* help us understand that, when we enter into conversations, especially crucial ones, we do not share the same pool. As the authors argue, leaders "who are skilled at dialogue do their best to make it safe for everyone to add their meaning to the shared pool—even ideas that at first glance appear controversial, wrong, or at odds with their own beliefs."[139] The goal is to ensure that all ideas find their way into the open for consideration.

As the pool of shared meaning grows on our team, this shared meaning helps team members be engaged with one another, learn together, and grow together as they are exposed to more accurate and relevant information. According to research from the VitalSmarts laboratories, "the larger the shared pool, the smarter the decisions."[140] In the end, teams make better choices. In a very real sense, the pool of shared meaning is a measure of a team's intelligence quotient (IQ) and emotional quotient (EQ).

In summary, MFM practice leaders know the questions to ask their colleagues and staff to ensure clarity in work assignments, engagement of strengths, and passion for the practice's mission and vision. They also know how to create teams that are skilled at dialogue. They fill the pool of shared meaning. They engage their teams in conversations that matter by inviting dialogue on shared themes, ideas, and values. Leaders who engage in crucial conversations and hold themselves and others accountable are successful leaders. The 12 Questions and the pool of shared meaning are the birthplaces of engagement, synergy, and excellence.

## Lead with Influence

We are blind to many of the sources of influence available to us as leaders. During our careers in leadership, we find no skill more essential—or overlooked—for transformational leadership than knowledge, skills, and best practices in influence. Built on years of experimental research by Albert

---

[137] Available at www.vitalsmarts.com and http://www.crucialskills.com, respectively.
[138] Patterson et al., *Crucial Conversations*, 24.
[139] Ibid., 24.
[140] Ibid., 178.

Bandura and other social scientists, Kerry Patterson and coauthors capture this critical skill in their books *Change Anything: The New Science of Personal Success* and *Influencer: The Power to Change Anything.*[141]

In *Influencer* and *Change Anything*, the VitalSmarts authors organize influence into two broad categories: motivation and ability. Three domains of influence—personal, social, and structural (organizational)—complete the model to make a six-source model of influence. Table 5.2 is a visual representation of the six-source model of influence.

Generally speaking, the six sources of influence can be described as the following.

## Sources 1 and 2

The first two sources of influence are (1) personal motivation and (2) personal ability. These sources of influence are found within an individual and determine that person's behavioral choices (motives and abilities).

## Sources 3 and 4

The next two sources of influence are (3) social motivation (friends) and (4) social ability (the ability to know friends and to build "fences" around accomplices—who may draw a person off his or her success path). Sources 3 and 4 are influences that can be leveraged by allies, friends, and mentors to positively motivate, empower, and affect success.

The key to understanding sources 3 and 4 is that source 3 includes the social support necessary for success. Source 4 is the ability of the social circle (colleagues, staff, and others) to do the right thing—or the desired thing. As a change agent, surround others with "champions" who can teach, coach, and provide ability.

## Sources 5 and 6

The final two sources of influence are (5) structural (organizational) motivation and (6) structural (organizational) ability. These sources of influence encompass the role of nonhuman factors, such as recognition systems, physical space, cues, and technology. Source 5 might include deadline accountabilities and rewards for timeliness, while source 6 might include visual clues to support vital behaviors at critical moments—such as posting the vision, mission, values, and commitments to the team in a common work space.

When thinking about and planning sources of influence, tactics, and strategies, a key point for MFM practice leaders to remember is to help colleagues and staff clearly understand the desired behaviors required to achieve success. To that end, MFM practice leaders need to influence behaviors, not outcomes. Influence needs to be focused on specific behaviors that can be used to

---

[141] Kerry Patterson, Joseph Grenny, David Maxfield, Ron McMillan, and Al Switzer, *Change Anything: The New Science of Personal Success* (New York: McGraw-Hill, 2008); Kerry Patterson, Joseph Grenny, David Maxfield, Ron McMillan, and Al Switzer, *Influencer: The Power to Change Anything* (New York: McGraw-Hill, 2011). See also www.vitalsmarts.com.

leverage behavior in four or more of the six sources of influence. Armed with this basic understanding of the six-source model from *Influencer* and *Change Anything*, MFM practice leaders can focus their energy to achieve valued outcomes. Research has found that using four of the six sources of influence will have a tenfold increase in leaders' change efforts. VitalSmarts provides a description of each source of influence in a YouTube video about hand washing called "All Washed Up."[142]

### Table 5.2. Six sources of influence

|  | Motivation | Ability |
|---|---|---|
| **Personal** | **Source 1: Personal Motivation**<br>**Ask yourself:** Left in a room by yourself, would you want to engage in the behavior?<br>**Source 1 sounds like:**<br>"It's boring."<br>"It's noxious."<br>"I don't like it."<br>"It's not who I am." | **Source 2: Personal Ability**<br>**Ask yourself:** Left in a room by yourself, do you have the knowledge, skills, and strength to do the right thing even when it is hardest?<br>**Source 2 sounds like:**<br>"I don't know."<br>"I don't understand."<br>"I can't do it."<br>"I've tried and have fallen short."<br>"It's just too hard." |
| **Others** | **Source 3: Social Motivation**<br>**Ask yourself:** Are other people (1) encouraging the right behavior and (2) discouraging the wrong behavior?<br>**Source 3 sounds like:**<br>"Everybody does it."<br>"Someone told me to do it."<br>"Someone made fun of me when I told them no."<br>"I'm doing exactly what other people are doing." | **Source 4: Social Ability**<br>**Ask yourself:** Do others provide (or withhold) the (1) help, (2) information, (3) resources required—particularly at critical times?<br>**Source 4 sounds like:**<br>"He did not get me the data and files I needed."<br>"Someone did not teach me the new system."<br>"I needed someone's approval, but he/she did not sign off."<br>"I can't find anyone to watch the kids." |
| **Structure** | **Source 5: Structural Motivation**<br>**Consider nonhuman factors:** Are rewards, costs, and perks encouraging the right behavior or discouraging the wrong behaviors?<br>**Source 5 sounds like:**<br>"That is not what I get paid to do."<br>"The more I use my credit cards the bigger the prize at the end of the year."<br>"I paid for this and I am not going to leave any food behind." | **Source 6: Structural Ability**<br>**Consider nonhuman enablers, or "things":**<br>Do rules, distance, tools, or cues enable or disable your actions or performance?<br>**Source 6 sounds like:**<br>"I had the wrong tool."<br>"My exercise bike broke, so I stopped doing cardio."<br>"The credit card company increases my limit every six months."<br>"They moved my office right next to the vending machines." |

In summary, the evidence is clear and compelling: MFM practice leaders must engage influence strategies from four or more of the sources of influence. If multiple influence strategies are used in combination, leaders can exponentially increase success within considerable-change initiatives that the fields of health care, practice leadership, and talent management face within the office.

---

[142] A description of each source of influence is portrayed in a VitalSmarts YouTube video, "All Washed Up," 6:19, posted September 21, 2009. http://www.youtube.com/watch?v=osUwukXSd0k.

## Conclusion

MFM physician leaders have a choice. The practice of medicine faces incredible opportunities and challenges. Leaders can elect to continue in the "old story"[143] of leadership; this practice of leadership views the world as a "grand, clockwork machine," to quote Margaret Wheatley. Old-story leaders have a mechanistic view of people, teams, and organizations; they see workers as cogs in a machine who need to get things done, offices as workplaces, and organizations as places with mammoth power struggles at every turn.

Leaders who live in the "new story" help us understand ourselves differently through the way they lead. They trust our humanness, they welcome the conversations we bring to them, they are curious about our strengths, and they delight in our differences and in our inventiveness. New-story leaders nurture us and connect us. They trust that we can create wisely and well and that we seek the best interests of our team, organization, and the people we serve. Be a new-story MFM practice leader.

---

To develop further knowledge, skill, and best practices in MFM leadership, join the authors of this chapter at the SMFM Academy for Leadership and Development, Intensive Transformational Leadership course. This includes an initial three-day residential training in Denver, Colorado, in October, a six-month leadership practicum, a closing three-day residential training in Denver in April, and a two-day annual reunion in March. Check the SMFM website for specific dates and registration.

---

[143] Wheatley, *Finding Our Way*, 16.

# 6

## Physician Recruitment, Engagement, and Retention

Daniel F. O'Keeffe, MD

Recruitment and engagement are two of the most important jobs of a medical director (chair of a department) or a practice administrator. Performed incorrectly, this one task can severely damage a department or practice. Many people believe that running a recruitment and engagement program is an art, but actually there is a significant amount of science to this undertaking, including numerous articles that have been written on how to form an effective recruiting and engagement program. Medical directors and practice administrators can use the information in this chapter to develop a strong process, thus ensuring a better success rate in hiring and retention, rather than pursuing an emotional or instinctive approach.

## What Are the Costs of Hiring the Wrong Physician?

Let's start with morale. When physicians do not fit well in a practice and are disengaged with their colleagues, the effect is evident throughout the practice. The other physicians and staff will experience low morale, infighting, hard feelings, or the need to avoid the troubled physician, which all contribute to decreased patient satisfaction, staff turnover, and even team disintegration. Consequently, this environment causes other staff members to become disengaged; then productivity declines, providers seek employment elsewhere at a high cost to the practice, and the practice finds itself in trouble. A practice or division cannot tolerate this, so what can be done to improve the chances of a good hire?

### Make a Plan

Initial efforts should focus on the development of a strong recruitment and engagement plan. A focused team is necessary to oversee these efforts. This must be done with a physician and administrator, as both are needed. Excluding physician input from this important endeavor is an unforced error and decreases the plan's chance of success.

The plan needs to be *in writing* and cover the whole process of recruitment and engagement in detail. The overseeing physician and administrator need to understand their practice's specific needs and include detailed instructions for the new-hire physician's eventual role in the practice. Having a detailed plan will enhance the likelihood of getting the right person for the job. Your goal should be to have three to five candidates who may be of interest to the practice on file at all times; you should be prepared so that, if a difficult situation arises, you never hire because of being in a crisis. This process should be ongoing, and the practice should already have the plan in place.

The usual places to advertise or look for physicians are

- Maternal-fetal medicine fellowship programs;
- The Society for Maternal-Fetal Medicine (SMFM) job website;
- The journal *Obstetrics & Gynecology*;
- The *American Journal of Obstetrics & Gynecology*;
- Colleagues; and
- Recruiting firms (an expensive option).

Know what your financial offer will be, as it has to be competitive with the current market environment. You can obtain salary information from SMFM surveys, the Medical Group Management Association (MGMA), the American Association of Medical Colleges (AAMC), and consulting groups. Your job offer should attempt to provide unique opportunities that distinguish it from the recruiting efforts of your competition.

The basics of a job offer include the following:

- salary
- on-call details
- benefits
- moving expenses
- bonuses
- partnership
- supplemental incentives (e.g., four-day work week, flexible time, continuing medical education [CME], research/administrative time, malpractice tail coverage, sign-on bonus, loan repayment, one-year stipend to finish a fellowship)

## Set the Process

Select one point person who will have help from the recruiting team. You should narrow the candidates down to two to four people to interview. The vision, mission, values, and norms that your practice lives by should be sent to the candidates. Send a job description and strategic plan to the candidates as well. This will allow them to see your practice on paper and determine whether they will fit in with the practice culture. You should also extend your efforts to recruit the candidates' spouses, as new recruits have cited spousal dissatisfaction as one of their main reasons for leaving a practice after two to five years. Factors such as social engagement, spouse employment opportunities in their sphere of expertise, partner work hour requirements, schools, and real estate possibilities should be discussed, as appropriate.

Next, perform a phone interview with every candidate. See if they feel that they would fit in with the practice and whether you feel similarly. With mutual approval between your hiring team and the candidate, you can then arrange an in-person interview. You also need to execute a recruiting process for the spouse, who should be invited along on this visit. The spouse should have a separate program focused on employment opportunities, housing, recreation, schools, and community. Have an agenda for the interview and make sure all the staff members are involved. The administrators from the hospitals, your neonatal colleagues, and the staff should also be part of the interview. Make sure that these interviewers are the most positive members of your practice and staff, as well as the best salespeople. Teach them to interview, since most people do not possess this skill and have little past experience with it. Show candidates the excellence of your practice and its distinguishing characteristics. People want to work in an excellent practice with exceptional doctors and first-rate staff. If you have local competition, then you should concentrate on what sets your practice apart. Many candidates are looking to work within a specific region, and thus they are likely interviewing with your competition as well.

Here are six things that a recruiting committee should *not* do: (1) concentrate solely on the CV or résumé; (2) disregard the emotional intelligence (EI) of the candidate; (3) discount the social intelligence (SI) of the candidate; (4) fail to screen for the "dark triad" (narcissism, Machiavellianism, or sociopathic and disruptive tendencies); (5) overlook the candidate's employment history; and (6) ignore recruiting the spouse.

**Examine a Candidate's Character**

There are several ways to examine the character of a candidate:

- One can find out a person's strengths by doing the CliftonStrengths assessment, formerly StrengthFinder, a test administered by Gallup.
- The candidate's personality can be assessed by performing a DISC personality test (dominance, inducement, submission, and compliance), which is readily available online.
- The candidate's EI can be measured by using the emotional intelligence test, which can also be found online.

Your practice needs to hire the right person the first time—it is too costly and damaging not to perform the proper due diligence to prevent errors. Following the interview, you need to do the following:

- Decide if a second interview should be performed. Either the interviewee or the practice can decide whether further information is required.
- Set a distinct timeline for making a decision in order to provide clarity for the candidate and for your practice. This timeline will differ based on the circumstances of hiring within your practice.
- Follow up on the candidate's references and genuinely probe all options, such as by making calls to labor and delivery nurses and past referring physicians whom the doctor has worked with.
- Have a contract ready (the contract and all its details should have been discussed during the interview). A memorandum of understanding of key components of the offer should be readily available if a contract requires extensive work from your institution or practice.

- Do not rationalize or normalize any negative information you discover. Remember, the best predictor of future behavior is past behavior.

**Other Caveats**

First, hire only nice people. You can teach skills or you can give them knowledge, but you cannot teach people to be nice, smile, or want to serve. Second, never shortcut the process or hire the wrong person because your practice has an urgent need. Third, once an offer is made, 90 percent of those applicants who will eventually take the job will do so in the first forty-eight hours; be aware of this so you can make offers to other candidates if you have multiple excellent applicants. Finally, never compromise on a high hiring bar. Doing so will damage the practice immensely, and it will take you years to recover.

## After the Hire: Does the Process Stop there?

Certainly not. *Engagement is the key to retention.* An engagement plan is just as important as a recruiting plan—probably more important. Your physicians want to be treated like the providers you *want*, not the providers you have. An engagement strategy should be started immediately and continued each year if you want to retain your excellent physicians. Multiple practices desire excellent physicians, so it is in your practice's best interest to keep your physicians satisfied, engaged, and feeling appreciated. You must really re-recruit your physicians each year. Why is this so? Because it costs between 50 and 150 percent of a physician's salary to find a replacement for that physician. Hence, it will cost you well into the broad range of 200,000-$600,000 if somebody leaves your practice, not to mention the disruption to your practice's morale. Here are some of the *do*s once you and the recruit have verbally agreed:

- Get the contract done quickly.
- Have a checklist of things that need to be completed before the recruit starts and for the first three to six months after that.
- Have a formal orientation plan in place.
- Have one of your best MDs act as a mentor (i.e., the buddy system) to the new recruit for at least the first six months.
- Have recruit's equipment/working space ready when they arrive.
- Make sure the employee handbook is sent to new recruits.
- Meet with the physician every month for at least the first six months.
- Help recruits set up their work/life balance plan in the areas of work, personal life, community, family, and spirituality.
- You should meet with physicians every year regarding this work/life balance plan to make sure they are following it and to ask what they are going to do the following year to help improve it.

Physician engagement has been identified as having fifteen elements, as found from a survey conducted in 2013 by the Physician Wellness Group and Cejka Search. Let me say this again: engagement is the key to retention. Doctors have left practices because these fifteen things were left undone. If your system is set up to address these things, then your chances of having an engaged, loyal physician will skyrocket.

Physicians reported in the survey that they wanted the following, listed in order of importance:

- Respect for their competency and skills;
- To feel that their opinions and ideas are valued;
- Good relations with physician colleagues;
- Good work/life balance;
- A voice in how their time is structured and used;
- Fair compensation for their work;
- Good relationships with nonphysician clinical staff;
- A broader sense of meaning in their work over and above their day-to-day duties;
- A voice in clinical operations and process;
- Opportunities to expand their clinical skills and learn new skills;
- Opportunities for professional development and career development;
- Good relationships with administrators;
- To align with their organization's missions and goals;
- To look to the organization as a leader and innovator of patient care;
- To participate in setting broader organizational goals and strategies.[144]

Communication is one of the key successful elements in engagement. Providing immediate feedback, whether positive or negative, is essential. Attempt to catch your physicians doing something well and then praise their efforts. Find out their strengths (via a strength finder test) and put them in their areas of strength to give them a better chance to succeed and enjoy their jobs. Understand their personalities (via DISC tests) so they can be appropriately motivated and so the medical director can understand the best means of approaching them.

If physician hires are not working out or if they turn out to be disruptive, Machiavellian, narcissistic, or psychopathic, then they must be disengaged from your practice immediately. Do not prolong this process, for it is terribly damaging to the practice's morale and engagement. The leader of the practice will appear ineffective and lose authority if a response is not fair and swift. On average, after it is known that people are not a good fit for a job, it takes twelve to eighteen months for the leadership to get rid of them—at the most, it should take twelve to eighteen *days*. The damage done during those months of indecision may never be reversible. If you feel uncomfortable with termination, then obtain training or have a member who is experienced in this

---

[144] Adapted from Cejka Search, "Rules of Engagement: New Survey Reveals Drivers of Physician Engagement and a Disconnect with Administration." January 8, 2015. https://www.cejkasearch.com/pr/rules-of-engagement-new-survey-reveals-drivers-of-physician.

area perform the task. One of a leader's most important duties is to take rapid, immediate action after recognizing workplace issues and disruption.

## Conclusion

Recruiting and engaging physicians can be more science than art, but plenty of information is available on how to do it right. Excellence begets excellence; if you have an excellent practice, excellent physicians, and excellent staff, then excellent people will want to join you and stay with you.

# 7

## How to Set Up a New Associate in Your Practice

Nubia Sandhu, BS

After months of grueling research, recruitment, interviews, and negotiations, you have finally hired your dream candidate. This rising star, who specializes in your needed area, is set to take your practice to the next level and increase profitability, morale, and overall efficiency. After a victory jog up the steps like that fictional boxer in the movie, your excitement and thrill quickly turn into sudden panic and lead to the question, "What do I do now?" Well, to put it simply: There's a lot for you to do now. And you must do it quickly, accurately, and to its maximum advantage. This process includes credentialing your new hire, implementing a training schedule, assigning mentors to guide the new hire, and promoting your new employee to the market and industry.

The competition to hire a maternal-fetal medicine subspecialist is fierce, with many job applicants receiving multiple offers. You have passed the point of being a possible choice to being the applicant's selection. Your job has now switched from obtaining a new provider to retaining a new provider and enhancing that person's chance of practice success. In general, annual physician turnover approaches 7 percent. Physician turnover costs an average of $1 million per physician due to recruiting costs, wasted administrative time, decreased productivity, and lost revenue. The goal is not simply to recruit a physician but to recruit and retain a high-quality, engaged, productive, and happy physician. Proper onboarding will increase new physicians' immediate productivity, increase provider satisfaction, improve long-term retention, and enhance future recruitment.

## Credentialing

Although credentialing can be an overwhelming and cumbersome process, it is a key aspect of a successful medical practice. Before getting into the credentialing process, let's define it. Most people define *credentialing* as the process of verifying a health professional's experience, education, and current licenses. This process was initiated decades ago in the hopes of decreasing medical malpractice lawsuits. In addition to acting as a preventative measure against lawsuits, credentialing helps a practice build trust with the outside world. Prospective patients, referring practices, and the general community feel more comfortable dealing with a vetted specialized medical professional.

Now that we've discussed the benefits, lace up your boots—let's start the process of credentialing your new hire. Many practices have implemented a good habit of including a request for the necessary items for credentialing within the offer letter to a new physician or associate. This process should be replicated at all times, given that it takes time for payers and other organizations to process the credentialing paperwork. It is imperative that the provider who is joining your practice does not ignore or overlook your request for this information. Any mishaps that lead to delays during this process can present a large financial burden, as the providers cannot bill for their services. To avoid time delays and ensure that the new physician or associate gets credentialed, it is vital to get organized and plan ahead with a "needs" list. Table 7.1 demonstrates a checklist of key items that must be obtained prior to starting the initial credentialing process.[145]

| Table 7.1. Key items for initation of credentialing process | | | |
|---|---|---|---|
| Item | Responsible party | Date assigned | Date completed |
| Obtain state medical license | | | |
| Obtain National Provider Identifier (NPI) | | | |
| Obtain DEA number | | | |
| Obtain controlled substance certificate | | | |
| Complete malpractice application | | | |

Once all items on this checklist have been obtained, you can move forward with the initial credentialing process. During this step, you will be required to attain copies of multiple items (see figure 7.1).

After you have received all these items, you can move forward and start the contracting process with hospitals and insurance companies. The key during this process is to follow up regularly and to ask for weekly updates. You can formulate a spreadsheet of payers, hospitals, and other third parties that require updates and record the requirements for submissions and deadlines.

Another task during the credentialing process is to complete the CAQH Universal Provider Datasource, a universal credentialing database. Many insurance companies now utilize this database to credential physicians and associates. Be diligent and make sure that your providers regularly update and attest with CAQH. This step will save time and energy during the credentialing and re-credentialing process.

---

[145] Ibid.

### Figure 7.1. Initial Credentialing Checklist

- ☐ Completed credentialing application
- ☐ Signed and currently dated attestation and release forms
- ☐ Completed W-9 federal tax form
- ☐ Completed Authorization for Direct Deposit Form (if applicable)
- ☐ Current curriculum vitae with completed professional history in chronological order and no gaps
- ☐ Copy of medical school diploma and training certificate(s), internships, residency, and fellowship
- ☐ Current CME (CME activity for the past three years)
- ☐ Copy of ECFMG certificate (if applicable) or Fifth Pathway certificate (if applicable)
- ☐ Copy of NBME, FLEX, USMLE, or SPEX scores
- ☐ Copy of current board certificate
- ☐ Copy of all current active state license wallet cards
- ☐ Copy of current federal DEA and current state-controlled substance registrations or certificates
- ☐ Copy of any: BLS, ACLS, ATLS, PALS, APLS, NRP certificate(s)
- ☐ Certificates of all professional liability insurance coverage or declaration page (face sheet) of policy (if applicable)
- ☐ Third-party documentation (i.e., court documents, dismissals) for all malpractice/disciplinary actions or completion of appropriate explanation form attached (if applicable)
- ☐ Copy of current driver's license or passport
- ☐ Copies of current immunization records and most recent TB test results (if available)
- ☐ Hospital case logs from last twenty-four months (if applicable)

## Specialized Training: EHR and Ultrasound Reporting

Although training should absolutely be provided to all employees, some practices and companies fail to provide sufficient and consistent training. Failure to provide necessary training can lead to employee dissatisfaction, patient dissatisfaction, and loss of revenue. When adding new providers to your practice, dedicate the first week of employment to learning all systems, which should include electronic health records (EHR) and ultrasound reporting. Furthermore, schedule a vendor-led training that will optimize learning and ensure that all templates and pick-lists are correctly customized. If costs prohibit you from bringing in a vendor, make sure that your new provider is trained by a "superuser." Do not skimp financially in this area, however, as the new associate will be using your EHR and ultrasound systems extensively. A new associate who is not fluent with these systems may then choose not to document for services (thus leading to malpractice concerns and inability to bill), underdocument services (leading to malpractice concerns and decreased billing), or take excessive time to complete documentation (resulting in patient delay and dissatisfaction and new associate frustration).

During the initial transition to your practice, new associates should be set up with a schedule that reflects their previous training, experience with your documentation systems, and abilities. Giving new associates a full schedule starting on their first day of work is counterproductive. Instead, gradually increasing patient volumes over a period of two to three months will ensure that your providers can do the many things during the transition that will allow them to be successful in multiple areas of your practice, including:

- Developing templates and expertise with your EHR and ultrasound reporting systems;
- Coding appropriately;
- Calling and introducing themselves to referring providers after seeing patients;
- Developing important professional relationships with employees in the office;
- Asking questions regarding outside referral patterns and consultations;
- Finishing hospital requirements such as inpatient EHR documentation classes; and
- Reviewing and memorizing practice protocols.

## Specialized Training: Coding

As we all can attest, coding discrepancies lead to losses in revenue or possibly investigation of coding irregularities. Providers are responsible for ensuring that the codes they submit accurately reflect the services they provide. To avoid coding issues, practices should provide new physicians and associates with coding and documentation training.

Two valuable methods can prevent such mishaps in incorrect coding. The first is to send your providers to a coding and reimbursement conference, such as that provided by the Society for Maternal-Fetal Medicine (SMFM). The second approach is to regularly provide consultation from a knowledgeable biller (preferably a biller who has attended the SMFM coding conference) to discuss and evaluate CPT and ICD-10 codes for services provided. You should consider both methods, as most providers have limited knowledge in coding; consistent training and information sharing will ease the new associate's transition, prevent coding irregularities, and ensure proper billing.

## Mentoring

In addition to specialized training, it is important that your practice's plan for new providers includes identifying and assigning a senior provider to mentor the new hire. Mentoring provides an opportunity for the senior employee to instill the practice's philosophies, strategies, policies, procedures, and overall goals into the new hire. It is critical that the mentor regularly meets with new providers, observes their work, offers feedback, provides constructive criticism, and listens attentively to new providers' questions and comments. Mentors provide a less problematic path for their mentees to be the most efficient, profitable, and reputable health-care providers possible while also establishing the culture of the practice.

## Marketing Plan

Now that you have hired a new physician or associate, you should promote your hire and update all your marketing material. Start by having your practice liaison share the news with all referring physicians through various forms of communication. Continue with the basics: ordering business cards, scheduling a photo shoot, and updating your website to include content from the new associate's biography. This biography should be professionally done, featuring quotes from your new providers that provide a human element to their background and will engender them to future patients. Don't forget to share the news through social media, including Facebook and Twitter. Social media is an important communication channel that is often overlooked, but it is becoming more and more important. Schedule an open house after business hours in which you invite professionals from the local community. This is a great way for referring physicians to meet your new provider on a personal level in order to start building a professional relationship.

## Conclusion

Adding a new employee to your practice is an exciting event that provides the opportunity of growing your revenue, increasing efficiency, filling a long-term need, and better serving your patients. With this added excitement comes the responsibility of providing your new hires with all proper resources to achieve their daily objectives, duties, and responsibilities while meeting the overall goals of the practice. These resources, when used properly, should lead to a more positive work environment. A sample onboarding checklist is provided below in table 7.2.

| Table 7.2. Onboarding checklist | | | |
|---|---|---|---|
| **Credentialing and licensure** | **Responsible party** | **Date assigned** | **Date completed** |
| Obtain state medical license | | | |
| NPI number | | | |
| DEA number | | | |
| Controlled substance certificate | | | |
| Malpractice application | | | |
| Hospital privileges | | | |
| Insurance plan credentialing | | | |
| **Basic office and hospital items** | | | |
| Order name tags | | | |
| Change office wall signage | | | |
| Buy lab coats | | | |
| Tour office with practice manager | | | |
| Have discussion with billing department | | | |
| Review practice financial policy and collection procedures | | | |
| Review social media policy | | | |

## Table 7.2. Onboarding checklist (cont.)

| Basic office and hospital items (cont) | | | |
|---|---|---|---|
| Apply for membership in local, regional, and national societies | | | |
| Give employee manual | | | |
| Review and apply for benefits (medical insurance, retirement plans) | | | |
| Complete tax forms | | | |
| Office keys or key fobs | | | |
| Set up and train for voice mail | | | |
| Parking decals and pass | | | |
| Arrange for cell phone with local number | | | |
| Create e-mail address | | | |
| Hepatitis B vaccination and TB testing | | | |
| Form office schedule templates in EMR | | | |
| Obtain hospital security badge | | | |
| Forms for direct paycheck deposit | | | |
| Have dinner with employee and significant other at end of first week | | | |

| Important procedures and training for hospital and office | Responsible party | Date assigned | Date completed |
|---|---|---|---|
| Set up training and passwords for office EMR and PACS | | | |
| Set up training for hospital EMR(s) | | | |
| Complete dictation system training for office/hospital (if applicable) | | | |
| Train with office telephone system | | | |
| Complete OSHA training | | | |
| Share compliance policy | | | |
| Give contact information to call service and hospitals | | | |
| Review patient management protocols | | | |
| Arrange ultrasound machine support from vendor and lead sonographer | | | |
| Review billing and coding procedures | | | |

| Advertising and promotion | | | |
|---|---|---|---|
| Order business and appt cards | | | |
| Add name to office stationary | | | |
| Schedule professional photos for website and other ads | | | |
| Add bio and photo to website | | | |
| Announce addition on social media | | | |
| Announce to referring physicians: e-mail/meet and greet | | | |
| Consider speaking opportunities | | | |
| Update physician online profile on rating sites | | | |

# 8

# Common Personnel Issues That Require Expertise in Human Resource Management

## Dina Costanzo, CMOM

Human resource (HR) management is a person or department within your practice responsible for recruitment, orientation, employee benefits, payroll administration, conflict resolution, disciplinary process, termination, safety-risk management, and record keeping. We will explore each of these areas and what you will need to know to create a successful employee-oriented practice. Employees are one of your greatest assets, and handling HR management correctly will cultivate the culture of your practice.

## Recruitment

Before you can start recruiting, you first need to conduct a job analysis. The questions below will help you to determine what is required for the position you need to fill. This can also be used as an outline for your job posting or advertisement (see the appendixes at the end of this book for common job descriptions and requirements).

1. What position are you hiring for?
   Physician, nurse practitioner, practice manager, HR, departmental manager, sonographer, medical assistant, front desk staff, scheduler, medical coder, billing specialist

2. What are the job requirements?
   Type and length of education, language requirements, computer skills, licenses, certifications

3. What are the wage requirements?
   Hourly position, salaried position, exempt or nonexempt position (be sure to review the current wage scale in your area)

4. Do you have a job description for the position?
   Create an accurate job description that is ADA (Americans with Disabilities Act) compliant. Job descriptions should include required skills, training, and education as well as specific duties and responsibilities. Outlining expectations will help ensure that you hire the right candidate. Sample job descriptions can be found online at the Medical Group Management Association (MGMA) website, the Society for Human Resource Management (SHRM) website, and other societies' websites.

Now you're ready to recruit! Next, you will need to identify where you want to advertise your job opening. Some options are your local newspaper, professional society websites, local medical society, career colleges, word of mouth, or a headhunter. The website www.indeed.com is an example of a free job-posting option. Something to keep in mind is that candidates are more likely to apply if they know the company they are applying for, along with some of the details of your benefit package. Keeping all information confidential can be a deterrent.

Evaluating résumés and selecting the proper candidates can be a time-consuming process, and it is best to review them when you can dedicate time just for this task. Once you have selected candidates who match your requirements, start narrowing down your possible applicants. Call the selected applicants to set up an in-person interview.

The in-person interview should involve at least two members of your staff (i.e., HR and an immediate supervisor). Each interviewer should have different sets of interview questions and should interview the candidate separately. This will allow for each interviewer to form an opinion about the interviewee. Interview questions can range from inquiries about past work experience to behavioral questions. At the interview, have the applicant fill out an application, which you will keep on file regardless of whether the candidate is chosen for the position. Set clear expectations by reviewing the job description and having the applicant sign the form. Depending on the number of qualified candidates, you might have to conduct two rounds of interviews to find the ideal candidate who meets your objectives: a qualified employee—one with the proper amount of experience and educational background as well as a professional demeanor and welcoming personality—who best suits the position, the company, and the existing culture of the practice.

Once you have completed all interviews, you will select your top candidate. Upon conducting a satisfactory background and reference check, contact the candidate and extend a conditional job offer. Background checks should be completed in the same way for all candidates; using a background-check service can be beneficial. A large selection of such services is available online to choose from; they will make sure that you are following all state and federal laws, along with supplying the consent forms.

After you have finished the background checks, you are ready to make the candidate an offer. Call the candidate and extend the job offer. Upon acceptance, let the candidate know that you will either e-mail or mail a job-offer letter that will confirm the details of the offer of employment. Include in the letter the job description, salary, benefits, work schedule, and details on paid time off. Ask the candidate to sign and return the letter in order to accept the position.

Call or send a rejection letter or e-mail to all candidates who were not chosen, but keep all résumés, applications, and letters on file. Thank all considered candidates for their time throughout the interview process and for their consideration of your practice for employment. Your thoughtful efforts toward the applicants will send a positive message about your practice culture, which can be very helpful if any of these candidates are considered in the future.

# Orientation

Before your employee arrives on the first day, prepare all log-ins for all the programs the employee will use. Decide on where her work space will be and make sure it is clean and ready for her to start. Prior to her first day, inform the employee to bring direct-deposit information (e.g., a canceled check) and acceptable forms of identification to complete I-9 paperwork. Have a new-employee packet printed with everything you will need for the orientation meeting. A new-employee checklist can help you keep track of all the items that will need to be completed during a new employee's orientation. Items that can be included on the checklist include all preemployment paperwork, a welcome e-mail to staff, returned payroll and benefits paperwork, enrollment in payroll and compliance programs, system accesses, signed policies, Office of Inspector General (OIG) search, state new-hire reporting, documentation of licenses and past training, and updated employee lists and databases.

It's best to have a plan for how you will handle the employee's first day, for example by taking him on a tour of the facility, introducing him to staff, completing compliance training, and holding an orientation meeting. Regardless of whether you have a human resource department or are managing a private practice, the new employee will receive job-specific training in the first days/weeks/months of beginning the job, but the first day of work should be focused on the employee and making him feel welcome.

Greet your new employee on her first day and take a tour of your facility. Show her the employee areas (break room, lockers, employee bathrooms, and the like). As you are touring, introduce the new employee to management and staff members and explain the different departments. Compliance training should be completed on the first day of work, following introductions. An outsourced compliance program will provide the most up-to-date training, including HIPAA (**Health Insurance Portability and Accountability Act**), OSHA (Occupational Safety and Health Administration), and CMS (**Centers for Medicare and Medicaid Services**) employee orientation and supplemental options. All completed training documentation will be securely located in the program. Using a compliance program is highly recommended to ensure that your practice is staying compliant and to keep the employee informed. The orientation meeting will follow compliance training.

The orientation meeting should have its own checklist to keep you on task and to make sure that the employee receives an informative orientation. Orientation should include a review of the facility and emergency action plans, personnel paperwork, a review and signing of the policies/employee handbook, completed payroll paperwork, a review of compensation and benefits, and distribution of keys and accesses. Discuss the mission of the practice, the chain of command, and performance appraisals. Let the employee interact and be part of the orientation. She is receiving a lot of information at once, so make sure she knows that you are available after the orientation for any follow-up questions she may have forgotten during the orientation.

## Reviewing Employee Benefits

Employee benefits will vary from practice to practice. Health benefits can include medical, dental, vision, and health-care-flexible spending accounts. Your practice may also offer other benefits such as short- and long-term disability, life insurance, supplemental insurance, retirement plans, or tuition assistance. A benefit packet listing all benefits, plan and cost information, and broker contact information is a must-have.

The HR department needs to communicate with employees about any changes in the cost of health benefits or in the health-benefit plan. They set up either enrollment meetings or online enrollment for employees to select or waive their benefits. After open enrollment is closed, all payroll deductions need to be updated to reflect the changes.

Supplemental insurance (such as AFLAC) can be coordinated with a representative from the insurance company, who will hold individual meetings with the employees and relay any payroll deductions that need to be added for the employee. A monthly bill will come to the practice to be paid.

Having retirement plans will benefit both your practice and your employees. A retirement plan can attract employees and help with employee retention. Human resources should facilitate open enrollments, education sessions, change in payroll deductions, and distribute all plan changes/disclosures.

## Details on Payroll Administration

Payroll administration means managing everything that involves payments, withholdings, personal time off, payroll deductions, direct deposits, and W-2s. Payroll is a small part of HR, but it is one of the most crucial areas to be correct. You input and maintain employees' schedules, time reporting, personal time calculation rules, withholdings, amount of pay, payroll deductions, and direct-deposit information. All payroll information is obtained at employee orientation. Payroll should be processed according to your pay schedule (weekly, biweekly, etc.).

# Conflict Resolution

Conflict resolution is an opportunity to hear and resolve employee complaints. When an employee presents a complaint, the complaint needs to be investigated, documented, and resolved. Most conflicts can be resolved at an employee supervisory level and will not require further intervention. The goal is always to resolve the situation and to retain a good employee, but conflict cannot always be avoided. Below are a few steps the supervisor or HR department can take when faced with employee conflict:
- Meet with the employees involved. Ask the employees to provide a summary of what they view as the disagreement or conflict. You are there to mediate; if one employee attacks another, it is your job to intervene. This is meant to be productive, and employees attacking one another is not going to achieve the goal.

- Ask the employees to provide a few detailed suggestions about what they would like to see changed to resolve the situation.
- Request commitment from all parties involved. Each employee needs to commit to making a change to arrive at a resolution. This does not mean that each employee necessarily will get his or her way, but you can settle on middle ground. The terms need to include a commitment from each employee to respect the other and to determine how much change each employee will work toward.
- Remain impartial and make sure the employees know that you are confident that they can continue to work on resolving their differences.
- Document all conversations and set up a follow-up meeting.

## The Disciplinary Process

Practices need to have a corrective action policy, which should be signed by all new employees during orientation. This will inform your employees of the practice's expectations for following certain work rules and standards of conduct. Employee handbooks should also include a corrective action section that mirrors the corrective action policy. Corrective action should be progressive. Before corrective action begins, it is in everyone's best interest to mentor and coach the employee in question, if the circumstances warrant. If the employee has been mentored and coached with no improvement, then it is time to move forward with corrective action.

The usual sequence of corrective actions includes an oral warning, a written warning, probation, and finally termination of employment. The corrective action process should be well documented; the disciplinary process paperwork should contain all details that pertain to the infraction, written with facts only, and should include an action plan; this needs to be reviewed with the employee. The employee should sign at the bottom of the disciplinary process document, and the original should be filed into the employee's personnel record. If the employee refuses to sign, then write "Employee refused to sign" on the signature line. Give the employee a copy of the corrective action document. If the disciplinary process progresses to termination, then your documentation will be extremely important; you will need to submit it to the US Department of Labor for unemployment rebuttals. The key is to document, document, document.

## The Termination Process

Termination can be a resignation, involuntary termination, or layoff. Regardless of the type of termination, be sure to conduct an exit meeting, the goal of which is to make the employee aware of postemployment information such as last paycheck, COBRA (Consolidated Omnibus Budget Reconciliation Act) notice, retirement plan information, and severance agreements. Collect keys and company property, and be sure to terminate any IT permissions and network access. Keep the meeting brief—conduct the meeting with empathy if the termination is due to involuntary reasons, and if for a resignation, offer the employee encouragement for any future endeavors. Just as with employee orientation, having an exit checklist or employment termination checklist will allow a safe and seamless transition for the former employee and your organization.

## Safety-Risk Management

Safety in the workplace can easily be achieved if the employees are educated to practice prevention. The workplace should be a safe environment for all employees. Implementing an injury and illness prevention program is one way to educate all staff members on your practice's safety procedures. If your practice does not have an injury and illness prevention program in place, then check with your state to see if they offer a free consultation to help you create one. It is the practice's responsibility to maintain OSHA injury and illness records.[146] Continued training for employees will help reduce potential safety incidents.

If injuries in the workplace occur, you may need to create a workers' compensation claim. If such an injury happens at your practice, you will want to contact your worker compensation insurance carrier to create a claim. They will provide advice on the next steps to take in the claims process.

## Record Keeping

Proper record keeping is essential to avoid potential penalties by various government agencies. Personnel files, background checks, completed I-9 forms, employee benefit documents, employee medical documents, workers' compensation files, and Family and Medical Leave Act (FMLA) files should be kept separate and in locked cabinets. An example of what each file should contain is listed in table 8.1 below.

---

[146] For more detailed information on the requirements, please refer to www.osha.gov.

| Table 8.1. Recommended human resource file contents | | |
|---|---|---|
| **Personnel file** | **Background checks file** | **Medical files** |
| • Job description<br>• Résumé<br>• Employment application<br>• Employee verifications<br>• Signed policies<br>• Performance reviews<br>• Disciplinary documents<br>• Unemployment records<br>• Termination records<br>• Emergency contact information<br>• W-4<br>• Changes in personal data form<br>• New-hire reporting<br>• Training requests/conferences<br>• Documentation of training<br>• Documentation of certification/licenses | • Background checks<br><br>**I-9 file**<br><br>• Completed employee I-9s<br><br>**Benefits file**<br><br>• All health, dental, and life enrollment documents<br>• FSA/HSA enrollment documents<br>• 401(k) forms and correspondence<br>• Direct deposit documents | • Workers' compensation file<br>  - Documentation on workers' compensation claims<br>• FMLA file<br>  - Completed FMLA forms<br>• Employee medical file<br>  - OSHA non–workers' compensation related documents<br>  - Hepatitis B documents<br>  - PPD documents<br>  - Flu documents<br>  - Mandatory inoculations and screenings |

Using record retention timelines is as important as knowing how to keep your records organized. These timelines can vary because of differences in federal, state, and local statutes. General timelines exist, but best practice is to verify all documents on a regularly scheduled basis.

## Conclusion

HR management encompasses a wide variety of areas that will affect your practice, and its demands are always changing. You may find it helpful to become a member of an organization such as the Society for Human Resource Management; these organizations provide resources that can help guide you through new situations you may encounter. They also have excellent templates and examples for checklists, policies, and forms. Local, state, and federal agencies can also aid in answering any law-related questions you may have. Most important, remember that your employees are one of your greatest assets.

# 9

## The Importance of Evidence-Based Medicine, Value, and Protocols in the MFM Practice

Vanita D. Jain (MD) and Anthony C. Sciscione (DO)

In April 2015, the American College of Obstetricians and Gynecologists (ACOG) published a committee opinion titled "Clinical Guidelines and Standardization of Practice to Improve Outcomes." In this opinion they note that protocols should be recognized as a guide to the management of a clinical situation or process of care that will apply to most patients.[147] ACOG encourages obstetrician-gynecologists (ob-gyns) to be engaged in the process of developing guidelines and presenting data to help foster stakeholder buy-in and to create consensus among physicians. Though this committee opinion was published fairly recently, the authors' practice has been creating and developing protocols to improve physician consensus since 2007. The use of checklists in medicine has been published in reading material for the nonmedicine population and is rapidly becoming common practice. In Atul Gawande's book *The Checklist Manifesto*, the author recounts story after story of how the use of checklists and protocols has saved lives, both in and out of the operating room.[148] In this chapter we will discuss the reasons why the use of protocols will improve how you practice; we will also provide a few examples of various clinical protocols that you can use as a starting point from which to develop your own management strategies.

## Why Use Protocols?

The use of protocols and checklists has been shown to reduce patient harm through improved standardization and communication among providers.[149] Creating protocols for the management of complex disease can be challenging in our field for two reasons: (1) evidence-based medicine (EBM) is often absent to support clinical decision-making, and (2) standardization can be difficult considering the wide variation of practice within the field of obstetrics.[150] Creating protocols should not necessarily be considered an insurmountable challenge, however. While variation in practice and lack of EBM in the field of obstetrics is problematic, attempting to create a protocol can at least reduce the risk of errors that everyone is subject to making, especially when running a busy ultrasound suite, performing consultations, and potentially even managing inpatients at the same time. The elimination of variation in processes can ultimately serve to improve performance and reliability.[151] Obviously, the motivation for the use of protocols is to ensure high-quality and safe practice. Though standardization is not driven by economics, as noted in the committee opinion, such standardization often results in significant economic savings.

---

[147] American College of Obstetricians and Gynecologists, "Committee Opinion: Clinical Guidelines and Standardization of Practice to Improve Outcomes," committee opinion no. 629, April 2015.
[148] Atul Gawande, *The Checklist Manifesto* (New York: Picador, 2010).
[149] "Committee Opinion: Clinical Guidelines and Standardization."
[150] Ibid.
[151] Ibid.

## What Is EBM in the MFM Practice?

Evidence-based medicine, in brief, refers to the rating system for a hierarchy of evidence for intervention/treatment questions. The hierarchy starts with the highest level of evidence, which is apparent from systematic review or meta-analysis of all relevant randomized control trials, and continues to the lowest level of evidence, which represents the opinions of authorities or reports of expert committees. Not that these lower levels of evidence do not have value, but when choosing how to create/generate protocols, the goal is to choose the papers or methods of management that are supported by the highest level of evidence.

In EBM, clinical research findings are systematically reviewed, appraised, and used to aid in the delivery of optimum clinical care to patients.[152] EBM is really a complex process that assures clinical effectiveness by producing evidence through research and scientific review, disseminating evidence-based clinical guidelines, implementing these guidelines, and then evaluating compliance with these guidelines. The Society for Maternal-Fetal Medicine (SMFM) Publications Committee has accepted the Grading of Recommendations Assessment, Development and Evaluation (GRADE for short) working group's recommendations, which is a reasonable place to start when developing protocols for your practice (see table 9.1).[153]

---

[152] W. Rosenberg and A. Donald, "Evidence Based Medicine: An Approach to Clinical Problem Solving," *British Medical Journal* 310 (1995): 1122–26.

[153] Adapted from G. H. Guyatt et al. and GRADE Working Group, "Going from Evidence to Recommendations," *British Medical Journal* 336, no. 7652 (2008): 1049–51.

### Table 9.1. GRADE recommendations

| Grade of recommendation | Clarity of risk/benefit | Quality of supporting evidence | Implications |
|---|---|---|---|
| **1A** | | | |
| Strong Recommendation | Benefits clearly outweigh risks and burdens, or vice versa. | Consistent evidence from well performed randomized, controlled trials or overwhelming evidence of some other form. Further research unlikely to change our confidence in estimate of benefit and risks. | Strong recommendations, can apply to most patients in most circumstances without reservations. Clinicians should follow strong recommendations unless clear and compelling rationale for alternative approach is present. |
| **1B** | | | |
| Strong recommendation, moderate quality evidence | Benefits clearly outweigh risks and burdens. | Evidence from randomized, controlled trials with important limitations (inconsistent results, methodological flaws, indirect or imprecise) or very strong evidence of some other research design. Further research (if performed) is likely to have impact on our confidence in estimate of benefit and risks and may change the estimate. | Strong recommendation and applies to most patients. Clinicians should follow a strong recommendation unless a clear and compelling rationale for an alternative approach is present. |
| **1C** | | | |
| Strong recommendation Low quality evidence | Benefits appear to outweigh risks and burdens, or vice versa. | Evidence from observational studies, unsystematic clinical experience, or from randomized, controlled trials with serious flaws. Any estimate of effect is uncertain. | Strong recommendation, and applies to most patients. Some of evidence supporting base recommendation is however of low quality. |
| **2A** | | | |
| Weak recommendation High quality evidence | Benefits closely balanced with risks and burdens. | Consistent evidence from well performed randomized, controlled trials or overwhelming evidence of some other form, further research is unlikely to change our confidence in estimate of benefit and risks. | Weak recommendation, best action may differ depending on circumstances or patients or societal values. |
| **2B** | | | |
| Weak recommendations Moderate quality evidence | Benefits closely balanced with risks and burdens, some uncertainty in estimates of benefits, risks and burdens. | Evidence from randomized controlled trials with important limitations (inconsistent results, methodological flaws, indirect, or imprecise) or very strong evidence of some other research design, further research (if performed) is likely to have impact on our confidence in estimate of benefit and risks and may change estimates. | Weak recommendations, alternative approaches likely to be better for some patients under some circumstances. |
| **2C** | | | |
| Weak recommendation, low quality evidence | Uncertainty in estimates of benefits, risks, and burdens; benefits may be closely balanced with risks and burdens. | Evidence from observational studies, unsystematic clinical experience, or randomized, controlled trials with serious flaws. Any estimate of effect is uncertain. | Very weak recommendation, other alternatives may be equally reasonable. |

## Why Incorporate EBM into Your Practice?

The use of EBM is important to your daily outpatient or inpatient MFM practice for a variety of reasons. As the authors of a 2014 article in *Preventative Medicine* have noted, "One provision of the Affordable Care Act is the requirement that new private health plans eliminate cost-sharing for a variety of preventive services, including those recommended by US Preventive Services Task Force (USPSTF) with an 'A' or 'B' rating."[154] As current US government insurance plans develop, reimbursement will likely be tied to performance outcomes, which will be determined and judged by adherence to evidence-based guidelines. Not only should physicians practice EBM, but groups should also reach consensus in how they carry out medicine for their patients. Consider this: What do referring doctors, patients, and families hear when MFM physicians in the same group disagree with one another? Referring doctors may initially wonder, "Perhaps there's no consensus, or there's no right answer," but this may lead to the thought, "I can then do whatever I want," which may not be the right answer. Or they may assume that the MFM physicians don't like or respect one another or the patient, which may lead to the thought that the doctors are motivated by charges, not evidence.

Obviously, the latter considerations are not what we want our referring providers to believe. From the patient and family perspective, again, when physicians in the group can't agree on a method of practice, often families think something like, "They don't know what they're doing. One of these doctors is recommending these complicated tests because of money. There must be no consensus, no right answer, so then I can just save money and not have these tests performed." Again, when looked at in this light, it is clear that patients could actually jeopardize their health because of a lack of standardization among the physician group.

If instead the MFM physicians followed a protocol and presented a unified message to referring doctors, perhaps what these doctors would then infer would be a more satisfactory deduction: "There is a consensus. There may not be one right answer, but at least these physicians have agreed on the best answer based on the evidence available." Providers might then also suspect, "If I did whatever I wanted to do, then I'd be deviating from a consensus of MFM physician recommendations and perhaps harming my patient." Ultimately we hope that our referring physicians will then take our recommendations based on clinical evidence as a sign that (1) we respect one another and our differences, but (2) we have agreed on at least one reasonable method of practice, and (3) we are motivated to treat the patient to the best of our ability based on the available evidence.

## How Should You Develop Protocols for Your Practice?

The process of protocol development should be collaborative. Often, in addition to including physician parties, you may also choose to include nurses or sonographers in your decision-making. You should take your individual practice setting into account. All physicians in the group should

---

[154] M. Saraiya, V. Bernard, and M. White, "A Need for Improved Understanding about USPSTF and Other Evidence-Based Recommendations," *Preventative Medicine* 60 (2014): 1–2.

be involved, as well as the practice manager and any other staff members who may be affected by the implementation of the protocol. All physicians should be informed when a new checklist or protocol is instituted or updated. The following example in figure 9-1 shows a typical decision-making process:

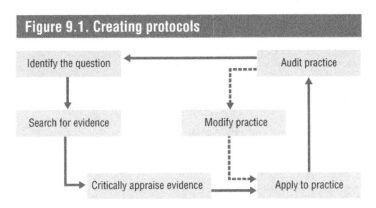

In the authors' practice, protocols are typically generated from two sources. First, a staff member may raise an issue with one of the physicians. For instance, if a sonographer notes a wide variation in the follow-ups the physicians recommend for a certain disease process or in their recommendations for ultrasound surveillance of a specific maternal or fetal condition, then the sonographer may bring this up with one of the physicians. Second, if a new practice bulletin or new SMFM guideline is published that would change the way the practice follows patients, then the physicians may initiate a meeting about protocols.

Another approach is to start with the most common reasons for referral to your practice. Have your billing manager provide you with the top ten ICD-10 codes your practice billed the previous year. Then consider what you see most during your ultrasounds and consultations as well as the most common inpatient diagnosis at your practice. Next, search for the evidence for these top ten conditions. You can either assign one person to do all the research or assign different topics to different people in the group. Later the researchers will bring their findings back to the group and have someone act as the facilitator for discussion.

In the authors' large group practice, one physician member typically culls the available data/evidence regarding the topic for which a protocol is to be generated. That physician then reviews this data and creates a viable protocol—whether it be a standard ultrasound testing schedule, lab work to be offered, or a follow-up plan. This protocol is then presented to the other physicians for review and input. During the discussion, a facilitator generates questions and prompts the physicians to consider opposing views. Once this has occurred, the protocol is then presented at an operational meeting, where managerial staff (including the lead sonographer, practice manager, nursing manager, and lead genetic counselor) are present. The decision is documented, and everyone is given adequate time to think about the new protocol and provide feedback.

Once this input is added and changes are made, the final protocol is presented to the physicians for one last review. Once approved by all physicians (in the past via signature on paper, now via electronic signature through e-mail), any changes to the ultrasound testing plan are uploaded into the dropdowns for our ultrasound reporting system. (See figure 9.2)

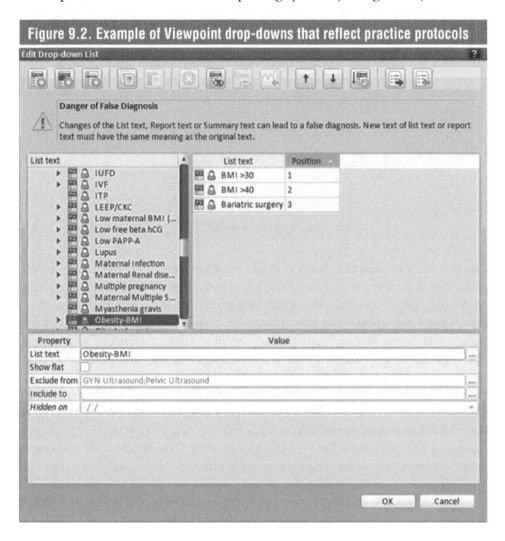

Figure 9.2. Example of Viewpoint drop-downs that reflect practice protocols

The final protocol is also uploaded into the shared drive as a sample drop-down/quick text, which is loaded into the ultrasound reporting system and when downloaded into a report the text is displayed to the referring physician (figure 9.3). The information is then disseminated to all staff through e-mail, and then again in person at the monthly staff meetings. In general, the protocols will include the appropriate references to the evidence-based journal article that was used to support the practice management style. These references are included in ultrasound reports as a resource for our referring physicians. Periodically protocols will need to be reviewed and guidelines updated. Protocols must also be audited at least every one to two years, and modifications should be made as necessary.

**Figure 9.3. Sample of Drop-Down or Quick Text within the Ultrasound Reporting System**

> Obesity in pregnancy is associated with an increased risk of adverse pregnancy outcomes. This risk is highest in those patients with a BMI > 40 kg/m2 (class III obesity). Their fetuses are at increased risk for neural tube defects, spina bifida, congenital heart defects, and omphalocele. However, the ability of ultrasound to detect fetal anomalies in patients with class III obesity is decreased. These patients should be screened carefully for signs of chronic hypertension and preeclampsia as they are at increased risk for these antenatal complications in pregnancy. In addition they are at increased risk for cesarean section and anesthetic complications surrounding delivery. An anesthesia consultation upon admission to labor and delivery (prior to admission if BMI >50 kg/m2) should be considered. These patients should receive compression boots for cesarean section and in in the immediate postpartum period. There is also a reported increased risk for stillbirth (Catalano 2007; ACOG Committee Opinion #315; Weis 2004) Due to the diagnosis of class III obesity, we recommend antenatal testing in the third trimester.

## Conclusion

In any field, in order to improve performance and accountability, one must have a shared goal that unites the interests and activities of all the stakeholders.[155] Within a practice, this can be difficult to do, as multiple interests need to be united: access to services, but also profitability; high-quality care, but also cost containment; safety, but also convenience; patient-centeredness, but also provider satisfaction. In the end, achieving a high value for patients is the overarching goal of health-care delivery.[156] Value depends on results, however, not on the volume of services delivered. The use of protocols, guidelines, and practice standards can contribute to predictors of outcomes and ultimately lead to better results.

To summarize:

- Protocols can improve care within an MFM practice.
- Having standardization of care within the practice and among physicians is important to the referral community and to patients.
- Protocol and checklist development founded on evidence-based care is an important component in developing an ideal environment for optimal outcomes and value care.
- The use of long-term, evidence-based practice protocols may be associated with reimbursement.

---

[155] M. E. Porter, "What is Value in Health Care?" *New England Journal of Medicine* 363 (2010): 26.
[156] Rosenberg and Donald, "Evidence Based Medicine," 1122–26.

# 10

## How to Operate an Efficient Outpatient Ultrasound Practice

Brian K. Iriye (MD) and Elizabeth Williams (RDMS)

Despite maternal-fetal medicine (MFM) practices sometimes having a focus on high-risk obstetrics in the inpatient setting, 70 to 80 percent of revenue is typically generated from their outpatient practices. Operating an efficient outpatient ultrasound practice is key to an MFM group's survival from both a clinical and financial perspective.

Outpatient profitability allows the practice to purchase equipment, hire high-performing employees, maintain the IT infrastructure, afford medical education, and permit adequate time off work to avoid physician burnout. Each of these components affects efficiency and the delivery of high-quality medical care. Yet most provider practices focus solely on medical matters while neglecting the importance of financial matters on clinical care. Managers or physician leaders who wish to create an efficient outpatient ultrasound practice should focus on eliminating waste, reducing costs, and avoiding unnecessary or duplicated effort.

## Lean Office Design

To create an efficient space that eliminates waste and improves efficiency, numerous medical practices have turned to Six Sigma and lean processing principles.[157] Attention to workflow is an important concept in any industry. Within a medical office, workflow inefficiency creates increased wait times for patients, unnecessary effort for personnel, and frustration and burnout for providers. A process called value stream mapping (VSM) can help visualize any roadblocks and redundancies. A VSM follows a process or procedure from beginning to end to visualize its flow. VSM is an important process to visualize the delays in your office processes, to find duplication of efforts, and to identify steps that might be integral to improving care.

When documenting the steps of any process, involve all sectors of your practice to make certain that no steps are omitted. Forming a team composed of staff members from all affected departments rather than a team composed of one or two selected experts will ensure investment in the project and produce the changes necessary for improvement.

One specific type of VSM is called *spaghetti mapping*. To create a spaghetti map, the physical path through the office from check-in, genetic counseling, vital sign assessment, provider visit, ultrasound, antepartum testing, lab draw and processing, and checkout is drawn and then analyzed. A similar process can be performed for the provider workflow during patient encounters by illustrating the interactions with multiple departments and systems. Each place in which the patient

---

[157] See chapter 4 for an in-depth discussion of this topic.

or provider moves throughout the office is plotted as a line on the map (see figure 10.1). This visual representation allows for the easy identification of workflow inefficiency and waste. Once these inefficiencies are identified, the team can then work together to streamline the process, which will result in enhanced organizational performance.

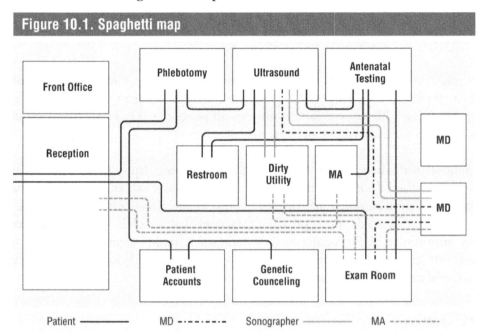

## Information Technology

Unlike practices of the past, the modern practice is now heavily reliant on technology as a tool to increase efficiency. Most offices have electronic medical records (EMR) and ultrasound reporting technology with a picture archiving communication system (PACS). These different systems often do not communicate with one another, which can result in redundant data entry of the information in multiple systems. An advanced application interface (API) or HL-7 interface is required to allow information to be shared across systems. This eliminates duplication of effort, such as adding patient demographic information in multiple systems.

These interfaces are also useful for transferring images and imaging reports into the EMR system without the need for additional clerical assistance. Clinicians often need information from different software systems while evaluating a patient's history, analyzing ultrasound images, and entering information into the ultrasound reporting system. Another technological aid is a dual-screen setup, which enables providers to view multiple systems at once and removes the need to toggle between systems. Large computer monitors with high pixel density are preferable for looking at multiple ultrasound images at the same time. Voice-recognition software allows providers to enter their findings via dictation and speed up reporting beyond basic template development for both EMR and ultrasound reporting systems. Taking advantage of technology and automation can save time and effort across all departments.

## Auxiliary Personnel

Timely communication with patients is a critical component of high-quality medical care and is the main driver of patient satisfaction. Phone-call volume in an MFM practice can be relatively high because of the nature of the specialty. To address patient inquiries promptly and professionally, communications (either by e-mail or phone) should be directed to auxiliary personnel as a first-tier response. Auxiliary personnel such as medical assistants, licensed practice nurses, or registered nurses can escalate a patient issue to the physician when deemed medically appropriate, based on predetermined practice protocols.

Developing a patient-care coordinator position, the main function of which is to communicate with patients and address concerns, can also enhance patient-practice interaction by giving patients a readily available resource without the need to involve physician providers for lower-acuity issues. A care coordinator is usually a registered nurse who has the education and training necessary to properly triage calls, thus decreasing the liability of having nonclinical staff members performing this task. When problems reach a care coordinator, he or she should have protocols to quickly triage information. In addition to handling phone calls, care coordinators can also screen laboratory test results and contact patients with normal results. Tasking the care coordinator with contacting patients with laboratory results not only provides the timely communication of the results but also alleviates the workload for overburdened providers. Ideally, normal lab results can be communicated with patients via a patient portal after the providers sign off on making this process completely automated. Practices should take the initial time and effort to encourage patients to sign up for EMR results available via a portal system.

Nursing staff may also be used to accomplish the time-consuming task of refilling prescriptions. By using a preset practice protocol, nurses can then refill various low-risk medications such as prenatal vitamins and thyroid medications; the physician will then only be involved for the much less time-consuming responsibilities of laboratory and record review and sign off.

All encounters with patients, either in person or by phone, should be documented in the EMR for clinical and legal reasons. The use of automation tools for chart documentation should also be considered. Whether this is a template that is created in the EMR system and/or by voice-recognition capability, having automation in place will significantly assist staff members with chart entry. The use of auxiliary staff will enable both nonphysician providers and physician providers to practice "at the top of their license," as the saying goes.

## Advanced Practitioners

The nonphysician provider is another key team member who can function as an addition to the role of the physician. Nurse practitioners, physician assistants, certified nurse midwives, and genetic counselors can all play a role in providing high-quality medical care, which may result in a significant reduction in the cost of providing these services.

The median MFM subspecialist salary in 2014 was $402,859 per year.[158] The average advanced practitioner earned $104,610 per year as of June 2016.[159] These practitioners should have adequate support and training from your practice to consistently perform at the top of their license. These practitioners may serve in various functions within inpatient and outpatient settings. The role of these practitioners is explained further in chapter 11.

## Ultrasound Quality-Management Program

Having a focus on imaging in the outpatient setting is essential for a practice because of the high costs associated with an ultrasound department and, more importantly, the effect that quality has on a practice's reputation. Sonographers must understand fetal anatomy, recognize abnormalities, identify normal variants, understand syndromes, make correlations, and solve problems. In the ultrasound setting, the goal of a quality management program should therefore be focused on efficiently producing a consistent, high-quality product. This includes communicating standards, formally measuring performance, and holding staff accountable by linking performance to compensation. Quality leads to patient safety and satisfaction. A team of physicians and sonographers should set the goals and expectations for an ultrasound quality-management program.

The first step in implementing an ultrasound quality-management program is the orientation and training of a newly hired sonographer. Orientation should cover all aspects of the job responsibilities, in addition to the position's imaging duties. Figure 10.2 shows a sample orientation checklist.

**Figure 10.2. Orientation checklist**

| Facility Orientation | Technical Orientation |
|---|---|
| ☐ Employee entrance | ☐ EMR training modules |
| ☐ Employee bathroom | ☐ EMR meaningful use |
| ☐ Lockers | ☐ PACS report building |
| ☐ Break room | ☐ Clinical protocols |
| ☐ Emergency exits | ☐ Coding documentation |
| ☐ Work area | ☐ HIPAA training module |
| ☐ Introduction to coworkers | ☐ OSHA training modules |
| ☐ Log-ins and passwords | ☐ Disaster preparedness |
| ☐ Time clock | |

In addition, observation of front- and back-office positions can be helpful in understanding how the sonographer's role is affected by and affects other roles in the practice. After orientation, the new sonographer will begin formal training with a period of shadowing an

---

[158] See practice-management benchmarking at www.smfm.org.
[159] US Department of Labor Bureau of Labor Statistics, "Occupational Employment Statistics," May 2016. Accessed July 18, 2017, https://www.bls.gov/oes/current/oes_nat.htm#29-0000.

experienced sonographer. After a predetermined period of observation, the new sonographer will perform ultrasound examinations with the trainer in the room. The trainer will assist with proper image acquisition and equipment utilization and will observe interactions with the patient.

Next, the new sonographer will be expected to scan independently, but with the trainer reviewing the images via the reading room or PACS. Sonographers should receive feedback about all aspects of their performance. Once training is complete, new sonographers should submit a sample of normal and abnormal exams to the trainer and physician staff for evaluation of image quality and sign-off. (Figure 10.3 shows a sample imaging checklist.) Only then will the newly hired sonographer be cleared to work independently, with the trainer available for assistance or backup as needed. A formal training program with documented evaluation and feedback will quickly detect and correct any technical deficiencies, eliminate poor habits, develop consistency between sonographers, and create a culture of accountability.

**Figure 10.3. Imaging procedures checklist [number of exams]**

- ☐ BPP [30]
- ☐ NST
- ☐ First trimester complete [30]
- ☐ First trimester screen [30]
- ☐ Second/third trimester complete [45]
- ☐ Second/third trimester detailed [60]
- ☐ Transvaginal cervical length
- ☐ MCA Doppler
- ☐ Umbilical artery Doppler
- ☐ Uterine artery Doppler

- ☐ Fetal echocardiography [90]
- ☐ Amniocentesis guidance
- ☐ CVS guidance
- ☐ PUBS guidance

**Upon completion of training:**
- ☐ Ob-gyn board certification

**Within three years of hire:**
- ☐ Fetal echo board certification

Beyond the training period, a sonographer's performance should be evaluated on an ongoing basis, and that data should be included in annual performance reviews. An annual performance review should include all the performance objectives, including exam length, number of exams per day the sonographer is expected to perform, image quality, utilization of PACS and EMR, documentation (including coding), customer service, teamwork, and any other responsibilities that are important in your practice. A 2013 Association for Maternal-Fetal Medicine Management (AMFMM) benchmarking study released the following data on the number of scans a sonographer typically performs in an eight-hour shift:

If performing BPPs:
Average—11.4
Median—10.5
25th percentile—9
75th percentile—12

If BPPs were not performed:
Average—9.84

Median—9
25th percentile—8
75th percentile—12[160]

By setting clear expectations that performance will be directly linked to annual compensation, sonographers will be held accountable. This accountability can incentivize average performers to improve their work and will keep high performers engaged by recognizing and rewarding their efforts.

To incorporate the quality-management program's data into annual performance reviews, perform a retrospective evaluation of a sampling of cases approximately one to two months prior to a sonographer's annual review. A sonographer who is undergoing assessment will select two to four cases for submission by evaluating staff, using selection criteria such as number of suboptimal images, gestational age, and BMI to ensure consistency between sonographers. The previously identified team of physicians and sonographers will also randomly select another two to four new studies to review. Sonographic criteria for evaluation are listed in figure 10.4. In addition to image quality, documentation accuracy should also be assessed. Any elements that are performed by physicians should not be included or attributed to the sonographer.

A scoring system can also be created to quantify the evaluation. Below-average scoring will require that the sonographer's performance be reevaluated in three months. A scoring cutoff should be developed that would require remediation with a retraining period and a review of all images. Reevaluation occurs for this latter group after an approximately three-month period; if the sonographer has demonstrated no improvement by that time, then termination should be considered.

---

[160] Society for Maternal-Fetal Medicine (SMFM), *40 Years of Leading Maternal and Fetal Care Our Journey Together* (Washington, DC: SMFM, 2013), 119–26.

**Figure 10.4. Sample sonographic criteria for ultrasound quality evaluation, second and third trimester**

**Images**
- Time study began
- Time study completed
- Clearly visualized LUS
- Clearly visualized placental location
- Placental cord insertion appropriately evaluated. Three-vessel cord documented
- Fetal position clearly documented
- Amniotic fluid index appropriately obtained
- Adnexa imaged
- Basic fetal biometries (BPD/HC/AC/FL)
- Appropriate head anatomy measurements (lateral ventricles, cerebellum, cisterna magna)
- Appropriate nuchal fold measurements
- Facial views (orbits, lens, profile, nose/lips, palate)
- Fetal spine (transverse/sagittal)
- Fetal heart views (four-chamber view, LVOT, RVOT, three-vessel trachea view)
- Appropriate thoracic cavity views (lung fields, heart positioning, ribs, diaphragm)
- Fetal abdominal cord insertion views
- Appropriate imaging of gastrointestinal tract (stomach, bowel, GB)
- Appropriate imaging of genitourinary tract (kidneys, bladder, renal arteries)
- Appropriate fetal gender imaging
- Appropriate views measurements of the long bones, hands/fingers, feet/toes, and
- Appropriate Dopplers as indicated anatomy/measurements appropriately entered into PACS?
- Each image evaluated based on AIUM guidelines:
  - E = Excellent [2 points]
  - A = Adequate [1 point]
  - S = Suboptimal [0 points]
- Calculate quality score (average of ten cases)
  - 60–45 points = 1% raise
  - 44–30 points = 0.5% raise
  - Less than 29 points = 0% raise

**Documentation**
- Were indications for study correct on report?
- Were all the anatomy/measurements appropriately entered into PACS?
- Was the report summary appropriately formatted?
- If performed, were Dopplers or BPP included in the summary?
- Was the MD discussion topic or the basic discussion dropdown included?
- Was the discussion time included in report?
- Was the tech/MD listed on the report?

Incorporating the score from the quality-management program into the metrics of the performance review links the quality of sonographers' work to their compensation. Since image quality is not the only performance criterion, other areas of competency, such as customer service and efficiency, should be included as well. Each area of competency is then assigned a value, which will result in the overall score of the performance review. Figure 10.5 shows a sample customer service performance requirements and merit raise percentage system.

### Figure 10.5. Sample customer service performance requirements and merit raise percentage system

1. Customer service: has detailed understanding and reflects in actions (Yes)
2. Patient interaction: demonstrates courtesy, compassion, and respect (Yes)
3. Responsibility: takes full responsibility for own actions without excuses (Yes)
4. Group dynamics: works well with all, sought out to work with (No)

Calculation is 3/4 = 75% section score for customer service performance = 0.5%
    90% and above = 1% raise
    50–89% = 0.5% raise
    Less than 50% = 0% raise

Figure 10.6 shows efficiency service requirements.

### Figure 10.6. Sample efficiency service requirements

1. Productivity: high producer (Yes)
2. Images: is able to obtain all images without assistance (Yes)
3. Time management: stays on or ahead of schedule. (No)
4. Critical thinking: gets appropriate additional views in anticipation of being asked (No)

Calculation is 2/4 = 50% = 0.5%
    90% and above = 1%
    50–89% = 0.5%
    Less than 50% = 0%

Table 10.1 shows sample three-part performance evaluation for purposes of quality and pay.

### Table 10.1. Sample performance evaluation for purposes of quality and pay

| Three-part performance review | Possible | Actual |
|---|---|---|
| Quality of work | 1% | 1% |
| Customer service and professionalism | 1% | 0.5% |
| Efficiency | 1% | 0.5% |
| Performance-based pay increase | 3% | 2% |

## Conclusion

Numerous tools can be utilized in MFM outpatient settings that can significantly reduce waste and improve efficiency. Adopting improved design, technology, personnel, and quality-management processes will likely lead to increased revenue and the efficient delivery of medical care.

# 11

## Utilization of Advanced Practitioners in MFM—Nurse Practitioners, Nurse Midwives, and Genetic Counselors

### Brian K. Iriye, MD

Advanced practitioners can play a key role in the ongoing efforts to provide value care. The relative shortage of maternal-fetal medicine (MFM) subspecialists limits patients' access to qualified providers for high-risk obstetrical care, while the presence of qualified advanced practitioners facilitates the provision of care in areas with provider shortages. Simultaneously, more and more patients with elevated risk require MFM services because of higher levels of patient comorbidities such as diabetes, obesity, and hypertension. A practice that appropriately uses its advanced practitioners allows timely access to care, thus improving patient satisfaction, although utilizing MFM subspecialists for care in instances of low or moderate risk increases the cost of care at times when an adequately trained and lower-cost advanced practitioner can instead provide that care.

Risk during pregnancy should be considered as a spectrum and not a categorical variable. Patients are not either low or high risk but have various gradations of risk. The point where care by advanced practitioners becomes valuable depends on the providers' skills, training, education, and practice support. Nonetheless, the mantra of "practicing at the top of your license" allows a practice to provide need-appropriate care at reasonable cost and efficacy.

The scope of practice of different advanced practitioners, including physician assistants, nurse practitioners, and certified nurse midwives, allows each to have distinct advantages and disadvantages when being utilized. The qualities and use of physician assistants is discussed in chapter 12. Nurse practitioners are initially trained in a nursing model with a focus on evidence-based approaches in physical, social, and behavioral issues to promote long-term wellness. Most nurse practitioners have either a master's or doctorate degree, which requires an additional two to three years of study after obtaining a nursing degree.

In many states, nurse practitioners can practice with independent licensure. The ability of nurse practitioners and certified nurse midwives to practice independently offers certain advantages over physician assistants. Certified nurse midwives follow an initial track of nursing study similar to nurse practitioners but have a different track of graduate study that focuses solely on pregnancy. Most services of nurse practitioners and physician assistants are billed at 80 percent of contracted charges. An advantage of certified nurse midwives is their ability to provide delivery coverage and also the usual billing of 100 percent of provider charges. National and regional data on pay for all these occupations can be found on the US Department of Labor Bureau of Labor Statistics website.[161]

---

[161] United States Department of Labor Bureau of Labor Statistics, "Occupation Employment Statistics." Accessed December 29, 2017. https://www.bls.gov/oes/current/oes_nat.htm#31-0000.

# Successful Integration of Advanced Practitioners in MFM

The inability to integrate advanced practitioners into a practice is more often the practice's problem, not the advanced practitioner provider's. These providers need to be seen as an asset to your practice, not as an add-on to services. It is important that pejorative terms such as "physician extender" or "midlevel provider" not be used; instead, use the term "advanced practitioner." As previously mentioned, nurse practitioners and certified nurse midwives have trained in their initial nursing programs prior to earning their advanced degrees and hence are well educated in a culture of team-based care.

Mentorship will play a key role in these providers' continued development and the solidification of their role within your team. The training of an MFM subspecialist includes four years of college, four years of medical school, four years of ob-gyn residency, and three years of MFM fellowship. In total, upon finishing an MFM fellowship, an MFM subspecialist will have approximately eleven years of experience in patient care, with seven years specifically in women's health. In contrast, an advanced practitioner will have a fraction of this experience in care. Understanding this difference in advanced practitioners' backgrounds and training is important so that you can assign them patients whose risk level is appropriate to their clinical development, provide proper oversight, and give them opportunities to focus on specialization within specific clinical areas within MFM to gain knowledge mastery, personal comfort, and confidence. Just as MFM subspecialists need opportunities for continuing education, advanced practitioners should also be afforded continuing medical education for further development.

One common mistake that practices make is to utilize an advanced practitioner as an overflow provider for MFM subspecialists. Tasking an advanced practitioner in this role is counterproductive for a few reasons. First, an advanced practitioner will not know the patients she will see during the day, which will inhibit her from preparing for a distinct patient. Second, the patient is not notified ahead of schedule and assumes she will be seeing the MFM subspecialist, having been told initially that her care was at a high enough risk level to see the MFM subspecialist. Upon arrival, when she finds out that she is now seeing the advanced practitioner because of time constraints, she may become dissatisfied. Third, this role does not treat the practitioner as a full team member but instead as a provider who primarily helps with patient bottlenecks, scheduling problems, or MFM provider inefficiency. To show that advanced practitioners are considered valuable team members, they should have their own patients of appropriate risk, be able to prepare for their patient visits, work with patients with follow-up, and set appropriate patient expectations for office visits.

The role of the advanced practitioner within your practice is not one size fits all. Much like your MFM providers, the successful advanced practitioner may find increased job satisfaction many different avenues. These providers should be afforded leadership opportunities within your practice and system to strengthen their voices and roles in care within your practice's sphere of influence. Some advanced practitioners can play a key role in educating students, residents, and fellows—not only do advanced practitioners introduce them to learning opportunities, but they also demonstrate their expertise as key components of team-based and value-oriented medical care.

Payment incentives and bonuses of advanced practitioners should be based upon driving realization of the mission of the practice or system, not based solely upon a relative value unit–based (RVU-based) incentive system. RVU-based incentive systems set an inappropriate impression that only production is valuable; they do not prioritize the attainment of other important goals such as research, patient satisfaction, medical education, or participation in hospital committees.

Compensation based primarily on RVUs can also cause the following problems:
- *Inadequate compensation.* Practices may be unable to adequately compensate advanced practitioners for prenatal care for lower-risk patients under global obstetric care payments that may not allow proper work attribution.
- *Lowered team morale.* RVU-based compensation can create animosity between MFM subspecialists and advanced practitioners. Because MFM subspecialists would be seeing higher-risk patients—whose visits take more time—this means that the MFM subspecialists would receive decreased compensation in comparison to the advanced practitioners, as their lower-risk patients' quicker visits allow for increased volume.
- *Mistrust between practice and practitioner.* RVU-based compensation can engender mistrust between the system or practice and advanced practitioners in regard to the veracity of the RVU data on which compensation is based: information that is extremely difficult for the provider to collect and track.
- *Upcoding and unnecessary services.* RVU-based compensation encourages providers to upcode or to bill additional services instead of providing quality and value.

## Identifying Areas within a Practice for Advanced Practitioners

The Medical Group Management Association (MGMA) has found that high-performing ob-gyn practices have a 1:1 ratio of advanced practitioners to ob-gyn physicians. In the current era of value medicine and the stated goal for providers to practice at the top of their license capability, this ratio easily could be more. Most MFM practices are not close to a 1:1 ratio and, in many instances, do not utilize advanced practitioners at all. The multiple advantages that advanced practitioners give to a practice include improved patient access, increased time for patient education, and possibly improved patient satisfaction; all these advantages allow MFM subspecialists more time to spend on complex risk-appropriate patients, improve the MFM physician's workload (which increases work satisfaction and decreases the possibility of burnout), and benefits the practice through the revenue advantages produced by a lower-cost provider. The average yearly salaries of an MFM subspecialist versus nurse practitioner, physician assistant, and certified nurse midwife as of 2015 to 2016 are listed in table 11.1.

### Table 11.1. Salaries of MFM subspecialists and advanced practitioners

| Provider type | Average/median | 25th Percentile | 75th Percentile |
|---|---|---|---|
| MFM subspecialist | $454,000 / $410,000 | $311,611 | $525,000 |
| Certified nurse midwife | $102,390 / $99,770 | $85,750 | $119,690 |
| Nurse practitioner | $102,390 / $99,770 | $86,970 | $120,450 |
| Physician assistant | $102,090 / $101,480 | $86,130 | $121,420 |

The near 4:1 cost from the salary of an MFM subspecialist to advanced practitioner provides an important avenue of reducing the cost of MFM care within at least the outpatient setting. A downside argument against nurse practitioners is that they cannot equally replace MFM subspecialists for night call for patients at the highest risk within hospitals.

Finding a proper role for advanced practitioners within a maternal-fetal medicine practice is an important step within your practice. Your practice should examine its current patient loads and needs and determine whether it would be appropriate to add advanced practitioner care to your services to address those needs. Within the outpatient setting, an ideal role for advanced practitioners may be in the setting of diabetes care. Diabetes care is often disjointed in many practices, with counseling for diabetes teaching and nutritional counseling done at a separate site from the MFM subspecialist's office, where medication care and glucose follow-up is performed. Hiring advanced practitioners for this role offers the advantage of keeping all these things within the MFM office for greater supervision and improved management. These practitioners can become certified diabetic educators (CDE) as well and have the advantage of being able to bill for these services as a provider with more appropriate reimbursement, as compared to a CDE alone.

In addition, the care of these patients can be somewhat time consuming, as it includes insulin education, glucose follow-up (often uncompensated, since it is performed by phone), and the occasional patient with poor compliance. Advanced practitioner care becomes much more cost effective in these circumstances and also allows specialization and mastery in one area of an MFM practice. This will allow you to market and extend services to preconception and postconception care, give instruction in insulin-pump therapy and continuous glucose monitoring when needed, and improve rapid access to care within your practice. The reputation of services provided by your practice can be further enhanced by obtaining American Diabetic Association certification.

Many practices miss revenue generation and lack documentation of care from advice and treatment provided within their prenatal diagnostic centers. Your prenatal diagnostic center may benefit from having a distinct area for maternal medical issues for evaluation and follow-up to improve care. Patients at moderate risk for hypertension, rheumatologic disorders, thyroid disease, morbid obesity, asthma, and many other disorders can have improved follow-up performed by advanced practitioners. The improved documentation will enhance communication with referring physicians and assist in reducing medical malpractice risk.

Within your testing center, patients often require care that is again undocumented and uncompensated. Frequent issues that are present at visits within a testing center include basic workups for glucose follow-up, hypertension management, and preterm labor or contractions; documenting the care that is provided is essential to mitigate risk and capture billing that is often lost. Total OB care for prenatal visits may be performed by advanced practitioners, and deliveries, of course, may be done by certified nurse midwives. Advanced practitioners can perform basic genetic counseling for low-risk patients, and they can receive additional training in the area by completing the genetic education module provided by the Perinatal Quality Foundation.[162] This care is uncompensated when performed by genetic counselors; in lower-risk cases, however, it can be performed by adequately trained advanced practitioners, as well as being reimbursable.

Within the inpatient realm, advanced practitioners also can become valued members of team-based care. For practices with a busy inpatient service, advanced practitioners can provide a huge boost from rounding on basic moderate-risk patients with premature rupture of membranes (PROM), preterm labor (PTL), hypertension, and so on. On labor and delivery, these providers can improve workflow and waiting times prior to evaluation, assist with notes and order entry, triage patients to labor and delivery, and in some cases act as first assistant for cesarean deliveries.

Advanced practitioners who work in the inpatient setting should consider pursuing fetal monitoring credentialing through the Perinatal Quality Foundation. To increase their capability and education in the field of critical care obstetrics, advanced practitioners can take the online critical care course via the Society of Maternal-Fetal Medicine.[163] Nighttime call triage can also be performed for low-risk or non-emergent calls, with triage to the MFM subspecialist for more difficult concerns. This will provide an enormous boost to morale and reduction of work stress for the clinically busy MFM subspecialist.

Although the SMFM recommends accreditation of MFM practices for performance of obstetric ultrasound, there are clearly some instances where accreditation is hindering value care and advanced practitioners may provide adequate services. Limited ultrasound for fetal position and biophysical profile assessment are two areas where advanced practitioners may play a role. Obtaining CLEAR certification (cervical length education and review) by the Perinatal Quality Foundation may also be a means for advanced practitioners to receive their certification in transvaginal (TV) sonography for cervical length, which would allow them to provide services in both the inpatient realm for PTL evaluation and the outpatient environment for the assessment of risk of preterm birth or cervical incompetence. Organizations need to collaborate to build guidelines for advanced practitioners and allow for their accredited role in obvious circumstances.

---

[162] See https://www.perinatalquality.org.
[163] See https://www.smfm.org/education/criticalcare.

## Genetic Counseling

It is clear within the subspecialty of MFM that in most practices, genetic counselors are needed for their expertise and also for how they increase the efficiency of the MFM provider. Most payers, however, do not compensate genetic counseling by a certified genetic counselor. If possible, your practice should attempt to obtain reimbursement for genetic counselor services within all your contracts. Within a university system, genetic counseling services are usually provided by one of the departments, such as pediatrics. Because of lack of reimbursement by payers, however, this service has become difficult to provide and may cause conflict among departments. Within community systems, this service is either absorbed by the practice or hospital system or is instead contracted out to laboratory companies.

Some of the advantages of this arrangement are that the laboratory absorbs the cost of providing the service and also maintains the training and education of the counselor, but contracting out services to a laboratory company can be problematic for several reasons.

First, because the counselor is not an employee of the practice, the counselor's hours and availability may be limited by the laboratory and be based on the practice's volume of ordered services. This may then create an incentive for a provider to increase the number of laboratory service orders to sustain genetic counselor availability; this action may also extend to counselors themselves so that they can maintain employment in a practice or locale.

Second, counselors who are employees of specific labs may primarily order laboratory tests from their own labs, which may not offer the tests with the highest detection or be the most cost-effective test for the patient or the payer. The patient may complain about the cost of the services. With payers, this may inflate the cost per patient and could affect your apparent efficiency in contrast to your competitors, both in the region and against national averages. This cost per patient cannot be dismissed and can result in having to engage in difficult conversations with your payers and in future contract negotiations.

Third, because the counselor is not under your practice's control, any employee problems need to be referred to a laboratory and are not adjudicated by your practice. Your practice will have the ability to discuss this scenario, but if you have low volume of lab services, you may have a decreased say in the eventual outcome, which could be dismissal and replacement or the issuing of verbal or written warnings.

## Conclusion

Overall, the addition of advanced practitioners to an MFM practice should be considered a huge asset in the move toward improving access, increasing affordability of care, and possibly increasing patient and employee satisfaction. Many groups lack success or financial returns with these practitioners because of the lack of a consistent utilization strategy or a culture that prevents respectful integration. Groups must set reasonable expectations on return on investment (ROI) and look toward the accomplishment of the practice's mission with the hiring of advanced practitioners. Having these providers be respected team members will help alleviate difficulties such as internal squabbling over team roles.

These providers and the MFM subspecialist must consistently work toward the "top of the license" mentality for care. Increasing an advanced practitioner's autonomy and initial specialization will increase patient access and improve provider workflow for the provider team. Continuing education and mentorship of advanced practitioners are the keys to obtaining maximal contribution and job satisfaction. Compensation of advanced practitioners should not be solely based on RVU but on the practice's mission. The combined goals of an advanced practitioner/MFM subspecialist team will eliminate incentives that drive these two provider types apart, enabling them instead to work as a team. Advanced practitioners, as members of the provider team, should be engaged in committees and leadership roles to foster practice engagement, reduce conflict, and share insights into their important issues. When set up in a practice with this respectful give and take, advanced practitioners and MFM subspecialists' efforts will result in a harmonious, fruitful, and successful working relationship.

## 12

**Physician Assistants in the MFM Practice**

Daniel Thibodeau (MHP, PA-C), Erin McCartney (MPAS, PA-C),
Aleece Fosnight (MPAS, PA-C), and Alfred Abuhamad (MD)

The twenty-first century has seen a rapid increase in the utilization of physician assistants (PAs). As one of the fastest-growing professions in the health-care workforce, PAs have become indispensable in several areas of medicine. Maternal-fetal medicine (MFM) is in its infancy in utilizing PAs in clinical practice. Within the practice of MFM, PAs can actively participate in clinical care in several areas, such as office practice, inpatient consultations, and labor and delivery (L&D). Considerable growth and a greater need for clinical help have created an environment that can allow greater usage of PAs in this field.

## Education and Licensure

The United States has 196 accredited PA programs as of 2017; the overwhelming majority of these programs are entry-level master's programs. While a small percentage of programs award either a bachelor's degree or certificate, the uniqueness of this profession is that all programs must comply with the same accreditation standards. In 2009 the profession convened a summit to evaluate the possibility of a clinical doctorate for PA education. At that time the master's degree was determined to be the terminal degree for the profession, since no benefit was found to be discernible from increasing the number of hours, amount of tuition, and labor it would take to achieve a doctorate degree. The master's degree remains the terminal degree for the profession. Applicants to a PA program usually have a minimum of a bachelor's degree from an accredited college or university and on average have a minimum of two thousand hours in the health-care employment field. Many will have some type of certification (RN, EMT, or paramedic, for example) along with their clinical experience.

A typical PA program is twenty-eight months long and is broken down into sixteen months of didactic classroom instruction, followed by twelve months of clinical rotations. Students gain more than two thousand hours of clinical exposure prior to graduating. Typically the didactic phase of the program consists of anatomy with cadaver lab, pathophysiology, a minimum one hundred hours of pharmacology, history and physical exam skills, clinical medicine, and surgery. Students are also instructed in clinical skills and coursework related to clinical reasoning, patient counseling and education, and medical writing.[164]

The clinical phase of the program consists of clinical rotations in core medical concentrations. All programs are required to have students rotate through internal medicine,

---

[164] American Academy of Physician Assistants, "Becoming a PA." Accessed December 28, 2017. https://www.aapa.org/career-central/become-a-pa/.

general pediatrics, family medicine, general surgery, women's health, and emergency medicine. The remaining time for the clinical year is in electives and specialty practice rotations.

All graduating PA students must take a national certification exam in order to practice in the United States. The National Commission on the Certification for Physician Assistants (NCCPA) administers the Physician Assistant National Certification Exam (PANCE) to all graduates. This one-day 360-question test covers all aspects of PA education and training to ensure the public's protection by proving that the graduate has met the requirements for practice.

To maintain the certification, all PAs must take one hundred hours of continuing medical education (CME) every two years. As part of their certification maintenance, 20 percent of their work must be done in their field of practice. In addition, all PAs must take the Physician Assistant National Recertification Exam (PANRE) every ten years to remain current.[165] Licensure for PAs is available in every state and the District of Columbia. Each state has different methods of governance for PAs, but all are listed under the state board of medicine and licensure. Most states will have a PA advisory board that also governs the profession.

## PAs in the Workforce

As of 2016, over one-hundred and six thousand PA jobs were filled. According to the US Bureau of Labor and Statistics, the PA workforce was projected to grow over 37 percent over the next decade from that time and to add approximately forty thousand jobs in total.[166] The PA is listed as one of the fastest-growing professions in the United States. The success of the profession has caught on in other countries, including Canada, which has utilized PAs for several years.[167]

The majority of PAs within health care are employed in primary care. Because of the general medical model of education, PAs are ideal for use in all fields of medicine. The flexibility of the profession allows graduates to consider working in almost any area that is available to them.

According to the American Academy of Physician Assistants, the median age of a PA was thirty-seven, with women making up 67 percent of the PA population. Most PAs were employed by a single-specialty physician group practice or solo physician practice office. The percentage of the workforce working in obstetrics and gynecology is approximately 2 percent.[168] Because of the flexible nature of the profession, women tend to favor working in this field for various lifestyle reasons. Job satisfaction rates are also very high and have remained high for several years. Flexibility, autonomy, and the ability to have a rewarding career are all factors in this profession's success.

---

[165] National Commission on the Certification of Physician Assistants, "About PANCE." January 1, 2015. Accessed August 15, 2015. http://www.nccpa.net/Pance.

[166] Occupational Outlook Handbook. Bureau of Labor Statistics. Accessed January 22, 2018. https://www.bls.gov/ooh/healthcare/physician-assistants.htm.

[167] US Bureau of Labor and Statistics, "Occupational Outlook Handbook." January 8, 2014. Accessed July 31, 2015. http://www.bls.gov/ooh/fastest-growing.htm.

[168] American Academy of Physician Assistants, *2013 AAPA Annual Survey Report* (Alexandria, VA: AAPA, 2014).

**Scope of Practice**

PAs practice medicine and provide a broad range of medical services that otherwise would be provided by physicians. They work under the concept of team-based care and have a working agreement with supervising physicians. The utilization of PAs in clinical practice typically falls under the concept of "performance-delegated autonomy." This concept, first described in the 1970s, allows PAs to increase their autonomy as they gain more experience in a working relationship with their supervising physicians. As the PA grows into the practice, more value and trust is placed in that provider.

In all fifty states and the District of Columbia, the physician is not required to be on site, so supervision can be done via telecommunication. This can allow a practice to manage patients in multiple settings, such as hospitals and offices, at the same time. PAs are granted medical staff privileges in hospitals and in ambulatory surgery centers. They can perform procedures, assist in surgery, and perform visits in skilled nursing facilities. Most states have provisions to allow PAs to perform certain invasive procedures once approved by the supervising physician. In some states, the performance of a specific invasive procedure must be documented and qualified by the state's medical board.

**Reimbursement**

Medicare recognizes PAs as enrolled ordering and referring providers. They can and do provide position Part B services, but they must not be included in Part A costs. Specific to Medicare benefit policies, "PAs may furnish services billed under all levels of CPT [the AMA's Current Procedural Terminology] evaluation and management codes, and diagnostic tests they furnished under the general supervision of a physician." PAs may provide evaluation and management services to new patients as well as established patients with new problems in the Medicare program. A PA who performs these encounters should be billed under the PA's national provider identification number for Medicare; reimbursement will be at 85 percent of the physician rate.[169]

## The Role of PAs in MFM

PAs may see a wide variety of patients in a maternal-fetal medicine practice, including both the outpatient and inpatient settings. Given that the PA practice is based on the concept of performance-delegated autonomy, we recommend an orientation period for PAs who join an MFM practice during which education and training is performed by the supervising physician(s). The PA is thus exposed to all facets of the MFM practice and over time acquires the skills and knowledge to care for high-risk pregnancies in the outpatient and inpatient settings.

---

[7] US Department of Health and Human Services, *Medicare Information for Advanced Practice Registered Nurses, Anesthesiologist Assistants, and Physician Assistants* (Washington, DC: CMS, 2015), 25.

A handful of fellowships currently exist for PAs who desire to expand their knowledge in women's health care. Based on the experience of the authors, an orientation period of about four to six months is recommended in order to enhance the knowledge and skills of the PA in MFM and to become familiar with the established protocols and guidelines of the specialty and practice. During the orientation period, progressive autonomy in practice will be provided based on ongoing competency assessments.

## The Outpatient Setting

The PA can play a major role in the outpatient setting of an MFM practice. This includes antenatal and postpartum care, MFM consultations, basic ultrasound examinations, and office procedures. With expanded knowledge and training, the PA can progress to providing supervised care to a host of medical and surgical complications in pregnancy, including those found in table 12.1.

The office practice can be structured in a way that will allow the PA to see established pregnant patients, which will free the MFM physician to focus on office consultations, co-management of complicated pregnancies, and new visits. Certain office procedures fall within the scope of practice for PAs, such as IUD placement, cerclage removals, and others. State and office practice regulations should be considered in this regard.

| Table 12.1. Conditions typically seen by physician assistants in MFM |
|---|
| Chronic hypertension/preeclampsia |
| Diabetes (pregestational and gestational) |
| Insulin pump management |
| Thyroid management |
| Infectious disease (i.e., HIV) |
| Recurrent miscarriage |
| Multiple gestation |
| Preterm labor (cervical insufficiency) |
| Fetal anomalies |

Performing ultrasound examinations requires additional training and competency evaluation. Acquiring skills in ultrasound requires knowledge, hands-on training, and continued medical education. It is therefore important for PAs who wish to become proficient in obstetrical ultrasound to acquire the necessary education and training and to dedicate a significant portion of their practice to ultrasound in order to maintain proficiency over time. As of 2017, a recognized pathway for the reliable establishment of education guidelines and the demonstration of proficiency for advanced practitioners does not exist. Establishing a national scope of practice of PAs and other advanced practitioners in obstetrical ultrasound, along with curriculum development for education and training (in collaboration with the American Institute of Ultrasound in Medicine), would be an optimal way to ensure the safety and quality of ultrasound practice.

## The Inpatient Setting

PAs can also provide substantial support to an MFM practice in inpatient settings. Following training and competency evaluation, PAs can help with labor and delivery, antenatal testing units, triage units, and antepartum/postpartum wards. Inpatient procedures include amniotomy, fetal scalp electrode placement, perineal repairs, nonstress testing, and others. In the authors' practice, PAs help to cover inpatient units on busy days and days when the residency team is on academic leave. PAs are also trained to provide surgical assistance in the operating suites.

## Conclusion

PAs can play a major role in an MFM practice and thus can increase efficiency and enhance safety and quality of care. The authors have employed PAs in their clinical practice for several years now and have found that they have integrated fully into MFM care and have become an irreplaceable component of high-risk pregnancy care.

On a national level, the number of PAs who currently practice in MFM is small. The annual census taken by the profession does not break down the specialty of women's health into MFM, so the actual number of PAs who work in this field remains unknown. Because the physician assistant profession is in its infancy, and this field of medicine is relatively new to PAs, much of the work that will be done in the coming years will determine the efficacy of using PAs in the MFM setting. More discussion will be necessary to determine and define the scope of practice. This will include extensive discussion of the education and training of PAs in ultrasound, prenatal testing, and high-risk obstetrical care. Discussion within the PA profession and its educational arms is ongoing to determine the best approach to educating PA students in the use of ultrasound for several different fields of medicine. We strongly believe that PAs can play a significant role in high-risk pregnancy care in partnership with MFM physicians and can work collaboratively to provide high-quality, safe, and efficient care.

# 13

## Improving Clinical Process Efficiency within Your MFM Practice

Thomas Lee (MD, MBA)

Health care is a business. Businesses require the application of business strategies in order to deliver their products or services to their consumers. In general, all businesses rely on processes and workflows to produce or deliver these end products. In the case of your MFM practice, your business exists to deliver your end product: high-quality perinatal services. Unfortunately, most MFM practices are inherently complex, with numerous interdependent departments (e.g., ultrasound, laboratory services, genetics, nursing, MFM, antenatal testing, nutrition, and social services) operating under one roof. Improving and coordinating the processes that will allow your practice to deliver its perinatal services can lead to greater practice efficiency, patient and staff satisfaction, profitability, and care quality.

These statements, though, are not meant to demean the altruistic motivations that undoubtedly led each of us to pursue a life dedicated to the practice of medicine. But the reality is that our ability to provide high-quality health care to our patients has been and continues to be assaulted by the economic, social, and political forces of our times. The fiscal pressures of practicing medicine in the current age of health-care reform demand a better understanding of business strategy and process improvement by the practitioner. Most corporate health-care systems and insurance companies adopted this approach decades ago. As author Frank Cohen has written in *Lean Six Sigma for the Medical Practice*, they "figured out how to deliver services, control costs, increase efficiency, and generate huge profits through the use of process technology."[170] Unfortunately, most health-care providers and groups have been either unable or reluctant to do so until recently. The truth is that business management, for most of us, was never part of our medical training.

The intent of this chapter is to present a basic approach to process improvement along with various tools and techniques taken from the business playbook with which you can start to improve the efficiency of your own MFM practice and enhance its ability to provide high-quality care to your patients. By streamlining your process workflows and reducing the amount of time you currently spend troubleshooting an inefficient care-delivery system, you will have more time available to focus on clinical care and relationships with your patients—which is why we went into this business in the first place.

---

[170] Frank Cohen, *Lean Six Sigma for the Medical Practice* (Phoenix, MD: Greenbranch Publishing; 2010), 15.

## How Do I Start?

*The journey of a thousand miles begins with one step.*

—Lao Tzu

As with most endeavors, the first step always seems to be the most difficult and the most important. Before you begin your journey of process improvement toward greater clinic efficiency, take some time to set your trajectory. In the words of the oft-quoted Yogi Berra, "If you don't know where you're going…you might not get there." Unfortunately, most health-care organizations are bad at planning, and taking on a "Just do it!" mentality is likely to lead to failure. This is where a little bit of strategic planning can go a long way.

Strategic planning does not have to be complicated. Indeed, for some organizations, a formalized process may be beneficial, especially when large-scale projects are undertaken. But if your clinic has decided to move forward with a process and efficiency improvement initiative, then coming up with a formal strategic plan is probably a bit daunting and likely unnecessary. The goal here is to create at least a rudimentary plan or road map toward your imagined future state. You can accomplish this by merely addressing a few basic questions that may help better define your approach to making your clinic more efficient, as suggested in table 13.1.

### Table 13.1. Basic strategic planning questions

| Question | Example answers |
| --- | --- |
| What is the process that we are trying to improve? | Registration and check-in<br>Ultrasound workflow<br>Genetic counseling visits<br>Communication back to referring providers |
| What are we trying to fix within this process? | Decrease in operating costs<br>Increase in patient capacity / volume<br>Higher quality of care<br>Improvement in patient satisfaction<br>Improvement in provider or staff satisfaction |
| What are the resources that we can dedicate to the project? | Paid clinical staff and administrative staff time<br>Clinical provider time<br>Financial resources<br>Outside consultants |
| Who will support or not support the potential changes that will result from the process improvement efforts? | Organization<br>Clinical providers and staff<br>Support staff<br>Patients<br>Referring providers |

Once you have defined a high-level view of an imagined future state and confirmed that you have both the resources and buy-in to feasibly complete the journey, it is time to take the next step: choosing your traveling companions, a.k.a. the project team.

## The Multidisciplinary Team

The project team is the crucible from which efficiency improvements will emerge. The team's mission is (1) to identify areas of process inefficiency and (2) to develop effective solutions to improve the clinic's workflows. In general, the optimal team size (frequently referred to as Dunbar's number) is typically somewhere between six to ten core members. Having too few members can lead to insufficient perspectives and input, while having too many members may result in a team that ends up being ineffective at making and executing decisions.

The members of the team should provide a diversity of operational perspectives from within your clinic. The potential benefits of a multidisciplinary team approach are that (1) it creates a unified interdepartmental vision of the future state, (2) the care delivery process can be standardized and coordinated throughout the entire patient experience, (3) the ripple effects of any considered changes can be vetted prior to rollout, and (4) the workflow needs between departments can be coordinated and made more efficient (see table 13.2).

| Table 13.2. Benefits of a Multidisciplinary Project Team |
| --- |
| Unified interdepartmental vision of the future state |
| Standardization and coordination of the care delivery process throughout the patient experience |
| Potential ripple effects of proposed changes can be vetted prior to deployment |
| Coordination of workflow needs between departments |

For instance, imagine an all-too-common scenario in which a well-intended workflow change made in isolation within one part of your clinic has had significant unintended consequences on another department's workflow. This scenario can frequently lead to dramatic reactions that can disrupt clinic flow, impact patient care, and disgruntle staff and providers. Creating a multidisciplinary project team to collaboratively work together to create complementary processes and provide feedback prior to going live with any operational changes will help to avoid these unintended downstream effects.

The team can also help improve overall clinic efficiency by better coordinating downstream needs. Later in this chapter, we will see that relatively simple changes in workflow and documentation at the time of patient scheduling can reap substantial benefits in quality and efficiency when the time comes to actually see the patient in the office. It is within the confines of the multidisciplinary project team where clinic needs are discussed, inefficiencies become apparent, and solutions that work for the entire clinic as a whole are developed. The potential core team members for a multidisciplinary project team for an MFM practice may include those found in table 13.3.

The core team itself, however, does not need to be all-inclusive—and inherently shouldn't be. As questions outside the scope of the team's expertise arise, subject matter advisers (e.g., IT support and marketing) can be brought into the project to help assist when needed.

**Table 13.3. Example project team**

| |
|---|
| Practice manager |
| MFM physician |
| Genetic counselor |
| Laboratory services coordinator |
| Ultrasound coordinator / sonographer |
| Perinatal nurse / medical assistant |
| Medical receptionist |
| Patient accounts specialist |
| Medical records coordinator |

## Lean and Six Sigma

As a greater emphasis on health-care efficiency has emerged at the forefront of everyday clinical practice, references to the perhaps unfamiliar concepts of lean and Six Sigma (briefly discussed in chapter 10) have more frequently come up within administrative discussions. While an extensive review of each of these process-improvement approaches is beyond the scope of this chapter, gaining a basic understanding of the general philosophies of both lean and Six Sigma can serve as a foundation for your approach to improving efficiency within your practice.

### Lean

Lean production was initially developed by Taiichi Ohno at Toyota after World War II and originated from the company's just-in-time production practices. The "Toyota Production System" was studied by researchers at MIT and first widely documented in the book *The Machine That Changed the World* in 1990.[171] The lean production approach has since become widely adopted by many fields of manufacturing and has also spread to health-care process improvement.

In a nutshell, lean's objective is to create a seamless flow within the production process by reducing wasteful steps that contribute to inefficiency. Within the lean system, waste (known as *muda* in Japanese) can take numerous forms (see table 13.4).

When lean process improvement is applied to health care, the steps involved in care delivery are individually examined as to whether they (1) add value to the end goal or (2) are wasteful and do not add value to the process. The ultimate goal of lean process optimization is to eliminate those steps that do not add value to the delivery of care in your clinic—thus leading to a more streamlined, efficient clinic workflow.[172]

---

[171] J. P. Womack, D. T. Jones, and D. Roos, *The Machine That Changed the World: Based on the Massachusetts Institute of Technology 5-Million Dollar 5-Year Study on the Future of the Automobile* (New York: Rawson Associates, 1990).
[172] D. B. McLaughlin and J. R. Olson, *Healthcare Operations Management*, 2nd ed. (Chicago: Health Administration Press, 2012).

| Table 13.4. Types of waste in healthcare | | |
|---|---|---|
| | **Definition** | **Example** |
| **Overproduction** | Producing more than is demanded or before it is needed to meet demand | Printing imaging reports or labels when they are not needed |
| **Waiting** | Time during which value is not being added to the product or service | Providers waiting for a staff member or patient |
| **Transportation** | Unnecessary travel of the product within the system | Movement of patients or equipment from one area of the clinic to another |
| **Inventory** | Holding or purchasing raw materials, work-in-process, and finished goods that are not immediately needed | Excess inventory of supplies and pharmaceuticals |
| **Motion** | Actions of operators that do not add value to the product | Unnecessary movement of the staff to obtain supplies |
| **Overprocessing** | Unnecessary steps and procedures that do not add value to the service | Unnecessary EMR documentation |
| **Defects** | Production of a part or service that is scrapped or requires rework | Incorrect documentation by sonographer on imaging report |

**Six Sigma**

Six Sigma was initially developed in the 1980s at Motorola as the company's in-house quality improvement initiative. The Six Sigma approach has since been adopted by many other organizations such as GE and IBM as part of their business strategies to improve product and service quality. Six Sigma has also found a niche within many health-care organizations as part of their quality improvement programs.[173]

The underlying philosophy behind Six Sigma process optimization in general is the elimination of defects through the removal of variance within manufacturing and business systems. In contrast to lean, Six Sigma's techniques for quality improvement place a much greater emphasis on data, statistical analysis, and mathematical modeling. In fact, the term *six sigma* itself comes from the mathematical concept that maintaining six standard deviations of variation within the confines of the process tolerance limits will nearly eliminate products that fail to meet required specifications (with the goal of no more than 3.4 defects per million opportunities). Formal Six Sigma methodology also incorporates the use of a martial arts–like hierarchical ranking system

---

[173] J. K. Bandyopadhyay and K. Coppens, "Six Sigma Approach to Healthcare Quality and Productivity Management," *International Journal of Productivity and Quality Management* 5, no. 1 (2005): V1–V12.
http://www.isqpm.org/2005%20Journal/Six%20Sigma%20Approach%20to%20Health%20Care1%20Quality%20Management-revised-1%20by%20Jay%20Bandyopadhyay%20and%20Karen%20Coppens.pdf.

(e.g., champions, master black belts, black belts, and green belts), along with specialized training and certification to define the roles that each individual plays within the Six Sigma process.

**The Best of Both Worlds**

Undoubtedly, much of how all this business theory applies to health care may be quite overwhelming to a clinician or practice manager who does not have formal training in lean or Six Sigma. The truth is that there is actually a substantial amount of overlap between the two approaches. Many organizations have advocated the concurrent use of lean and Six Sigma philosophies and tools in tandem into what is known as lean Six Sigma. In this author's opinion, the lean Six Sigma approach is well suited for use within health care, since it simultaneously brings together the goals of lean's reduction of waste with Six Sigma's reduction of process variability.

Figure 13.1 provides a conceptual illustration of how these two systems can be used together in the clinical realm. Imagine that points A and B represent the beginning and end of a clinical process such as performing a routine fetal ultrasound. The steps involved in completing the study are represented by each oval (check-in, notifying the sonographer, reviewing the orders, retrieving the patient, performing the study, completing the documentation, etc.). Each step in the process is characterized by an "amplitude" that represents the variability that exists within your clinic for that specific step, since each staff member is likely to have a slightly different way of completing that task. In order to improve efficiency, lean techniques can be used to eliminate wasteful (or non-value-added) steps and thereby reduce the overall length of the process. Six Sigma techniques can also be brought to bear on the process to reduce the workflow variation among the staff members (through work standardization), which is represented by a reduction in the amplitude of the step. The end result is a more streamlined, less wasteful workflow for completing the ultrasound study—which is the ultimate goal of your efficiency improvement efforts.

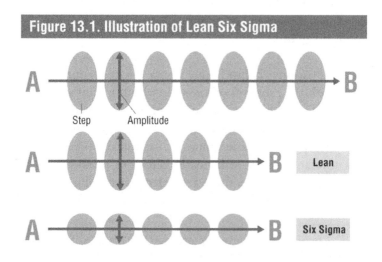

Both the lean and Six Sigma systems contain a wealth of suggested tools and techniques that can be used to accomplish these tasks—a handful of which will be highlighted later in this chapter. Suffice it to say that numerous resources are currently available in the modern literature that can provide a more in-depth review.

Define-Measure-Analyze-Improve-Control (DMAIC)

A number of different approaches to process improvement are available. A commonly used tool that comes from the Six Sigma lexicon is the Define-Measure-Analyze-Improve-Control (DMAIC) cycle, which will form the framework for this chapter's discussion (see figure 13.2).

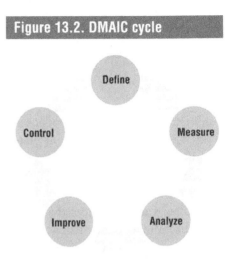

The DMAIC cycle is composed of the following phases:

- **D**efine: understand the problem to be solved or the process to be improved.
- **M**easure: understand how the current state is meeting the clinic's requirements.
- **A**nalyze: examine collected data to determine the influential variables.
- **I**mprove: identify and implement solutions.
- **C**ontrol: hardwire the changes to maintain the gains you achieve.

Using this series of steps will allow your team to systematically gain an understanding of the process that you are trying to improve and then work toward a sustainable solution. While DMAIC may seem somewhat rigid at first, the utility of the DMAIC process will become evident rather quickly as you navigate through this. As with most skills that you have been formally trained in over the course of your career (such as doing your first amniocentesis or cesarean section), the use of DMAIC will become more automatic and less formal as you continue to use it over time.

A similar method is the frequently used Plan-Do-Study-Act (PDSA) cycle, developed by the engineer and statistician W. Edwards Deming. Tools such as these can serve as a guide for your efficiency improvement journey.

**The Define Phase**

Selecting the right process for your practice to focus on for efficiency improvement is important. Given the changing landscape of advancing technologies, alterations in clinical protocols, and administrative/regulatory requirements, more and more pressure is being applied to practices to adjust and change accordingly. As such, there never seems to be a shortage of opinions as to which workflow requires attention first. But resources, including time and financial funding, are scarce, so separating the wheat from the chaff is critical. This requires an initial assessment of which processes are currently working well in your practice, which are in most need of your attention, which ones are superfluous, and which processes, if improved, will have the highest return on investment (ROI)—either from a financial perspective or in regard to clinical care.[174]

For the remainder of this chapter, let us use a relatively straightforward example of a routine MFM office visit comprised of an ultrasound study followed by an MFM consultation to examine patient flow. This is a process that is performed numerous times a day in most MFM clinics, and any improvements in patient flow efficiency could have a significant impact on a myriad number of quality and financial metrics.

## The Measure Phase

### Process Mapping

Understanding the current process (or workflow) that exists within your practice is one of the first tasks within the measurement phase. Simply put, a process is the sequence of events or actions that occur in order to accomplish something. Typically, existing processes have historically come about as a patchwork of adjustments over time due to the changing clinical needs that arise in day-to-day office practice. Conducting a high-level analysis of your practice's current process is a relatively straightforward activity that can be collectively accomplished by the members of your multidisciplinary team using a process map, which is essentially a graphic representation of the workflow process. Conducting process mapping forces the team to think about and account for the steps involved in the process, along with its inputs and outputs. Figure 13.3 presents a basic process map for our MFM patient visit example.

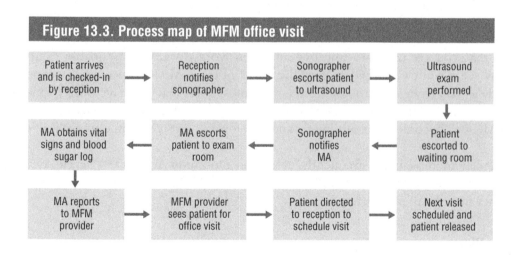

---

[174] D. A. Shore, *Launching and Leading Change Initiatives in Health Care Organizations* (San Francisco: Jossey-Bass, 2014), 42–59.

Starting off with a formal exercise in process mapping has several additional benefits. Process mapping:

1. Helps to identify from the very beginning where there may be inherent and unrecognized variations in clinic workflow from one staff member to another;
2. Provides a global perspective and a common starting point for all members of the multidisciplinary project team—some of whom may not truly be aware of the process in its entirety;
3. Prevents the project team from jumping to immediate solutions based on anecdotal experiences and preconceived notions.

Once the project team has a clear understanding of the current process within your clinic, it's time to move on to collecting some efficiency data about the workflow.

*Metrics of Efficiency*

Understanding the efficiency of your clinic relies on examining appropriate measures of process performance. In the words of quality improvement guru H. James Harrington, "Measurement is the first step that leads to control and eventually to improvement. If you can't measure something, you can't understand it. If you can't understand it, you can't control it. If you can't control it, you can't improve it."[175] It is imperative that the metrics your clinic is tracking provide relevant feedback regarding both the practice's strengths and the areas in which it has opportunities for improvement. This involves understanding ahead of time what is actually being measured, why it is being measured, and how this knowledge will be useful to the practice.

The metrics should also be accurate, timely in their collectability, and not cost prohibitive. The potential pitfall of examining inappropriate metrics is that the organization may come to incorrect conclusions that can lead to changes that will then have significant negative effects on the practice. Table 13.5 presents a few commonly used process metrics that are frequently used in the health-care setting.

---

[175] H. J. Harrington, *Business Process Improvement: The Breakthrough Strategy for Total Quality, Productivity, and Competitiveness* (New York: McGraw-Hill, 1991), 164.

### Table 13.5. Frequently used process metrics in health care

| | Definition | Example |
|---|---|---|
| Process capacity | Maximum possible amount of output from a process | Number of NSTs that can be performed in a day |
| Capacity utilization | Percentage of time that a resource or process is actually busy producing or transforming output | Percentage of a sonographer's total work time spent in patient care |
| Cycle time | Total time from the beginning to the end of a process | The time a patient spends in ultrasound |
| Percent value-added time | Percentage of time in which value is actually added to the process | Percentage of total visit time that the patient spends with either staff or a provider |
| Motion | Actions of operators that do not add value to the product | Unnecessary movement of the staff to obtain supplies |
| Wait time | Time that is spent waiting to be processed | Patient waiting in an exam room for staff or a provider |
| Errors | Number of errors or defects | Omissions or errors on ultrasound report |

In our MFM office example, because we are focusing on patient flow, it seems appropriate to examine time metrics. Process-improvement authorities frequently advocate the use of time metrics in health-care settings—especially patient wait times. Why focus on patient wait times? As Aneesh and Carolyn Suneja suggest in their book *Lean Doctors*, "Amidst all the mind-boggling information that is available in healthcare, wait times are refreshingly simple. After all, wait times are easy to understand, and there is no arguing with them."[176] Using patient wait times as your key metric in assessing your clinic's patient flow has numerous advantages as outlined in table 13.6, and is a recommended metric with which to start.

That being said, numerous other efficiency-related metrics can be analyzed, including data on resource allocation, constituent satisfaction, and care quality, but in general these metrics tend to be more indirect by-products of operational processes and less a direct reflection of process efficiency. Regardless of which metrics your practice examines, being proactive and clear about the purpose and execution of your data-collection process

### Table 13.6. Advantages of using patient wait times as a metric

| |
|---|
| Powerful metric of workflow inefficiency |
| Patient-centered |
| Common single assessable metric within all departments |
| Easy to understand by everyone |
| Emotionally removed from the provider-patient relationship |
| Significant driver of patient dissatisfaction |

---

[176] Aneesh Suneja and Carolyn Suneja, *Lean Doctors: A Bold and Practical Guide to Using Lean Principles to Transform Healthcare Systems, One Doctor at a Time* (Milwaukee, WI: ASQ Quality Press, 2010), 29.

will increase the likelihood of obtaining useful information to help guide operational changes.

**Figure 13.4. Example of a time data collection tool**

PLEASE DO NOT FILL OUT THIS FORM  This form is being used to help improve our patient flow.
Please carry this form during your visit and you will be asked for it by our staff. We appreciate your help- *Thank you*

PROVIDER: ☐ BF  ☐ MT  ☐ PW  ☐ MW  ☐ TL  ☐ MOD  ☐ WB  ☐ KH  ☐ JM

**Front Desk ONLY**

DATE _____  FIRST APPOINTMENT TIME: _____  ARRIVED: _____

CHECKED IN: _____  ☐ US  ☐ LAB  ☐ NST  ☐ RN  ☐ GC  ☐ MD

INTERPRETER: ☐ PHONE  ☐ IN PERSON  PATIENT ID:

**GC**

Genetic Counselor IN _____

READY _____  MFM IN _____  OUT _____

Genetic Counselor OUT _____

☐ MFM not available  ☐ Add-on

**NST**

NST IN _____

READY _____

NST OUT _____

☐ Awaiting NWP MD
☐ Awaiting WHA MD
☐ Additional monitoring  ☐ Add-on

**LAB**

Patient IN Lab _____

READY _____  MFM IN _____  OUT _____

Patient OUT Lab _____

☐ SEQ1
☐ SEQ2
☐ cffDNA
☐ 1hr GTT
☐ Other Studies
☐ Delay: Prior Patient
☐ Awaiting MFM
☐ Back-up MFM Required
☐ Order Clarification

**US**

Patient IN Ultrasound _____

READY _____  MFM REVIEW _____

MD/GC IN _____  OUT _____

RN/MA IN _____  OUT _____

Patient OUT Ultrasound _____

☐ Amnio / CVS
☐ Anatomy Survey
☐ Anatomy Follow-up
☐ BPP
☐ Dating/Viability
☐ Doppler Studies
☐ Echocardiogram
☐ Endovaginal
☐ Growth Follow-up
☐ Limited
☐ Sequential Screen
☐ GYN  ☐ SIS
☐ Multiple Pregnancy
☐ Phoenix Summary
Unavailable
☐ Add-on
☐ Abnormal Finding
☐ Awaiting MD
☐ Delay: Prior Patient
☐ Mentoring
☐ Order Clarification
☐ Prep Issue
☐ Scheduling Issue

**MD/RN**

RN IN Exam Room _____

RN OUT Exam Room _____

☐ Awaiting US Report
☐ Assisting Other Patient/Provider
☐ Interpreter Involved
☐ Phone Call
☐ Awaiting Records

MD IN Exam Room _____

MD OUT Exam Room _____

☐ Awaiting US Report / RN
☐ Assisting Other Patient/Provider
☐ Interpreter Involved
☐ Provider Communication
☐ Awaiting Records
☐ Follow-up NST / US

RN IN Exam Room #2 _____

RN OUT Exam Room #2 _____

☐ Assisting Other Provider
☐ Interpreter Involved
☐ NST / Monitoring
☐ Patient Education
☐ Blood Draw / Injection
☐ Care Coordination

**Front Desk ONLY**

PRE CHECKOUT  ☐ MSW Consult  ☐ Patient Accounts  ☐ Patient Private Time  ☐ Social Visit

Patient IN Scheduling _____  ☐ Orders Unavailable  ☐ Time Unavailable

FINAL CHECK OUT _____

PLEASE GIVE THIS FORM TO CHECK OUT AS YOU LEAVE

*Data Collection*

Developing a strategy for collecting your data will depend on your individual practice and the metrics you are examining. However your clinic decides to approach this, it is important that a predetermined methodology is developed and communicated to your staff—just as if you were performing a formal research study. Data collection is data collection, regardless of the setting, and the methodology of data acquisition should be rigorous. The potential consequences of not doing so are either that you will have unusable data or that you will have data that directs you to incorrect conclusions and interventions.

If you decide to use time metrics, these data can be collected either prospectively or retrospectively. Prospective time data collection can be performed through the development and deployment of a time data collection tool. Figure 13.4 presents an example of a collection tool that we have used in our own practice that has come to be known as the Patient Passport. This form was maintained by the patient and filled out by the staff members and providers that she encountered throughout the entirety of her office visit.

Alternatively, time data can potentially be retrospectively collected using time stamps from EMR status changes, data entry, and ultrasound images, although these tend to be limited in their ability to accurately reflect the course of the patient experience. Using a process of prospective data collection is generally recommended.

## The Analyze Phase

Up to this point, your clinic's efficiency project has assembled your team, assessed your process workflow, and gathered data to understand your current process. It is now time to bring these together and apply some of the aforementioned lean and Six Sigma tools in order to improve your process efficiency.

*Value Stream Mapping*

As noted in chapter 10, value stream mapping (VSM) is a powerful lean tool that combines both process mapping and time data into a single view (figure 13.5). VSM is used to list the individual steps within the overall process in order to identify value-added steps and non-value-added steps that will contribute to individual process cycle times and their associated wait times. This also involves breaking down each step (process 1, process 2, etc.) into its specific subprocesses. Figure 13.6 presents a VSM generated in our MFM office example.

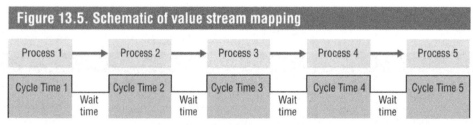

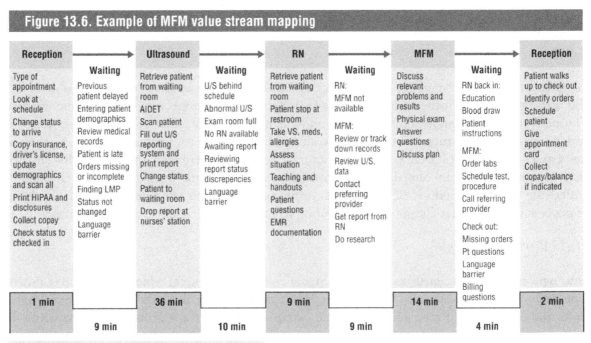

Figure 13.6. Example of MFM value stream mapping

AIDET= Acknowledge, Introduce, Duration, Explanation, and Thank You

In our example, at a high level we can see that the workflow associated with seeing a patient in the clinic involves several steps, which include the patient passing through interactions with reception, ultrasound, nursing, and MFM. VSM then directs the team to identify the various subprocesses involved. For instance, as part of the ultrasound process, we can see that this involves activities such as retrieving the patient from the waiting room, performing introductions, scanning the patient, completing reporting documentation, changing the patient status in the EMR, taking the patient to the waiting room, and delivering the report to the nursing station. We can also identify factors that can contribute to delays in handoffs both before and after the ultrasound process.

When these subprocesses are reviewed in conjunction with time data that provide efficiency relevance, the targets for process and efficiency improvement efforts become apparent. As your team engages in this exercise, the VSM should facilitate discussion and raise questions such as:

(1) What actually is the process?
(2) Why are there variations among the staff?
(3) Are all these steps necessary?
(4) How do these subprocesses contribute to the cycle times and wait times?

To reiterate, one of the key benefits of engaging in formal process mapping and VSM is that doing so helps to identify the actual problems in the current workflow, rather than relying on perceived anecdotal notions of what may be contributing to inefficient workflow.

*Root-Cause Analysis*

Gaining a better understanding of the processes and subprocesses that contribute to cycle times and wait times in your office workflows is a major step toward improving overall clinic efficiency. The next phase of analysis aims to better understand the factors that generate these non-value-added steps through structured techniques collectively known as root-cause analyses. As clinicians, this aspect of process-efficiency improvement may be the most familiar. In essence, this should be akin to what we do in our day-to-day activities as health-care providers in determining the underlying cause or diagnosis of the clinical symptoms with which our patients present. In the case of process analysis, what factors are contributing to prolonged cycle times and wait times?

## THE 5 WHYS TECHNIQUE

One type of root-cause analysis is the Six Sigma 5 Whys technique, which simply boils down to repeatedly asking the question "Why?" It is a way to peel away the layers of symptoms that can cover the root cause of a problem, since the ostensible reason for a problem will frequently lead you to another question.[177] Usually about five rounds is a good rule of thumb. An advantage of the 5 Whys technique is that it is a simple tool that can be used without having to conduct a statistical analysis. Let's present a simple example:

- **Problem:** A large number of patients are late to their appointments, which contributes to an inability for the clinic to run on time.

1. **Why** are patients late to their appointments?

    **Because** they underestimate the time that it will take to get to the clinic.

2. **Why** do they not know how long it will take them to travel to the clinic?

    **Because** they do not have good directions to our office.

3. **Why** do patients not have good directions to our office prior to coming?

    **Because** nobody has given them directions prior to their appointment.

4. **Why** hasn't somebody (like their referring provider's office) given them directions?

    **Because** we have not provided them with patient fliers with directions.

5. **Why** haven't we provided our referring providers with patient fliers with directions?

    **Eureka!**

The simplicity and power of the 5 Whys technique seem self-evident, although 5 Whys can also be somewhat limiting, since the assumption is that the effect will be attributable to a single cause at each level of questioning. Nonetheless, using 5 Whys is frequently a good place to start.

## CAUSE-AND-EFFECT DIAGRAMS

---

[177] iSixSigma, "Determine the Root Cause: 5 Whys." 2015. http://www.isixsigma.com/tools-templates/cause-effect/determine-root-cause-5-whys/.

Another type of root-cause analysis that goes beyond the 5 Whys technique is the cause-and-effect diagram, sometimes known as a fishbone diagram. Because a number of factors often contribute to a process, using a cause-and-effect diagram can be valuable in accounting for multiple inputs.

Returning to our example, let's examine the potential causes that contribute to the effects that increase wait times for our patient prior to her ultrasound. Figure 13.7 presents a cause-and-effect diagram that identifies numerous factors that can potentially affect the patient's wait time based on the subprocesses listed in our prior VSM exercise, such as a delay in the previous patient's visit or additional time spent by the sonographer reviewing medical records, clarifying orders, or entering patient data. From there, additional layers of cause-and-effect relationships can be determined.

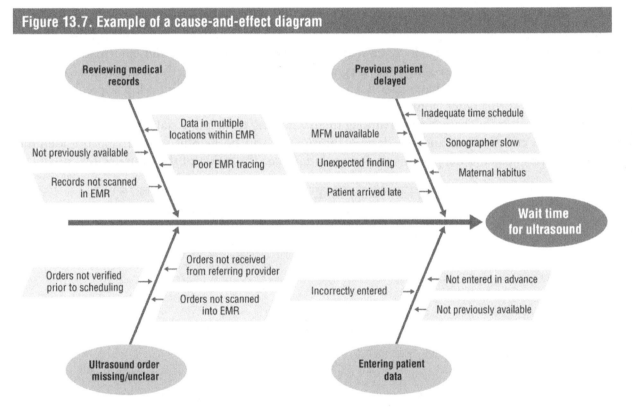

This exercise can be repeated for each of the steps and wait periods within the VSM. Again, the goal is to peel back the layers of the process in succession to identify potential sources of waste within the workflow—that is, getting to the root causes of inefficiency.

## The Improve Phase

*Developing Solutions*

This part of the DMAIC cycle is dependent on what your clinic identifies as major contributors to the inefficiency metrics that you choose. As part of this approach to improving clinic efficiency, remember that the lean-derived goal is to reduce unnecessary steps in the process, while the Six

Sigma–derived goal is to reduce variation within the remaining value-added steps. This does not imply that your team cannot add steps to the current process. The important thing to remember is that any additional steps need to add value to the new process and should theoretically replace a less efficient, wasteful series of steps in your existing process.

With that in mind, this is where your team needs to be a bit creative. You still need to be realistic, however, as to what your clinic can accomplish given the resources and capabilities you have at your disposal. The goal is to create an attainable vision of the future state of your clinic process—one that is efficient and standardized. Finally, ensuring that your team has a common vision as they undergo the task of creating and operationalizing this future state is essential to the change-management process that will ensue.

In our example, we have identified several key contributors to patient wait times for ultrasound through our VSM and root-cause analyses. Longer wait times arise from a sonographer's need to repeatedly review medical records, verify orders, and enter patient data. As you can see from the cause-and-effect diagram shown in figure 13.7, the root causes for each of these contributing factors have also been identified, which helps to develop a picture of your current state. At this point, your team needs to consider these factors together as a whole and then identify the common characteristics among them. Creating descriptive statements (as in table 13.7) of both the current state and the desired future state can be helpful in clarifying the identified efficiency problem and the parameters for a solution (i.e., the vision of the future state).

### Table 13.7. Examples of current state and future state

| | Characteristics |
|---|---|
| **Current state** | A significant amount of staff time is spent searching for different types of information (medical records, orders) that is either unavailable or located in multiple varying locations—these all contribute to patient wait times prior to the study. |
| **Future state** | A standardized process in which incoming information (medical records, orders) is retrieved, verified, and entered into the EMR in a single location. |

Let us imagine that the team decides that the solution is a process that would be centered on a standardized review process of incoming information into the clinic. While this process may add steps to the global process as a whole, the process is anticipated to reduce the multiple inefficient steps that contribute to the patient wait-time metric. Once your multidisciplinary team has developed the future state vision, a few additional questions need to be answered:

1) Who can do this, and do we have the staffing for this?
2) What will the workflow for information and communication need to look like?
3) What technical resources do we need?
4) How do we communicate this process change to our staff and referring providers?
5) Do we believe that we can accomplish this?

The answers to these questions will need to be individualized to your clinic's capacity and resources. As your team collaboratively works through the reengineering of the process, the solution that you eventually design needs to be well documented and communicated. Figure 13.8 presents an example of a multilane process map developed in Microsoft Visio that can be helpful in the design phase and subsequently used as a communication tool for the new process workflow.

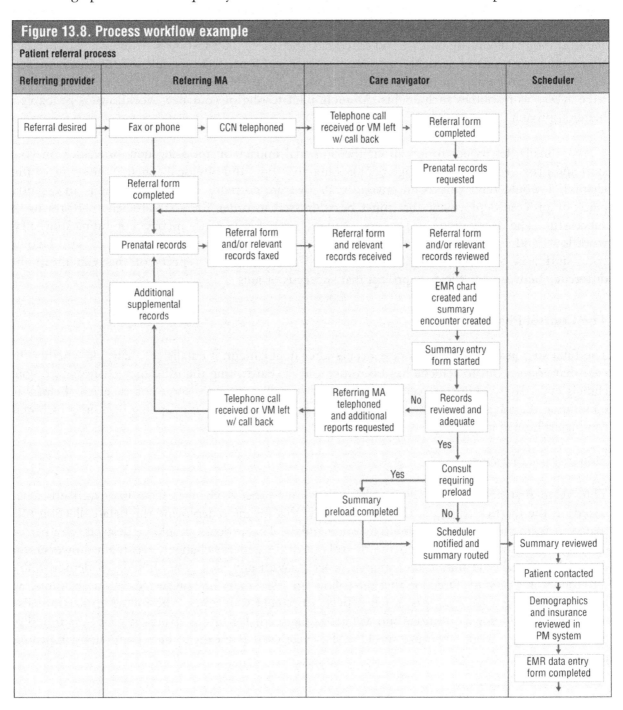

*Implementation*

Once you have devised your efficiency solution to address this aspect of your office flow, you will need to test your new process before deploying it in the rest of the organization. For this, pilot simulations of the workflows are likely the best strategy in a clinic situation. These small-scale trials can be performed using a handful of patient encounters and staff to test the waters and identify any unanticipated hiccups within the process. Because we are dealing with processes that can have significant impacts on patient care and outcomes, the use of pilot testing is strongly recommended. While other methods of predeployment testing such as Monte Carlo simulation (the mathematical modeling of probability distributions of outcomes) do exist, most organizations are unlikely to have access to resources such as this. As such, pilot testing of your new workflows is probably a better approach.

Finally, let us not forget about the potential impact of imposing new processes on your staff and providers. Change management is a massive topic and obviously outside the scope of this chapter. I would refer you to the myriad texts that are currently available.[178] This is an essential piece of process deployment that must be addressed in order for your efficiency efforts to be successful. The facilitation of process changes goes far beyond merely communicating new workflows and setting a date for going live. You will be "moving people's cheese," and helping your staff and providers navigate the technical and emotional aspects of this can mean the difference between an efficiency project that succeeds or fails.

## The Control Phase

The final step in the DMAIC process occurs after deployment; it entails (1) analyzing whether the goal that you set out to achieve has been met and (2) hardwiring the efficiency changes into your clinic's everyday workflow. Creating a system of surveillance and response is especially helpful in continuing the advances in efficiency that your team has made, since slipping back into historical routines is human nature.

*Measuring and Monitoring*

Your team first needs to be able to show that your process changes have improved efficiency based on the metrics you have chosen. Typically, this means redeploying the data-collection tool that your team initially used to obtain its original data. This process should be delayed for a period of time so that the dust can settle from the rollout of the process changes; eventually, however, the data collection should mimic the original process. With any luck, you should see demonstrable differences in a positive direction that the follow-up assessment has suggested. In our example, we hope to see a decrease in at least a few aspects of patient wait times. The follow-up data are also likely to raise additional questions and will act as the seeds for future efforts in your next round of process-efficiency work—because the DMAIC cycle itself is meant to be a continuous, repeating process.

---

[178] Shore, *Launching and Leading Change Initiatives*; D. E. Lighter, *Basics of Health Care Performance Improvement* (Burlington, MA: Jones & Bartlett Learning, 2013); J.P. Kotte, *Leading Change* (Boston: Harvard Business Review Press, 2012).

*Maintaining the Momentum*

Beyond this aspect, understanding and communicating the benefits of your efficiency project is important for continued buy-in from your staff and providers. Providing ongoing feedback and reinforcement will allow your clinic to hardwire the changes it has made. One method of providing this feedback is to develop a performance dashboard of some sort. Performance dashboards are useful in many areas of health care and are increasingly being used to track and assess individual performance among staff and providers. A dashboard can also be used for the clinic as a whole.

Demonstrating information about continuing improvements of process efficiency can provide significant positive reinforcement for the clinic, and such information should be shared with the staff on a regular basis. This does not need to be complicated: for example, the information can be a chart that is posted in the staff lunch area or as a part of a brief presentation at staff meetings. Figure 13.9 presents two examples that can provide this feedback to your staff. The point is to maintain the gains your team has made and create additional momentum and acceptance for the future efficiency projects that will undoubtedly emerge from your first round of DMAIC.

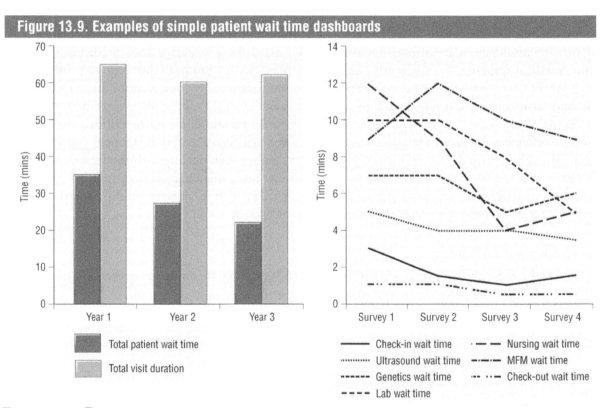

## Permanent Beta

I would like to end this chapter with a business concept that applies to all organizations that are undergoing change and can be appropriately applied to health-care systems and your MFM practice: permanent beta. David A. Shore conveys this rather well, and I would like to borrow this excerpt from his 2014 book *Launching and Leading Change Initiatives in Health Care Organizations*:

*Beta* is a term borrowed from the technology world, where it refers to products that are still in testing and hence not quite finished. Successful organizations realize that they are never perfect, and that virtually everything about them can always be improved. They exist in a state of permanent beta.[179]

Adopting and helping to instill the mind-set of permanent beta within your team, staff, and providers will likely have a lasting impact. Improving on process efficiency within your clinic is unfortunately not a once-and-done project, as suggested by the cyclical nature of the DMAIC structure. Without a doubt, the advances that you make within your practice after your first foray into process-efficiency improvement will uncover numerous future targets on which to focus your team's future efforts. Having a permanent beta mentality, when applied in a positive manner, can both lessen the initial anxiety associated with process change and eventually transform your clinic into one that actually drives and proactively seeks out more efficient processes at every level of the organization.

## Conclusion

The landscape of health care as we know it will continue to change with the perpetual introduction of new technologies and shifting environmental forces. As a maternal-fetal medicine specialist, your medical practice is inherently highly complex, with multiple different yet interrelated departments, which increases your susceptibility to inefficiency. As your practice strives to provide the highest-quality care to your patients amid the many changes taking place right now, the need for process efficiency within your everyday work will become even more critical. By applying process-efficiency business strategies such as lean and Six Sigma to your practice, you can focus more of your time on the actual care of your patients rather than dealing with the frustrations of an outdated and inefficient care-delivery system. With any luck, this chapter has provided you with a sampling of a number of tools that can be used to take that first step within your practice to improve its clinical efficiency and the care that you provide for your patients.

To summarize this chapter:
- Improving clinical efficiency within your MFM practice through the application of business strategies can improve clinical care quality, satisfaction, and profitability.
- Lean process improvement aims to eliminate wasteful steps that contribute to inefficiency.
- Six Sigma process improvement aims to minimize errors through the elimination of variance at each step.
- Having an effective multidisciplinary project team in place is critical to your success.

---

[179] Daniel A. Shore, *Launching and Leading Change Initiatives in Health Care Organizations: Managing Successful Projects* (San Francisco: Jossey-Bass, 2014).

- This chapter has presented the DMAIC approach to process-efficiency improvement as well as tools such as basic process mapping, value stream mapping, and cause-and-effect diagrams.
- Patient wait times are a recommended metric for measuring efficiency.
- The permanent beta mind-set should be imbedded within your practice.

# 14

## Performance Indicators for MFM Practices

C. Andrew Combs (MD, PhD) and Alan Fishman (MD)

Performance indicators (PIs) are standardized measures that summarize processes, outcomes, and progress toward defined practice goals. Key performance indicators (KPIs) are measurements of activities that are vital to the practice. In this chapter, we will introduce several PIs and KPIs that can help managers and providers evaluate their practice along several distinct but interrelated dimensions:

- *Clinical performance indicators.* The mission of a medical practice is to improve the health of its patients. Therefore, health outcomes are the "gold standard" measures of the success of the practice.

- *Patient accounts and financial performance indicators.* Profit is not the primary goal, but profit is necessary for the practice to stay in operation. A practice that continually loses money will not be able to pay its bills and will ultimately close.

- *Operational performance indicators.* Timely scheduling and efficient patient flow will optimize the indicators in other dimensions (clinical, financial, and patient satisfaction).

- *Patient satisfaction indicators.* If the medical care is flawless but patients are unhappy with their treatment, they will tell their referring providers and their friends, and then referrals will decline.

Simultaneously tracking key indicators in all these dimensions requires constant vigilance and significant effort. This is perhaps the most challenging aspect of the practice manager's job, but it can also be the most rewarding.

In this chapter, we will examine several key indicators in each of these dimensions, starting with patient accounts and financial PIs. We will provide a few examples to show how the evaluation of PIs can lead to changes in processes that will improve the functioning and efficiency of the practice. The tracking and periodic reporting of PIs serves several purposes:

- To view a snapshot of the performance of individuals or groups
- To summarize trends in performance over time
- To gauge the efficiency of various processes

- To identify areas for potential improvement
- To identify the root causes of problem areas
- To aid in setting goals and expectations for individuals or groups
- To compare actual to budgeted amounts for the current fiscal year
- To inform the budget for the next fiscal year

If you are in a small private practice, the manager will often be responsible for tracking and evaluating PIs. If you are part of a large institution, such as a university or multispecialty group, dedicated divisions of the institution may do the tracking and reporting. Even so, maternal-fetal medicine (MFM) practice managers should stay current on the PIs that are being reported to the administration, because PIs will often be used to determine how resources are allocated to the MFM division.

## Patient Accounts and Financial Performance Indicators

### The Revenue Cycle

Before tackling PIs and KPIs, it is helpful to understand the basic processes of revenue generation in medical practice. Patient encounters are the main source of revenue for most practices. To effectively bill and collect for a single patient encounter, many distinct steps are required. These can be summarized in a simple graphic commonly called the revenue cycle, an example of which is shown in figure 14.1. An Internet search of "revenue cycle images" will readily produce dozens of similar figures that differ primarily in the amount of detail, the number of steps they include, and the precise ordering of the steps. The concept of the revenue cycle is widely used throughout the health-care industry, especially in the management and financial arenas.

**Figure 14.1. Depiction of the health care revenue cycle**

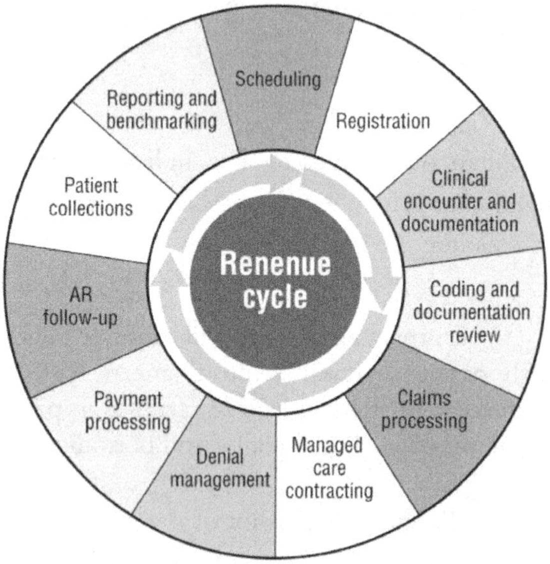

Modified from University of Michigan Health System.

One glaring problem with the concept of the revenue "cycle" is that many MFM patients are seen only once (for example, for a consultation and/or an ultrasound exam) and have no follow-up encounter. For such patients, the so-called revenue cycle is not a cycle at all but a linear timeline that starts at the Scheduling step and ends at the Reporting and Benchmarking steps.

### A Revenue Flowchart

The flowchart shown in figure 14.2 more accurately represents the flow of an MFM practice. This chart emphasizes that each patient encounter has a distinct beginning (the Scheduling step) and ending (the Collections step). It shows the intimate relationship between revenue processes and clinical documentation processes. The rotating circles (personnel, processes, technology) drive the flow and correspond roughly to front- office (scheduling, registration, and clinical) and back-office functions (billing and collections). The graphic also shows the subtle transition from "patient" to "consumer" after completion of the clinical encounter.

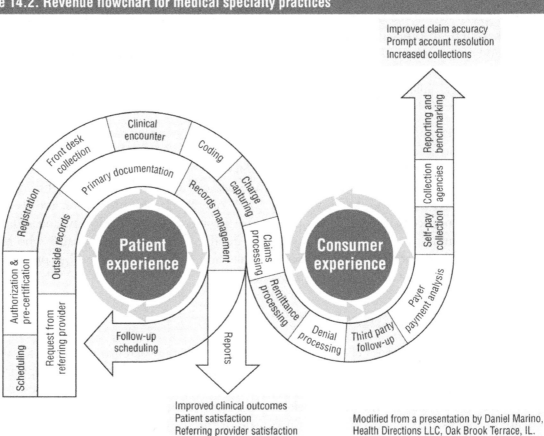

Figure 14.2. Revenue flowchart for medical specialty practices

Modified from a presentation by Daniel Marino, Health Directions LLC, Oak Brook Terrace, IL.

Each step in the flowchart can be divided into several processes, each of which must be optimized to facilitate efficient revenue collection. For example, an important process during the Scheduling step is to obtain detailed primary and secondary insurance information. In a separate Verification step, the insurance information should be verified with the payer before the encounter, any needed precertification or authorization should be obtained, and a determination should be made as to whether a copayment or deductible will be required from the patient. When the patient arrives for her visit, the Registration step will include processes such as obtaining a copy of the patient's identification and insurance cards, the patient's signature on assignment-of-benefits forms, and the collection of any required copayment. Every subsequent step in the diagram can be similarly subdivided.

Successful practices use a set of detailed written procedures to guide the employees who perform each step. Developing, maintaining, adapting, and improving these procedures should be an ongoing process, driven by the manager with input from those employees who actually perform the processes.

## Performance Indicators

Virtually every step in the flowchart can be measured in some way. In fact, it is critical to measure certain key steps in order to understand whether revenue collection can be improved. Table 14.1 lists several commonly tracked financial PIs in medical practices. We have designated KPIs with an asterisk (*). Routine periodic reports for most, if not all, of the KPIs can be readily generated from standard medical billing and collections software packages. These indicators are fairly well standardized across the industry.

The sheer number of PIs, KPIs, and subreports may appear daunting at first. It is a good idea to start using a few KPIs regularly and to increase the number of indicators that you track as you gain familiarity with them. Most often, you will track aggregate KPIs for the entire practice. If these show a trend that requires investigation, the use of subreports may be useful in which you break down the KPI by payer, by provider, by CPT code, by class of procedure, and so on. Which subreports are needed will depend on the precise problem that is being investigated. It is not necessary to routinely run all the subreports listed in table 14.1. In fact, a manager who tries to do so will be hopelessly bogged down in micro-details and will easily lose the big picture. We will focus on just a few key examples for this reason.

**Some KPIs Should Be Reviewed Daily**

Let's start by looking at gross charges. We recommend that the total gross charges for the whole practice be reviewed on a day-by-day basis. Table 14.2 shows a hypothetical report of gross charges for a one-week period. A quick inspection shows that the total gross charges were much lower on Thursday than on the other weekdays. An alert manager will look for system problems or process problems that might explain this. Did one of the providers forget to submit charges that day? Did a whole stack of fee tickets get inadvertently thrown in the trash? Did a computer problem prevent one of the billing clerks from entering charges? All these problems are much easier to identify and solve if they are caught immediately, rather than waiting until month-end.

## Table 14.1. Some financial and patient accounts performance indicators

| | Measure | Units | If needed, subreports by |
|---|---|---|---|
| * | Gross charges | Dollars | Payer, provider, procedure class, CPT |
| * | Adjustments | Dollars | Payer |
| * | Net charges | Dollars | Payer, provider, procedure class, CPT |
| * | Gross collections | Dollars<br>% of gross charges<br>% of net charges | Payer, provider, procedure class, CPT |
| * | Accounts receivable (AR), total | Dollars | Payer |
| | AR aging overall | Distribution of days | Payer |
| * | AR over 90 days | Dollars<br>% of total AR | Payer |
| | Average days in AR | Days | Payer |
| * | Time-of-service collections | Dollars<br>% of net charges<br>% of gross collections | Payer, procedure class, CPT |
| * | Encounters with no charges | Encounters | Provider |
| | Self-pay balances | Dollars<br>% of AR | Procedure class, CPT |
| | Sent to collection agency | Dollars<br>% of net charges | Payer, procedure class, CPT |
| * | Write-offs | Dollars<br>% of net charges | Payer, provider, procedure class, CPT |
| * | Insurance denials | Dollars<br>Number of denials<br>% of claims | Payer, provider, biller |
| * | Reason for denials | Number of denials by reason<br>Dollars denied, by reason | Payer, provider, biller |
| * | Paid versus contracted amount | Dollars paid for CPT code minus contracted dollars for that code | Payer and CPT |
| | wRVUs | wRVUs | Provider |
| | Charges per wRVU | Gross charges divided by total wRVUs | Provider |
| | Collections per wRVU | Gross collections divided by total wRVUs | Payer, provider, CPT |
| * | Charge entry lag | Days from DOS to charge entry | Provider, biller |
| | Claim drop lag | Days from DOS until claim dropped | Provider, biller |
| * | Days to pay | Days from DOS until payment received | Payer, provider, CPT |
| | Active accounts | Number of patients with open claims | |
| | Active accounts per worker | Active accounts divided by number of billing/collection personnel | |

\* Key Performance Indicator (KPI)  
wRVU—work Relative Value Unit  
AR = accounts receivables  
DOS—date of service  
Procedure classes are Evaluation & Management, Surgery, Laboratory, Imaging, Other

| Table 14.2. Daily gross charges (dollars) for one week—example report | | | | | | | |
|---|---|---|---|---|---|---|---|
| | Monday | Tuesday | Wednesday | Thursday | Friday | Saturday | Sunday |
| Procedure class | June 1 | June 2 | June 3 | June 4 | June 5 | June 6 | June 7 |
| Evaluation & management | 4,306 | 2,245 | 3,044 | 3,240 | 1,113 | 522 | 476 |
| Surgery | 926 | 1,224 | 8,250 | 0 | 4,515 | 0 | 1,845 |
| Laboratory | 0 | 0 | 146 | 73 | 0 | 0 | 0 |
| Imaging | 15,240 | 16,800 | 14,246 | 11,358 | 16,244 | 460 | 0 |
| Other | 0 | 0 | 45 | 0 | 0 | 0 | 0 |
| Total | 20,202 | 20,269 | 25,731 | 14,671 | 21,872 | 982 | 2321 |

In this case, let's say that the problem with Thursday was simply that one of the ultrasound techs called in sick, so ultrasound volume was down somewhat. Coupled with the lack of surgery-code procedures on that day (a coincidence), the low production on Thursday can then be explained. The manager will readily understand this if gross charges are reviewed daily. If this review waits until month-end, then the manager is unlikely to remember the particular circumstances on any given day.

But it is not enough to simply understand and explain away outlier days. If managers simply accept the results ("problem understood"), then they will miss an opportunity for improvement. In this case, the practice might want to pursue ways to have a back-up ultrasound tech available to cover on short notice in case a scheduled tech calls in sick. It might be expensive to have someone be on call for this, but the expense might be justifiable if it prevents losing revenue and having to cancel appointments.

Time-of-service collections is another KPI that should be reviewed daily. This includes payments made at the beginning or end of a patient visit, including copayments, deductibles, and self-pay payments, whether paid by cash, check, debit card, or credit card. It is much more efficient to collect a twenty-dollar copayment up front than to bill the patient later. Billing and collections will likely cost well over twenty dollars, considering personnel time, materials, mailing expenses, and write-offs for nonpayment. But money kept at the front desk is at high risk for theft and must be reconciled and deposited daily.

Encounters-without-charges is another KPI that should be reviewed daily. Did the provider lose the charge ticket? Is the provider still working on the documentation for the visit? Billing personnel should attempt to resolve these discrepancies as soon as possible so that claims can be filed in a timely fashion.

## Many PIs Should Be Reviewed Monthly

Again, let's use gross charges as an example. Table 14.3 is a hypothetical subreport showing charges by provider and by class of service for a given month, along with a running year-to-date tally. This report can be used to identify physicians who are not performing as expected. In this case, it is obvious that something is very different about Dr. Gray. Maybe she works only two days per week, while the others work five days. A separate report showing charges per provider per full-time equivalent (FTE) worked should resolve this issue. But if Dr. Gray works five days and is constantly forgetting to complete her charges, this is a major problem that needs to be fixed, pronto!

### Table 14.3. Monthly gross charges—example report

| Procedure class | Dr. White | Dr. Gray | Dr. Wong | Total |
|---|---|---|---|---|
| **Report for June** | | | | |
| Evaluation & management | 21,645 | 12,200 | 19,360 | 53,205 |
| Surgery | 15,332 | 7,004 | 18,360 | 40,696 |
| Laboratory | 2,188 | 0 | 1,835 | 4,023 |
| Imaging | 82,040 | 26,320 | 94,252 | 202,612 |
| Other | 0 | 0 | 45 | 45 |
| Total | 121,205 | 45,524 | 133,852 | 300,581 |
| **Recap of year** | | | | |
| January | 85,320 | 46,189 | 103,296 | 234,805 |
| February | 100,255 | 42,232 | 96,327 | 238,814 |
| March | 96,239 | 49,281 | 151,962 | 297,482 |
| April | 108,953 | 54,360 | 84,972 | 248,285 |
| May | 125,200 | 44,250 | 102,516 | 271,966 |
| June | 121,205 | 45,524 | 133,852 | 300,581 |
| Year-to-date | 637,172 | 281,836 | 672,925 | 1,591,933 |

The differences between Dr. White and Dr. Wong are relatively small. Maybe this is because they have similar skills, similar hours, and similar work habits. Dr. Wong bills slightly more, perhaps because he is slightly busier or perhaps because he performs a particular specialized ultrasound-based procedure that Dr. White does not. If the manager or the doctors are interested, they can generate a report that counts the number of encounters for each CPT code for each physician. It is doubtful that drilling down to this level of detail will prove useful in this particular case, however, because the difference between the two doctors is quite small. Doctors will often be very interested in their individual gross charges and gross collections reports, because their compensation or bonus often depends on their productivity.

Most of the other PIs and KPIs shown in table 14.1 are amenable to monthly reporting and tracking. In most cases, monthly reports should be based on the date of service (DOS), not the month of the report. For example, a collection that is received in January for a service that was performed in October should be accounted as applying to October's accounts receivable (AR). That way, any outstanding AR balances from October can be readily tracked. The only places where this payment should be accounted in January is on the bank account deposit slip and check register.

"AR over 90 days" is another important KPI, because the probability of successful collection goes down and the probability of denial or write-off goes up substantially as AR ages past ninety days. The whole practice should work aggressively to minimize AR over 90 days, starting with providers submitting charges on the DOS, billers dropping electronic claims to payers within one day, and billers and collectors working to clean up and appeal any denials within a day. As a hypothetical scenario, lets surmise that a practice put so much emphasis on AR over 90 days that they tied the manager's year-end bonus almost entirely to this number, with a maximum bonus when AR over 90 days was less than 5 percent. However, an unintended result was that the staff would simply write off claims that had not been paid at 89 days. This minimized AR over 90 days, but unfortunately it also decreased gross collections, which shows that you cannot rely on any single PI to gauge the performance of the practice. Each PI provides a different insight into the processes involved. Remember, AR over 90 days may be harder to collect, but it's not impossible. It should continue to be worked until no further collection is possible.

Rate of denials is another important KPI that should also be tracked monthly. A simple "run chart" (figure 14.3) will reveal if there is a trend toward increasing rates of denials. If a trend is found, then a subreport showing denials by payer may reveal that the problem lies with one particular payer. It may also be useful to drill down on the reasons for denials. Common reasons include (1) lack of prior authorization; (2) it is not a covered service; (3) failure to file claim in a timely fashion; (4) regulatory penalty; (5) claim not "clean" (i.e., incomplete or contradictory data); and (6) other denials.

These are all different than contractual write-offs, such as preferred provider organizations (PPO) discounts, and capitated patient write-offs (as in health-maintenance organization [HMO] payments), which are accounted in adjustments, not denials. Of course, adjustments are another important KPI that should be tracked, both by month and by payer.

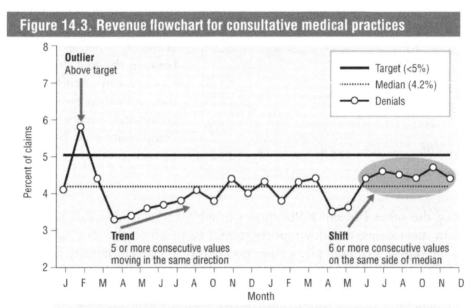

Figure 14.3. Revenue flowchart for consultative medical practices

This hypothetical practice has set 5 percent as the "maximum acceptable" target (double line). Any value above the target is an obvious cause for concern. But even though this practice is almost always within the target range, certain patterns may indicate need for improvement. A "trend" of five or more values moving in the same direction or a "shift" of six or more values on the same side of the median should be examined closely. These patterns may indicate a systematic problem because they are very unlikely to occur by random chance.

If a trend toward an increasing rate of denials is noted, a Pareto chart (figure 14.4) will reveal the most common reasons. In the example, because over 80 percent of the denials are due to "unclean" claims and lack of authorization, the most efficient approach to reducing denials will be to focus on these two issues. A subreport may show differences in rates of denials between individual billers. Billers with lower rates can be queried to learn best practices. Written procedures for all the billers can then be revised to reflect these practices.

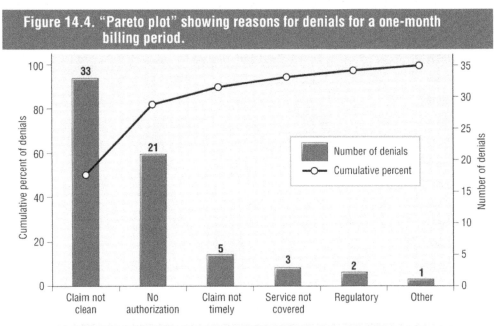

Figure 14.4. "Pareto plot" showing reasons for denials for a one-month billing period.

Bars show the number of denials of each type. *Line with dots* shows cumulative percentage of denials, moving left to right. *Claim not clean* accounts for 51 percent of the denials, *No authorization* accounts for 32 percent of denials, so these two categories cumulatively account for 83 percent of denials. These are the two areas where performance improvement is most needed.

**Some PIs Should Be Reviewed Quarterly or Every Six Months**

Table 14.4 is a hypothetical example showing collected versus contracted amounts for six ultrasound CPT codes for two payers. It takes a bit of study to understand the differences between the payers. The practice saw more patients insured by NumberTwoChoice than by NumberOneCare. NumberTwoChoice had a higher contracted rate of reimbursement, but it paid a lower percentage of the contracted amount. NumberTwoChoice also paid claims more quickly.

It will be important to understand this report when it is time to renegotiate the contracts with the two PPOs. The negotiations will hinge on mutual expectations of the practice and the payers: How many patients will be seen? How much will be paid? How quickly will the payments be made? Of course, the manager should not wait for contract renegotiations to troubleshoot problem areas. If NumberTwoChoice is paying less than the contracted rate, then the reasons need to be understood and addressed. A detailed investigation of NumberTwoChoice's denials and adjustments should be undertaken.

## Table 14.4. Payer performance review of closed 2nd quarter ultrasound claims—example report

| CPT | Number performed | Total collections | Collections per procedure | Contracted amount | Percentage collected | Average days to pay | Lost revenue |
|---|---|---|---|---|---|---|---|
| **NumberOneCare PPO *** | | | | | | | |
| 76802 | 35 | 7,968 | 227.66 | 248 | 91.8 | 65 | 712 |
| 76801 | 4 | 517 | 129.34 | 136 | 95.1 | 80 | 27 |
| 76805 | 148 | 42,105 | 284.49 | 290 | 98.1 | 68 | 815 |
| 76810 | 7 | 1,186 | 169.48 | 174 | 97.4 | 84 | 32 |
| 76811 | 137 | 47,957 | 350.05 | 372 | 94.1 | 73 | 3,007 |
| 76812 | 8 | 3,186 | 398.23 | 425 | 93.7 | 90 | 214 |
| Totals | 339 | 102,919 | 303.60 | | 95.5 | | 4,807 |
| **NumberTwoChoice PPO *** | | | | | | | |
| 76802 | 60 | 15,763 | 262.72 | 320 | 82.1 | 42 | 3,437 |
| 76801 | 5 | 792 | 158.36 | 185 | 85.6 | 50 | 133 |
| 76805 | 214 | 59,235 | 276.80 | 320 | 86.5 | 48 | 9,245 |
| 76810 | 10 | 1,467 | 146.74 | 166 | 88.4 | 51 | 193 |
| 76811 | 165 | 58,606 | 355.19 | 405 | 87.7 | 60 | 8,219 |
| 76812 | 15 | 5,033 | 335.54 | 380 | 88.3 | 68 | 667 |
| Totals | 469 | 140,896 | 300.42 | | 86.6 | | 21,894 |

We have barely scratched the surface of the wide range of financial and patient account PIs and how to use them. More comprehensive examinations are provided in the Additional Reading section. For now, it is important that you get started on measuring a few of the KPIs that reflect different steps of the billing and collections process. As you gain experience with these processes, you will quickly add others to track so that you will have a comprehensive view of the practice's revenue flow. In fact, you may find that you need to develop other PIs that are not shown in table 14.1 to get a handle on particular issues.

## Operations Performance Indicators

Several key operational steps in the practice flowchart (figure 14.2) are not tracked directly by financial PIs. These include scheduling issues (number of appointments, delays to obtain appointments), issues related to appointments not kept (no-shows and cancellations), and patient flow issues (wait times, time spent in various phases of the encounter). Some PIs and KPIs for each of these areas are shown in table 14.5. As with financial PIs, we recommend starting with a few KPIs and increasing the number tracked as you gain experience with them. Many of these can be tracked easily with modern patient-scheduling software systems. We will focus on a few key examples.

**Table 14.5. Some operations performance indicators**

| | Measure | Units | If needed, subreports by |
|---|---|---|---|
| | **Scheduling** | | |
| * | Requests from referring providers | Number of requests | Provider, referring provider, procedure class, CPT |
| * | Requests received but no appointment made | Number<br>% of requests<br>Tabulation of reasons † | Payer, provider, referring provider, scheduler, procedure class, CPT |
| * | Appointments scheduled | Number of appointments | Payer, provider, referring provider, scheduler, procedure class, CPT |
| * | Scheduling lag, new patients | Days from date of request until original scheduled date of service | Payer, provider, referring provider, scheduler, procedure class, CPT |
| | **Encounters** | | |
| | Encounters per day | Number of encounters divided by number of work days in reporting interval | Payer, provider, procedure class, CPT |
| | New patient encounters | % of total patient encounters | Payer |
| | Appointments kept | Number of appointments<br>% of scheduled appointments | Payer, provider, referring provider, scheduler, procedure class, CPT |
| * | Appointments not kept | Number of appointments<br>% of scheduled appointments<br>Tabulation of reasons ‡ | Payer, provider, referring provider, scheduler, procedure class, CPT |
| | **Patient flow** | | |
| * | Patient cycle time | Total minutes patient spent in office | Provider, procedure class, CPT |
| * | Patient wait time >15 minutes | Number of appointments<br>% of scheduled appointments | Payer, provider, procedure class |

\* Key Performance Indicator (KPI)
Procedure class = Evaluation and Management, Surgery, Laboratory, Imaging, Other
† Reasons for appointment not made = Patient did not call, unable to reach patient, patient declined, out-of-network, patient delivered, other
‡ Reasons for appointment not kept = Patient canceled, patient rescheduled, no show, our office canceled, our office rescheduled, patient delivered, other

## Scheduling

Because MFM is largely a consultative specialty, referrals from other providers are the lifeblood of the practice. It is critical to track the total number of requests for services by week, by month, and by quarter. Referrals from individual providers should be tracked at least quarterly and compared to historical rates. If referrals from Dr. Smith have dropped significantly from the prior quarter, then it will be important to understand why: Has Dr. Smith been dissatisfied with your service? Is she referring patients elsewhere? Has she been on extended vacation? Has her staff been steering patients away? A phone call from manager to manager or from doctor to doctor may help resolve any conflicts and restore referral volumes.

It is critical to track requests for services that do not result in patient appointments. Requests should result in patient appointments virtually 100 percent of the time. Referral requests languishing in the inbox, waiting for the patient to call, represent lost revenue for the practice.

Sometimes the patient never calls! A successful practice will take the initiative and call the patient to arrange for service. A run chart (such as was shown in figure 14.3 earlier in the chapter) can be useful for tracking the rate of requests without appointments, while a Pareto chart (such as figure 14.4) will show the common reasons; both should suggest processes to target for improvement.

## Appointments Not Kept

"Appointments not kept" is another KPI that should be tracked. Again, a run chart may be useful for tracking the rate, and a Pareto chart may be useful to show the common reasons. If the number of no-shows is high, then a system should be implemented to remind patients and confirm appointments via phone calls, text messages, or e-mails. This function can be done by practice personnel or can be outsourced to a specialized commercial service or software application. Such a system should decrease the rate of no-shows for reasons such as "I forgot the appointment" or "I had the wrong day." It is mandatory to follow up on every no-show appointment and to attempt to reschedule the encounter.

One issue that deserves special attention is the office itself canceling or rescheduling the appointment. This is sometimes necessary when unanticipated staffing shortages occur from illness, hospital emergencies, and the like. But it is a nuisance and inconvenience for patients to be canceled and rescheduled at the last minute, so this should be kept to an absolute minimum. If this is a frequent problem, then the practice should explore solutions.

## Patient Flow

Patients detest long waits. If your practice habitually makes patients wait for long periods, they will perceive (correctly) that you are not very well organized and that you do not sufficiently respect their time. Waiting time is a major driver of patient satisfaction, which we will discuss in the next section.

To start, we suggest tracking the percentage of patients whose waiting time is more than fifteen minutes, which is perhaps the upper limit of what many patients might consider acceptable. A run chart may be useful for tracking this. If your practice has succeeded in keeping this rate low, then you can consider adopting a ten-minute target, implementing changes as needed to make this happen. For starters, we suggest a simple name change. Most offices have an area in front called the "waiting room" (message: "Sit down and wait!"). Instead, call it the "intake area" (message: "We are taking you in!") and try to live up to the new name.

Patient times during encounters can be divided into distinct phases. Figure 14.5 is a hypothetical "cycle time" graph that breaks down a patient's entire time from entering the office until leaving. For this new-patient ultrasound encounter, the total cycle time was ninety-nine minutes (one hour and thirty-nine minutes), of which only twenty-one minutes was spent actually having the ultrasound exam (seventeen minutes with the sonographer, four with the physician). The patient spent thirty-four minutes doing other tasks (registration, intake, scheduling follow-up, and checkout) and forty-four minutes waiting (waiting for a room, for the sonographer, for the physician, and for documentation).

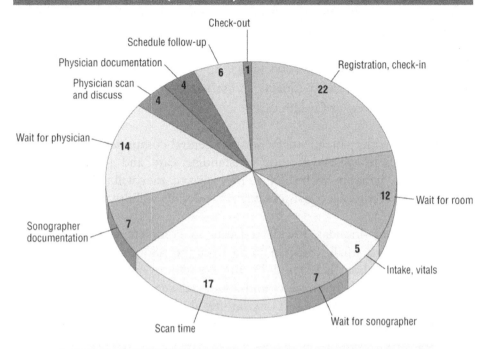

Figure 14.5. "Cycle time" analysis of a hypothetical new-patient ultrasound encounter (in minutes)

Cycle time is the total time the patient spends in the office, from actual arrival to physical departure from the office

A detailed analysis showing the precise allocation of patient time in the office can identify areas for performance improvement. In the example shown in figure 14.5, if the sonographer and the physician do their documentation in the patient room rather than in a separate work area, the patient may perceive this as part of the encounter time rather than as waiting time, thus reducing perceived wait time by eleven minutes. But this will not reduce the total cycle time. In this example, other key areas for improvement will be reducing the amount of time waiting for the room to open and (dare we say it?) reducing the amount of time waiting for the physician. Reducing these times will reduce the total cycle time.

To obtain detailed patient-flow data, the practice must invest personnel time or money. Time studies can be accomplished simply by having the staff use a flow sheet to write down the clock time as the patient moves through each step. This will be a labor-intensive process, so it can only be performed on a sample of patients. Also, handwritten times are subject to inaccuracies unless all clocks and watches are synchronized, and even that does not guarantee accuracy. Alternatively, automated tracking systems are available that will accurately record precise times when patients move through various steps. This will be less labor intensive and can be applied to 100 percent of patients, if desired, although the equipment and software systems to perform this function will cost money. Still, this might be a worthwhile investment for practices that experience patient-flow problems.

# Patient Satisfaction Performance Indicators

In 2008, the Institute for Healthcare Improvement introduced the "Triple Aim," which holds that health-care systems should simultaneously pursue three distinct goals:

- improve the health of the population served
- improve the patient experience (quality and satisfaction)
- reduce the per capita cost of health care

According to this framework, patient satisfaction is a central component of good health care. It is no longer good enough to simply provide outstanding care and to achieve excellent health outcomes. If patients are unhappy with the care they receive, they will tell their referring providers and their friends. If this becomes a consistent pattern, referrals will dry up and the practice will fail.

These days we are inundated with requests to complete a survey after almost every business transaction, big or small. Order a pizza over the phone, and "Now would you mind answering a few questions about how we did?" Buy something online, and then "Can you please be sure to post a review about the product and about our services?" Buy a new car, and (yikes!) you might be filling out surveys for the rest of your life, about the salesman, the dealership, the car, the service department. The reason why businesses invest millions of dollars in surveys, and why they risk annoying their clientele by doing so, is that your opinions teach them valuable information about improving their products and their services. At its core, a medical practice is just another business, and it can learn just as much by listening to feedback from its customers.

**Your Ratings on the Internet**

Patient feedback about your practice is already on the Internet, freely available to you and to the rest of the world. Consumer rating services like Yelp and health-care rating services like Healthgrades probably have a rating for you and your practice (generally a score from one to five stars) as well as narrative reviews from both satisfied and disgruntled patients. You should scrutinize this free information at least once a month, paying attention to areas where criticism can be turned into constructive change. As providers who work hard and generally do a great job, our natural response to criticism is to become defensive, to make excuses ("I remember that patient. Nobody could please her!"), and to rest on our laurels knowing that most patients are happy with our service. Maintaining a healthy skepticism about negative reviews will certainly protect our egos from becoming too badly battered. But we cannot emphasize enough that *negative reviews represent valuable opportunities* to do something better next time. We ignore criticism at our own peril!

We strongly recommend that you *do not respond* online to negative reviews. Physician responses usually appear defensive at best or hostile at worst. Such responses will actually reinforce the negative views the patients have expressed.

Online ratings from companies such as Yelp and Healthgrades may not represent a scientifically or statistically valid cross-section of your patients. You have no way to know basic data, such as the percentage of patients who post reviews or whether some posted reviews are not actually displayed online. You do not own the data; the ratings company does. In order to get a more reliable indication of patient experience, the practice may wish to conduct a more formal survey.

**Formal Surveys**

One type of formal survey is an exit survey. At checkout, the patient can be given a simple form with a few key questions. If she is willing to spend a minute or two, you can collect data on wait time, aspects of the care the patient liked or disliked, and suggestions to improve your service. We recommend that you keep this very brief, because time spent filling out surveys adds to the total "cycle time" for the visit. If you decide to do an in-house exit survey, you will need to commit personnel time toward entering survey results into a computer database so that they can be analyzed.

The Agency for Healthcare Research and Quality (AHRQ, an agency of the US Department of Health and Human Services) has developed a set of survey tools called the Consumer Assessment of Healthcare Providers and Systems (CAHPS). The CAHPS survey most relevant to MFM practice is the Clinician and Group Survey for Adult Visits (CG-CAHPS). The full survey has thirty-seven multiple-choice questions: twelve questions about patient demographics (age, race, education, general health, how long coming to the practice), ten questions about visits in the past twelve months, and fifteen questions about the most recent visit. Selected questions from the survey are shown in table 14.6. The full survey, the standardized multiple-choice responses, and detailed instructions can be downloaded for free at the AHRQ website.[180] If you are conducting your own in-house exit survey, you might start by selecting a few of the CG-CAHPS questions most relevant to problem areas in your practice.

If you decide to ask patients to complete the full CG-CAHPS survey, you will need to decide the best way to implement this. Full implementation will involve substantial time for data entry and analysis. You should consider that conducting and analyzing surveys is not your core business and not the area of expertise of your providers. Several commercial firms will conduct and analyze the CG-CAHPS survey for a fee. Considering the personnel time that you would have to invest in doing this, and considering that the commercial firms have economies of scale, standardized reporting, and expert analysis, paying the fee may be the most cost-effective way for you to get the feedback you need. Having an independent firm conduct the survey also assures patients that their responses will be anonymous, which will likely lead to more honest responses. Patients will be hesitant to give criticism if they believe that it might affect the care they receive at their next visit.

The AHRQ emphasizes that CG-CAHPS is a survey about patient *experience*, not patient *satisfaction*. Satisfaction can be influenced by factors such as amenities within the office, such as free coffee, public Wi-Fi in the intake area, or childcare services. It is also affected by how the practice handles insurance authorizations and claims disputes. While none of these are included in the CG-

---

[180] https://www.ahrq.gov

CAPHS survey, it does seem likely that patients who are favorably impressed by the amenities and the claims process will be more likely to provide favorable survey responses.

### Table 14.6. Patient experience indicators: selected questions from the CG-CAHPS Adult Visit Survey

**Questions about the last 12 months:**

| | |
|---|---|
| | How many times did you visit this provider to get care for yourself? |
| | Did you phone this provider's office to get an appointment for an illness, injury, or condition that **needed care right away**? |
| * | When you phoned this provider's office to get an appointment for **care you needed right away**, how often did you get an appointment as soon as you needed? |
| | Did you make any appointments for a **check-up or routine care** with this provider? |
| | When you made an appointment for a **check-up or routine care** with this provider, how often did you get an appointment as soon as you needed? |
| | Did you phone this provider's office with a medical question during regular office hours? |
| | When you phoned this provider's office during regular office hours, how often did you get an answer to your medical question that same day? |
| | Did you phone this provider's office with a medical question **after** regular office hours? |
| | When you phoned this provider's office during regular office hours, how often did you get an answer to your medical question that same day? |
| | How often did you see this provider **within 15 minutes** of your appointment time? |
| | How long has it been since your most recent visit with this provider? |

**Questions about the most recent visit:**

| | |
|---|---|
| * | Did you see this provider **within 15 minutes** of your appointment time? |
| | Did this provider explain things in a way that was easy to understand? |
| | Did this provider listen carefully to you? |
| | Did you talk with this provider about any health questions or concerns? |
| | Did this provider give you easy to understand information about these health questions or concerns? |
| | Did this provider seem to know the important information about your medical history? |
| | Did this provider show respect for what you had to say? |
| * | Did this provider spend enough time with you? |
| | Did this provider order a blood test, X-ray, or other test for you? |
| | Did someone from this provider's office follow up to give you those results? |
| | Using any number from 0 to 10, where 0 is the worst provider possible and 10 is the best provider possible, what number would you use to rate this provider? |
| * | Would you recommend this provider's office to your family and friends? |
| | Were clerks and receptionists at this provider's office as helpful as you thought they should be? |
| * | Did clerks and receptionists at this provider's office treat you with courtesy and respect? |

CG-CAHPS: Clinician and Groups Consumer Assessment of Healthcare Providers and Systems.
* Key performance indicator

Many providers' natural response to criticism found in formal surveys is similar to their response to criticism in online reviews: defensiveness, denial, and the making of excuses. "This is not a representative sample. Only patients who have complaints fill these things out. We're not that bad." The practice will not improve unless it is willing to face criticisms head on, with an attitude like "Even one dissatisfied patient is too many. Let's fix the things she's telling us about."

Of course you will not be able to fix everything all at once, so you should focus on those areas where the number of negative reviews is highest. A Pareto chart might be useful to help identify the most important areas.

## Clinical Performance Indicators

The Institute of Medicine defines "quality" in health care as "the degree to which health services for individuals and populations increase the likelihood of desired health outcomes and are consistent with current professional knowledge." [181] Accordingly, measurements of *actual health outcomes* are gold standard KPIs for assessing the quality of health care. But because MFM is largely a consultative specialty, we often do not have direct access to information about pregnancy outcomes. Few MFM practices have systems in place to systematically obtain delivery records for every mother who is seen for an ultrasound exam or consultation and fewer still to obtain newborn records. Such systems are very expensive and are resource intensive to maintain. Therefore, we often measure *processes rather than outcomes* as surrogate KPIs for clinical quality. In other words, we ask, "Did we do the right thing?" when we cannot reasonably get information about "Did we get a good result?"

**Continuous Quality Improvement (CQI)**

Several examples of outcome measures and process measures relevant to MFM practice are shown in table 14.7. This list is far from complete. The clinicians in the practice may readily think of other measures that might be worthwhile to track. Tracking any one of these will require some effort. Before investing that effort, the clinicians should discuss and agree on a formal CQI program for the practice, starting with one or two measures that represent key areas of practice activity, especially areas where the practice is concerned that improvement is likely needed.

Because it may seem difficult to justify the time and effort required to perform a formal CQI program in a private practice, especially when there is no regulatory requirement to do so, let's look at a hypothetical example to illustrate some of the possible benefits.

This variation in practice leads to confusion in the community. Referring obstetricians have no idea what to do, since they get conflicting recommendations from their MFMs. Furthermore, some of the MFMs recommend low-dose aspirin via a single weak sentence, "Consider low-dose aspirin," buried on page 3 of a four-page consultation report, while others ***Recommend Low-Dose Aspirin***—bold, italic, capitalized—reinforced with a direct discussion with the patient, a handout showing the dose and frequency, and a clear notice to the referring provider: "Low-dose aspirin (81 mg daily) is recommended because it has been clearly shown to reduce recurrence risk of preeclampsia by about 25 percent and also reduces the rate of fetal growth restriction. I told the patient to start this right away." It is no surprise that patients who receive the first type of recommendation are less likely to actually take aspirin.

---

[181] Committee on Quality Health Care in America, Institute of Medicine. (2001). Crossing the quality chasm : a new health system for the 21st century. Washington, D.C. :National Academy Press.

### Table 14.7. Some examples of clinical outcome and process measures relevant to MFM practice

| Target population | Outcome measures | Process measures |
|---|---|---|
| Patients referred for ultrasound fetal anatomy survey (detection of fetal anomalies) | False negative rate (% of detectable anomalies not detected)<br>False positive rate (% of anomalies detected by ultrasound but not confirmed at birth) | Suboptimal imaging, by organ, by gestational age (% of exams) |
| Patients referred for ultrasound fetal weight estimation at term | Rate of weight estimates within 10% of actual birth weight (% of ultrasound exams) | Image review confirms proper measurements (% of exams) |
| Patients with prior preterm birth | Rate of recurrent preterm birth (% of patients) | 17OHPC recommended (% of patients)<br>Actually received 17OHPC (% of patients)<br>Serial TVU cervical length (% of patients) |
| Patients with sonographic short cervix | Rate of preterm birth (% of patients) | Treated with cerclage, progesterone, and/or pessary (% of patients) |
| Patients diagnosed with fetal growth restriction | Stillbirth rate (% of patients)<br>Neonatal morbidity (% of patients)<br>Iatrogenic preterm birth (% of patients) | Doppler velocimetry performed (% of patients) |
| Patients at high risk for preeclampsia (prior preeclampsia, chronic hypertension, renal disease, autoimmune disorders, multiple gestation) | Rate of preeclampsia (% of patients) | Low-dose aspirin recommended (% of patients)<br>Low-dose aspirin taken (% of patients) |
| Patients with gestational diabetes | Rate of perinatal complications of diabetes (large-for-dates, birth trauma, cesarean delivery, as % of patients) | Large-for-gestational age fetus on ultrasound (% of patients)<br>Treatment with insulin or oral hypoglycemic agents (% of patients) |
| Patients with gestational diabetes | Rate of postpartum diagnosis of impaired glucose tolerance or type 2 diabetes (% of patients) | Postpartum GTT recommended (% of patients)<br>Postpartum GTT actually performed (% of patients) |
| Patients with twin pregnancy | Perinatal morbidity and mortality (% of patients) | Early ultrasound report establishes amnionicity and chorionicity (% of patients)<br>Fetal echocardiogram for performed (% of patients with monochorionic twins)<br>Serial assessment of fetal growth performed for all twins (% of patients)<br>Serial assessment for signs of twin-twin transfusion (% of patients with monochori- |

After receiving several phone calls from referring providers asking why the MFMs all have a different approach, they decide to come to a consensus. They have a contentious meeting to review the literature and argue their positions. Ultimately, they agree that there is insufficient evidence to show that any one approach is clearly better than the others but that the variation is confusing to patients and the community providers. To minimize the variation, they pick one of the methods and all agree to abide by it. They agree on a standardized text template to put in their electronic health record (EHR) that will strongly ***Recommend Low-Dose Aspirin*** for patients who meet the agreed-on criteria.

A medical assistant is assigned to track medication adherence and pregnancy outcomes for all patients for whom low-dose aspirin is recommended. When the patient is at about twenty-five weeks of gestation, the assistant makes a phone call to the patient to ask whether she is taking the aspirin. Shortly after the anticipated delivery date, she makes a phone call to the referring provider's office to obtain the date of delivery and to ask whether the patient developed recurrent preeclampsia. This data is then collated and reviewed annually.

Some of the immediate potential benefits of having such a CQI program are: (1) better patient adherence to recommendations (a process measure), (2) fewer phone calls from referring providers requesting clarification (a process measure), (3) a higher likelihood of community doctors following the same protocol on their own (a process measure), and (4) lower rates of recurrent preeclampsia (an outcome measure). Another potential benefit may come when the practice is negotiating contract renewals with payers. A practice that can show added value by demonstrating improved outcomes obtained through its CQI programs may see improved contracted payments for its services.

**Ultrasound Quality Assurance**

Many MFM practices voluntarily choose to have accreditation of their ultrasound program through the American Institute of Ultrasound in Medicine (AIUM). Some payers will pay accredited practices at a higher rate than nonaccredited practices. A few payers will not contract with nonaccredited practices. A quality assurance program is required to obtain and maintain AIUM accreditation. The AIUM "Standards and Guidelines for the Accreditation of Ultrasound Practices" contains the following statement under the heading Quality Assurance:

> The practice must show ongoing monitoring of the clinical practice's ultrasound personnel performance, including all physicians and sonographers through regular, retrospective review. To assess diagnostic accuracy, the practice must obtain correlation of ultrasound diagnoses of normal and abnormal studies with clinical, radiographic, laboratory, surgical, and pathologic findings. The review must include normal and abnormal case studies to evaluate the following: Content, completeness, and technical quality of the images; accuracy and timeliness of final reports. When deficiencies are identified, the causes should be investigated and corrective action should be planned and implemented. Information obtained should be disseminated to both physician and sonographer personnel of the ultrasound practice in a timely fashion. A record of QA activities must be maintained and kept current.[182]

Whether or not a practice seeks AIUM accreditation, we believe that it is sound clinical practice to have a quality assurance program in place, similar to the one described here.

---

[182] American Institute of Ultrasound in Medicine, "Standards and Guidelines for the Accreditation of Ultrasound Practices." Last approved October 31, 2015. http://www.aium.org/officialStatements/26.

## Tracking Systems for Ordered Tests

Physicians frequently order tests to be performed elsewhere. Common examples include blood tests, Pap smears, cultures, and diagnostic imaging. Failure to follow up and act on abnormal results is a potential area of medicolegal liability for the practice, which needs to avoid several potential pitfalls, including the following:

- The practice does not log or track tests that are ordered.
- Tests are ordered but not performed.
- Tests are performed incorrectly.
- Test results are not returned to the physician.
- The physician does not review results.
- Test results are not entered into patient charts.
- Patients are not notified of all test results.
- Actions are not taken on abnormal results.

The tracking and following up of test results is a universal challenge for every MFM practice. Each practice needs a clear policy on how this will be done. There is no universal "turnkey" solution that will work for every practice. Some offices have EHRs that will automate most of this tracking. Others will need to dedicate personnel to manually log, track, and follow up on results.

AHRQ has a toolkit on "Improving Your Office Testing Process," which is available for free download. The toolkit starts with an assessment tool to help you evaluate your current practice and offers several suggestions for systems that will improve your performance.

## Medicare PRQS Program

The Physician Quality Reporting System (PQRS) is a program of the US Centers for Medicare and Medicaid Services (CMS) that encourages individual providers and group practices to report information on the quality of care. The "encouragement" consists of a "negative payment adjustment" (i.e., financial penalty) to providers who do not satisfactorily report quality data for physician services covered under Medicare Part B.

For most MFM practices, only a tiny percentage of patients are covered by Medicare, so failure to report PQRS measures will have little impact on their practice revenue. If your practice decides to report to the PQRS program, you should download the most recent implementation guide at the CMS website. The guide provides key details as to whether you should report by individual provider or as a group, how many measures must be reported, how often they must be reported, and acceptable mechanisms for reporting (certified EHR, a qualified registry, or a data-submission vendor). Each measure has strict definitions regarding which cases must be included in the numerator and which cases in the denominator. Table 14.8 shows a few of these Medicare PRQS measures.

## Table 14.8. Selected Medicare PRQS measures relevant to MFM practice

| | | PQRS # | Description | Domain | Measure type |
|---|---|---|---|---|---|
| **Pregnancy-Specific Measures** | | | | | |
| | Ultrasound determination of pregnancy location for pregnant patients with abdominal pain | 254 | Percentage of pregnant female patients aged 14 to 50 who present to the emergency department (ED) with a chief complaint of abdominal pain or vaginal bleeding who receive a transabdominal or transvaginal ultrasound to determine pregnancy location | Effective clinical care | Process |
| | Rh Immunoglobulin (Rhogam) for Rh-Negative pregnant women at risk of fetal blood exposure | 255 | Percentage of Rh-negative pregnant women aged 14–50 years at risk of fetal blood exposure who receive Rh-Immunoglobulin (Rhogam) in the emergency department (ED) | Effective clinical care | Process |
| | Epilepsy: Counseling for women of childbearing potential with epilepsy | 268 | All female patients of childbearing potential (12–44 years old) diagnosed with epilepsy who were counseled about epilepsy and how its treatment may affect contraception and pregnancy at least once a year | Effective clinical care | Outcome |
| | Pregnant women that had HBsAg testing | 369 | This measure identifies pregnant women who had a HBsAg (hepatitis B) test during their pregnancy | Effective clinical care | Process |
| | Maternity care: Elective delivery or early induction without medical indication at ≥ 37 and < 39 weeks | 335 | Percentage of patients, regardless of age, who gave birth during a 12-month period who delivered a live singleton at ≥ 37 and < 39 weeks of gestation completed who had elective deliveries or early inductions without medical indication | Patient safety | Outcome |
| | Maternity care: Post-partum follow-Up and care coordination | 336 | Percentage of patients, regardless of age, who gave birth during a 12-month period who were seen for post-partum care within 8 weeks of giving birth who received a breast feeding evaluation and education, post-partum depression screening, post-partum glucose screening for gestational diabetes patients, and family and contraceptive planning | Communication and care coordination | Process |
| **Screening and Prevention Measures** | | | | | |
| * | Preventive care and screening: Influenza immunization | 110 | Percentage of patients aged 6 months and older seen for a visit between October 1 and March 31 who received an influenza immunization OR who reported previous receipt of an influenza immunization. | Community/ population health | Process |
| | Preventive care and screening: Body Mass Index (BMI) screening and follow-up plan | 128 | Percentage of patients aged 18 years and older with a BMI documented during the current encounter or during the previous six months AND with a BMI outside of normal parameters, a follow-up plan is documented during the encounter or during the previous six months of the current encounter | Community/ population health | Process |
| | Documentation of current medications in the medical record | 130 | Percentage of visits for patients aged 18 years and older for which the eligible professional attests to documenting a list of current medications using all immediate resources available on the date of the encounter. This list must include all known prescriptions, over-the-counters, herbals, and vitamin/mineral/dietary (nutritional) supplements AND must contain each medication's name, dosage, frequency and route of administration. | Patient safety | Process |
| | Preventive care and screening: Screening for clinical depression and follow-up plan | 134 | Percentage of patients aged 12 years and older screened for clinical depression on the date of the encounter using an age appropriate standardized depression screening tool AND if positive, a follow-up plan is documented on the date of the positive screen. | Community/ population health | Process |
| | Preventive care and screening: Unhealthy alcohol use: Screening | 173 | Percentage of patients aged 18 years and older who were screened for unhealthy alcohol use at least once within 24 months using a systematic screening method | Community/ population health | Process |

### Table 14.8. Selected Medicare PRQS measures relevant to MFM practice (cont.)

| | | PQRS # | Description | Domain | Measure type |
|---|---|---|---|---|---|
| **Screening and Prevention Measures (cont.)** | | | | | |
| | Preventive care and screening: Tobacco use: Screening and cessation intervention | 226 | Percentage of patients aged 18 years and older who were screened for tobacco use one or more times within 24 months AND who received cessation counseling intervention if identified as a tobacco user. | Community/ population health | Process |
| * | Controlling High Blood Pressure | 236 | Percentage of patients 18–85 years of age who had a diagnosis of hypertension and whose blood pressure was adequately controlled (<140/90 mmHg) during the measurement period. | Effective clinical care | Intermediate outcome |
| | Preventive care and screening: Screening for high blood pressure and follow-up documented | 317 | Percentage of patients aged 18 years and older seen during the reporting period who were screened for high blood pressure AND a recommended follow-up plan is documented based on the current blood pressure (BP) reading as indicated. | Community/ population health | Process |
| | Hypertension: improvement in blood pressure | 373 | Percentage of patients aged 18–85 years of age with a diagnosis of hypertension whose blood pressure improved during the measurement period. | Effective clinical care | Intermediate outcome |
| **Diabetes-Specific Measures** | | | | | |
| | Diabetes: Hemoglobin A1c poor control | 001 | Percentage of patients 18–75 years of age with diabetes who had hemoglobin A1c > 9.0% during the measurement period | Effective clinical care | Intermediate outcome |
| * | Diabetes: Eye exam | 117 | Percentage of patients 18 through 75 years of age with a diagnosis of diabetes (type 1 and type 2) who had a retinal or dilated eye exam by an eye care professional in the measurement period or a negative retinal or dilated eye exam (negative for retinopathy) in the year prior to the measurement period | Effective clinical care | Process |
| * | Diabetes: Medical attention for nephropathy | 119 | The percentage of patients 18–75 years of age with diabetes who had a nephropathy screening test or evidence of nephropathy during the measurement period | Effective clinical care | Process |
| | Diabetes: Foot exam | 163 | Percentage of patients aged 18–75 years of age with diabetes who had a foot exam during the measurement period | Effective clinical care | Process |

PQRS—Physician Quality Reporting System
* Key Performance Indicator
Source: Selected from "PQRS 2015 Measure List_122314.xlsx" downloaded from cms.gov.

Even if your practice is not participating in PQRS, you would be wise to know about it and to consider taking steps to prepare for the possibility that PQRS may expand beyond Medicare. When CMS initiates programs like this for Medicare, it is often only a matter of time before Medicaid and private payers initiate similar programs of their own. At the very least, it is reasonable to consider adding some of the PQRS measures to your own practice CQI program, because they reflect fundamentally good care.

Of the 253 measures in PQRS as of 2015, only nineteen are relevant to pregnancy in general or to MFM practice in particular. Of the six measures that specifically mention "pregnancy" or "maternity care," two are process measures for the emergency department, one is relevant primarily to neurologists caring for nonpregnant women of childbearing age, and three reflect the care given by primary ob-gyn providers more than the care given by MFMs. Still, a handful of general screening and prevention measures are likely applicable to virtually all MFM practices, and a few measures are relevant to those practices that provide diabetes care during pregnancy. Practices that provide only ultrasound services are out of luck here: none of the PQRS measures are related to ultrasound quality assessment.

## Getting Started

We have covered several examples to show ways in which following KPIs and PIs in your practice and using them to guide performance-improvement activities can lead to improved financials, operations, patient satisfaction, and quality of care. The sheer number of items that can and should be tracked may seem overwhelming. As we have said, you should start by tracking only a few KPIs in each area, adding more as you develop comfort and expertise, and then adding more as new problem areas are identified. Also, you don't have to do this all alone. Help is available in a variety of forms:

- *Financial and accounting PIs.* Patient-accounts software packages should generate reports and subreports that cover virtually all the PIs we have outlined in this chapter. If your billing and collections are outsourced to a vendor, then your contract should specify which PIs they report to you and how often. If your software or vendor does not provide the information you need, then you should shop for different solutions.

- *Operations PIs.* Scheduling software should have reporting capabilities that will allow you to track many of the PIs we have discussed. If yours does not, you should shop for different solutions. Tracking patient flow is more problematic and may require investment in a dedicated tracking system if this is an issue in your practice.

- *Patient-satisfaction PIs.* Internet ratings sites such as Yelp or Healthgrades are free and may give you insight into any problem areas. If you want to do an in-house survey, use a few of the CG-CAHPS questions that are available for free download. Larger formal surveys might best be outsourced to a vendor with expertise in collecting, analyzing, and interpreting the results.

- *Clinical PIs.* The clinicians in the practice should design the CQI program, starting with one or two measures that cover areas where there is a concern about quality or variation in practice. The manager will work with the clinicians to decide whether to track processes, outcomes, or both.

The tracking of performance indicators is a continuous, never-ending process. Individual performance-improvement projects may have a finite life span, with specified start and end dates. But performance improvement in general is never complete. An MFM practice is a complex enterprise, and no complex system is ever perfect. No matter how good we get, we will always have room for improvement!

## Additional Reading

Agency for Healthcare Research and Quality. "The CAHPS Program." Accessed December 20, 2017. https://cahps.ahrq.gov/about-cahps/cahps-program/index.html. "Assessing Your Testing Process." Accessed December 20, 2017. http://www.ahrq.gov/professionals/quality-patient-safety/quality-resources/tools/office-testing-toolkit/officetesting-toolkit6.html.

Centers for Medicare and Medicaid Services. "2015 Physician Quality Reporting System (PQRS) Implementation Guide." Accessed December 17, 2017. http://cms.gov/Medicare/Quality-Initiatives-Patient-Assessment-Instruments/PQRS/Downloads/2015_PQRS_ImplementationGuide.pdf.

Cohen, Frank, and Owen Dahl. *Lean Six Sigma for the Medical Practice: Improving Profitability by Improving Processes.* Phoenix, MD: Greenbranch Publishing, 2010.

Institute of Medicine. "Crossing the Quality Chasm: The IOM Health Care Quality Initiative." Washington, DC: National Academies Press, 2001.

Israel, L. A. *Practice Management Handbook 2015: Practical Advice to Ensure Compliant Operations & Revenue Cycle Management Success.* Durham, NC: Coding Institute, 2015.

Woodcock, Elizabeth W. *Mastering Patient Flow: Using Lean Thinking to Improve Your Practice Operations.* 3rd ed. Englewood, CO: Medical Group Management Association, 2007.

# 15

# A Guide to Marketing Your MFM Business

Stewart Gandolf, MBA

Why marketing for a maternal-fetal medicine (MFM) medical practice? The quick answer is that communicating value—articulating benefits for patients and the public—is a sound business activity. Health-care marketing is vital to maintaining and growing a healthy and profitable enterprise.

Effective marketing is a planned process that educates the community, prospective patients, professional colleagues, and others about your expertise and about how an obstetrical specialty practice benefits people in need. In general, health-care marketing can

- Distinguish the practice in a competitive environment;
- Engender professional referrals from obstetricians, reproductive endocrinology and infertility (REI) doctors, and others;
- Inspire patient self-referrals and word-of-mouth patient referrals;
- Shape expectations for supportive care environments and patient experience;
- Enhance and manage professional reputation and community visibility;
- Maintain or expand market share or enter new service areas; and
- Expand personal, professional, and financial rewards.

## Unique Challenges of MFM Marketing

Maternal-fetal medicine, since it has a collaborative role in care delivery with professional colleagues, is unique in many respects. From a marketing and communications perspective,

- The work of MFM subspecialists is not widely understood by the public or younger couples in particular;
- High-risk pregnancy situations may be underdiagnosed by physicians who are in a position to refer or recommend others;
- Patient self-diagnosis, self-referrals, and high-risk pregnancy knowledge are low; and
- Traditionally, low-profile MFM marketing and limited direct-to-consumer advertising inhibit patient and physician awareness.

Consequently, the women who are most in need of the collaborative care of an MFM specialist, together with their obstetricians, may not have the benefit of an optimal plan for a successful pregnancy.

## MFM Marketing Audiences and Methods

MFM practices have four primary marketing audiences and methods:

1. *Professional referrals.* MFM practices have historically relied on referrals from general obstetrician or ob-gyn practices, as well as REI practitioners and their infertility clinics.

2. *Patient referrals and self-referrals.* Less frequently, new patients will be referred via word of mouth by patients who have had their high-risk pregnancies viable to term and who know other women who may have similar circumstances.

Both professional and patient audiences remain viable target audiences and pathways to MFM care. Education and awareness are mainstays of messaging for both groups. That said, traditional MFM marketing has changed in many markets. Change agents include dramatic health-care reform shifts, increased competition, and the influential role of the Internet and social media in patient decisions and provider selection. In addition, those who require care from MFM subspecialists belong to an age bracket in which people are frequent users of mobile technology and social media.

3. *Practice liaisons or practice representatives.* These representatives have an increasingly vital role. Specialty practices that rely on the flow of professional referrals for new business are vulnerable to shifting market conditions and competition. The once-reliable referral stream is neither "automatic" nor assured. These representatives ensure frequent communication from referring providers and their staff, which aids the collegial working environment.

Most MFM practices recognize the need to retain trained and experienced practice representatives and to manage systems that will establish and maintain relationships and foster professional referrals.

4. *Direct-to-patient marketing methods* have emerged as a means to reach and educate prospective patients and influence potential referral sources. Further, those areas with an absence of market education represent an opportunity to reach an underserved audience and become a recognized authority in the community.

But would direct-to-consumer advertising raise concerns with referring doctors? If MFM subspecialists desire a collegial relationship in patient care, they may address concerns (if any) by proactively informing referral sources in advance of an external media campaign. Nonetheless, the educational and public-service objectives that benefit the patient are also of value to other health-care providers. In an MFM practice that is principally consultation oriented, referral to loyal generalist providers for the delivery of self-referral patients will build further trust among the practices.

## Medicine Is a Profession, but Health Care Is a Business

As the health-care system in the United States has been reinventing itself, the purpose and benefits of marketing have become significantly different from the past. Medical practices—especially for MFM providers and other specialists—are seeing empowered patients in an atmosphere of greater health-care consumerism. Taking an old-school approach or putting in a token marketing effort—which may have been adequate in the past—is simply not a sound business approach today. Ignoring marketing or putting in minimal effort does not increase revenue, and it can endanger the present stability and future growth of the business. Marketing has become a practical and necessary part of sound business management that can increase revenue and profit, enhance image and reputation, inform professional colleagues, and educate prospective patients.

## Getting Started: A Marketing Plan Drives Success

A goal without a plan is just a wish. A physician approached me following a marketing presentation I had just given at a professional association meeting. "I've been in practice for nine years, and I don't do marketing," he said with some pride. This statement began a revealing conversation.

Fast-forward about an hour. Privately, I concluded that the doctor—a skilled professional with a good reputation—had not been in practice for *nine* years. He had been in practice for *one* year—nine times. His business was flat and fading. Competition was growing, and his business goals were vague at best. After some discussion, we agreed on two eye-opening lessons about marketing: (1) although practicing great medical care often wins and is a guiding principle, simply being a good clinician is no guarantee of success; (2) a well-considered and written marketing plan—with specific goals, strategies, and tactics—is often necessary to maintain and grow a successful health-care practice. Without having a plan, it's all wishful thinking.

### Goals and Objectives

Begin with the end in mind. At the outset—when the blank paper stares back at you—creating a comprehensive marketing plan can seem intimidating. Even for experienced practitioners who have a marketing plan in play, it can seem risky. Previous assumptions may have changed. The competitive environment is a moving target. Patients are increasingly "highly informed consumers," thanks to an ever-expanding digital landscape. On the upside, having a detailed plan—custom fit to your practice situation—reduces risk, protects and grows your market share, and guides the achievement of your personal, professional, and financial goals.

Although every marketing plan will be individualized, the "SMART goals" technique provides focus to the effort and protects limited resources. Following the acronym, goals must always be the following:

**S** = Specific, significant, systematic, and synergistic
**M** = Measurable, meaningful, and motivational
**A** = Achievable, agreed on, action based, and accountable
**R** = Relevant, realistic, responsible, results oriented, and rewarding
**T** = Tangible, time based, and thoughtful

**Know Your Target Audience**

A comprehensive marketing plan is likely to have more than one target—and the composition of the target audience may vary within service areas. Carefully and precisely identifying the audience is a critical factor for success. You need to know—in precise detail—whom you want to reach, what they like, what their values are, and what will be the most effective channel for speaking to them. The point is that you (1) likely have more than one target audience, (2) need to define each audience in detail, and (3) need to understand each audience deeply.

On the surface, it is relatively easy to identify audience characteristics such as age, gender, race, language, insurance coverage, and so on. But digging deeper, we can identify four primary descriptive headings:

1. *Geographic*: Exactly where is your target audience located? How does that match with the area(s) that you serve? Are there physical or psychological barriers between the audience location and your front door?

2. *Demographic*: In addition to the obvious, what is the target audience's family composition, occupational and educational profile, and household income?

3. *Psychographic*: How would you describe the target audience's lifestyle, personality type, interests, and/or typical activities?

4. *Behaviors*: What is the best way to describe the concerns, needs, wants, and/or desires of the target audience? Are particular consumer patterns evident? What is their "health and lifestyle IQ"?

Knowing and understanding the target audience—with a clear and well-defined picture—is fundamental to shaping a compelling marketing message. The more precisely you can define the target audience, the greater your ability to reach, engage, and attract members of that audience.

**SWOT Analysis**

Perhaps the single most powerful planning tool is a SWOT analysis, which helps you clearly identify your Strengths, Weaknesses, Opportunities, and Threats. For a proper outcome, your analysis needs to be two things: (1) *fresh*—do your analysis every six months, or no less than once per year; and (2) *objective*—research with a fresh perspective, and don't assume you know the answers. On a piece of paper, sketch the four quadrants with Strengths and Weaknesses above Opportunities and Threats (see figure 15.1).

**Figure 15.1. SWOT Analysis**

**INTERNAL**

**Strengths**
*Examples:*
Special expertise
Reputation
Cost advantages
Technology advantages

**Weaknesses**
*Examples:*
Limited service lines
Marketing deficiencies
Management or staff problems

**EXTERNAL**

**Opportunities**
*Examples:*
New technology
Lack of dominant competition
New markets or services

**Threats**
*Examples:*
New or increased competion
Insurance plan changes
Adverse demographic changes
Adverse government policies
Economic slowdown

Strengths and Weaknesses are internal matters, meaning that these are conditions that you control. Opportunities and Threats are external issues outside of your control. In all instances, be candid.

*Strengths:* List capabilities and resources that are or could become a competitive advantage. Which are most important or useful? These might include a unique expertise, technological advantages, or an extraordinary reputation.

*Weaknesses:* Where is improvement possible? What barriers should be removed? What changes are needed? These might include marketing deficiencies, staff problems, or poor location.

*Opportunities:* What external circumstances can be exploited or used to your advantage? These might include the availability of a new technology, or a capability or market vacated by a competitor.

*Threats:* What considerations are clear obstacles to your success? Don't overlook or minimize threats. Consider how you can deal with challenges. Threats could include new or increased competition, shifts in your professional referral stream, or economic pressures.

An insightful SWOT analysis will be specific, objective, and realistic. Keep it short and direct. Revisit and refine any entries that include vague generalities or are biased. Compare your notes with those of an informed third party.

## Competitive Review

Over the course of the past few years, nearly everything about the nation's health-care delivery system has changed—a little or a lot, for the better or not, either by design or by consequence. These ongoing seismic shifts have, along with many other things, seriously disrupted what was once a predictable competitive landscape. Conducting diligent research is necessary to evaluate how things have changed (even if you think you already know). This research, which requires an open mind and an investment of time and effort, will (1) reveal how your professional colleagues have adjusted, (2) identify short- and long-term trends, and (3) spot changes within the target audience. Mentally erase what you think you know. Competition is an ever-present consideration but is not always at the forefront of your mind. Using a clean slate and an unbiased view, look for the immediate issues as well as the forward-looking trends and anticipated moves in the market. Three useful techniques for gathering competitive intelligence are as follows:

*Online research*—potential patients often search the Internet for health-care information and resources. Using keywords and links, identify and study the websites and social media channels of direct and indirect competitors as well as current and prospective referral sources. Consider how your online presence compares to, or could positively differentiate you from, the competition.

*Traditional media research*—compile examples of competitive advertising as it appears in local newspapers, magazines, and elsewhere. In particular, identify the media that reaches your target audience.

*Ear-to-the-ground research*—make note of information from vendors, laboratory and drug company representatives, staff members, and others. The heard-in-the-hall method may be insightful…or not. Take this one with a grain of salt.

## Budget for Success

When the task is to create a realistic marketing budget—and the paper is blank—there are two high-level considerations:

- Effective marketing is an investment intended to produce a measurable return. Marketing is not an expense item. As long as you have business goals to achieve, marketing should not be considered as an optional item. An intelligent and well-thought-out marketing plan will not be a cost but instead will generate revenue. Marketing is not expensive if it generates a positive return on investment (ROI).

- An effective budget is goal driven. The right amount is not based on the prior year, a percentage of gross revenue, or most of the folklore formulas that float around. The sweet spot is the "just right" amount between insufficient and needlessly wasted resources.

- A realistic and practical marketing budget dedicates sufficient resources to the activities that will produce a return equal to or greater than the quantified goals.

## The Basic Marketing Budget Formula

The process of strategic planning does not have a simple answer. Plans and budgets will vary with individual circumstances. To create a time-tested starting point when there is no previous budget, or when the existing budget is out of touch with reality, use this four-step formula:

1. *Clearly quantify your goal(s).* Calculate the amount of incremental growth (in dollars) that you intend to achieve over the next twelve months. (There may be more than one revenue stream to consider.) Above and beyond your current annual revenue, how much do you plan to grow in the next twelve months? For this example, let's say $200,000 is the goal for incremental growth.

2. *Divide your goal by an ROI factor of four.* Some marketing efforts produce a stronger return than others, but experience shows that a return between 3:1 and 5:1 is reasonable for planning purposes. For this example, allow a middle ground of 4:1 ROI: $200,000 divided by 4 comes to $50,000 to meet the annual growth goal.

3. *Divide the total budget by twelve months.* For this example, the monthly budget becomes $4,100 per month (roughly). Consider that this allowance is not likely to be spent in a conveniently flat pattern. Monthly amounts will vary within the plan, and startup expenses may occur at the beginning. Nevertheless, use your "monthly" number as a point of reference.

4. *Adjust the goal and/or the budget if needed.* Reality may dictate a few adjustments, but maintain the ratio between the goal(s) and the budget. Increasing the goal or pulling down on the budget (or vice versa) will change the opposite side of the equation.

## Tracking and Return on Investment

The true measure of successful marketing is the ROI calculation. Simply, ROI is the revenue produced divided by the marketing investment. Let's say, for example, that a particular magazine advertising effort costs $3,500, and it produces nine new cases at $1,500 per case (which is the average value of a patient referral in a consultative MFM practice). That would be $13,500 in revenue divided by $3,500, for an ROI of about 4:1. The math is simple enough, but several critical elements shouldn't be neglected:

- *Tracking the source of new patients requires a reliable system.* There is no way to accurately assess the performance of any marketing, advertising, or referral system without having a reliable means to identify and attribute the source of each new patient.

- *New-patient tracking is best done at the time of the first call or contact.* Asking a tracking question any time later than this in the patient journey is likely to produce unreliable information or incorrect attribution.

- *Make tracking a priority.* A busy office is overflowing with tasks and distractions. Create a fail-safe office routine that accurately captures, records, and reports data early. Make tracking part of staff training and emphasize the value of the information that's collected.

- *Review tracking and ROI data often, and not just after the fact.* An ongoing assessment of promotional activities allows for crafting midcourse adjustments, if needed. For example, one of several ads that are running in rotation might be outperforming the others. Making schedule adjustments can boost results.

Here is an example of a quick-tracking question that is easy to use during the first phone call. Simply ask every prospective new patient: "Who may we thank for referring you?" It turns out that people like to be asked, and compiling their answers in relation to your marketing efforts is truly vital to measuring success.

## Health-Care Marketing Essentials

There are dozens of definitions of marketing. A few are a bit long-winded and academic, but most artfully describe it as "the process by which an organization communicates, connects, and engages a target audience to convey value and benefit and ultimately to deliver services at a profit." Health-care marketing connects professional medical service offerings with patients who are in need.

### Goals, Strategies, and Tactics

A marketing plan is a process roadmap for success that outlines various goals, strategies, and tactics with defined timelines, deadlines, tasks, resources, and responsibilities.

> **Goals** are the starting point—and the ending point. They are specific, measurable, tangible, and achievable business objectives. *Example: Increase professional referral stream by [amount] within six months.*
>
> **Strategies** identify one or more general pathways to achieving each goal. *Example: Engage [number] new referral sources and enhance relationship with existing sources.*

**Tactics** are the specific action items—usually several—that support strategies and must occur to achieve success. *Examples: Institute physician liaison program. Hire and train representative. Create new professional referral support materials.*

There are hundreds of strategies and thousands of tactics in a marketing toolbox. Effectively implementing a comprehensive program often requires obtaining experienced and professional assistance to define and manage a program while minimizing risk and maximizing potential return.

## The Six Fundamental Building Blocks

Although a multifaceted plan for growth can appear complex and confusing, at least six ways have been proven to market any health-care organization. These six essential elements provide a manageable starting point for any plan:

- branding
- external advertising
- internal marketing
- internet marketing
- professional referral marketing
- public relations/publicity

*Branding* is the tangible and intangible attributes of a product or service that collectively engender awareness, value, and influence. This includes virtually everything that you do, say, or present that differentiates you and your practice in the mind of the audience. What's more, meaningful and effective branding is part of your reputation. It does not occur without a deliberate effort to shape and express the right message at the right time.

*External advertising* is commonly referred to as traditional advertising; these channels are intended to reach prospective patients who don't know you. Visibility through traditional advertising channels such as television, radio, print, and outdoor ads reaches an audience that needs to know that you provide an answer for their specialized needs and concerns.

*Internal marketing* includes all the means by which you communicate with people who already know you—primarily current and previous patients. This includes proactive patient experience and customer-service programs. Collectively and individually, these can be a rich resource for inspiring referrals, creating demand for additional services, providing testimonials, entering ratings or reviews, and/or engendering word-of-mouth recommendations.

*Internet marketing* includes websites, blogs, social media, patient portals, paid search advertising, search engine optimization (SEO), and the other connecting points that collectively represent your online presence. Because prospective patients commonly use the Internet for health-care information, it has become a primary channel for marketing, advertising, and public relations.

*Professional referral marketing* is the business lifeblood of most MFM practices. A dependable and continuing stream of inbound referrals is neither automatic nor assured and, therefore, can never be taken for granted. In recent years, competition has increased; referring doctors and practices have aligned with groups, hospitals, or health systems, which can lead to similar dynamic changes in referral patterns. Preserving and growing professional referral sources requires a dedicated practice liaison staff and a proactive system.

*Public relations/publicity* includes activities, such as newspaper articles or broadcast interviews that extend visibility and awareness for the practice or the provider. The MFM environment lends itself to media story opportunities, such as high-risk pregnancy, with human-interest and female-audience appeal.

## Additional Words of Advice

Any investment in marketing—from modest to aggressive—requires company resources (time and money) and creates an expectation of a measurable return in the face of measurable risk. With that in mind, you must recognize what marketing and advertising *do not* include. Professional practices are often asked to buy ads in civic theater programs, sponsor Little League teams, or buy mugs or trinkets. Put any worthy contributions like this under "charitable giving." They are not part of the marketing budget or ROI calculations.

## Marketing Implementation Checklist

From a top-level perspective, a well-conceived marketing plan expresses four key elements. If each component of your plan does not clearly and specifically articulate these, then synergy and success are at risk. Being mindful that "performance precedes accountability by a narrow margin," confirm the following for every item on the plan.

*When* will this occur? Create a master calendar of events, including start and end dates. Allow for lead-up, creative preparation, or training time as needed prior to rollout. Adjust for holidays, staffing, or other variables. Include ongoing or long-term commitments.

*How* will this be done? What resources—time, people, money, outside help, and so on—are needed for each activity? New activities may need to be front-loaded in an initial or one-time preparation.

*Who* will be responsible? Tasks that are "everyone's job" are at risk without an assigned "champion" or specific individual who will be accountable to the task. Some assignments may require a team effort or a combination of internal and external people.

*What* results will be tracked and reported? Is a tracking system in place to monitor results, compare them with the goals/objectives, and facilitate frequent reporting? Using regular tracking and having feedback for ongoing activities can allow for making midstream adjustments. How will this be done? For example, new ads may have a different phone number for the referral that can be tracked. What is the ROI?

In addition, evaluate progress periodically as the plan and marketing activities unfold. Provide feedback channels to recognize the strengths and weaknesses of the plan and make adjustments. Finally, realize that marketing, advertising, brand building, and related programs need time to realize their full potential. In addition to the time it takes to create and implement elements, you can expect that some of the strategies and tactics will have a relatively rapid ROI, while others will require repetition over a longer term.

**Success Is in the Details**

It's important for everyone in the organization to be aware of the big picture, even if they play an incidental role. As a quick reference, perhaps as an addendum to the marketing calendar, include these action items: (1) create an overview summary of the current situation (see the SWOT analysis), (2) list the main marketing objectives (see the SMART goals), (3) summarize the main strategies for achieving goals, and (4) identify reasonable benchmarks for assessment.

Add or subtract from the following checklist and use it as a framework to create your own implementation system.

### Preparation and setup
- Create a marketing calendar, including critical deadlines and milestones.
- Establish a unique value proposition.
- Develop campaign concepts, positioning, and brand message.
- Create media plan (for external media).
- Create marketing materials, ads, brochures, etc.
- Design protocol for testing, tracking, and reporting.
- Conduct staff orientation and training.
- Define evaluation measurements.

### Identification of internal resources and responsibilities
- Assess current personnel workload, including the need for new hires.
- Evaluate current and estimated staff time demands.
- Consider knowledge, experience, and skill sets for assignments.
- Assess computer hardware/software needs and acquire appropriately.
- Document sources of internal funding.

### Identification of external resources and responsibilities
- Advertising agency and creative support
- Vendors for printing, mailing, supplies
- Vendors/resources for website, IT, SEO, etc.

- Additional creative resources (consultants, designers, writers)
- Sources of external funding

**Assignments and responsibilities**
- Identify primary and secondary oversight responsibilities.
- Clarify tasks, cooperative efforts, and reporting lines.
- List how and when the plan will be monitored and measured.
- Install analytics for monitoring and reporting.

A marketing plan will inevitably include dozens of large and small details…all of which are important to minimize risk, preserve available resources, and maximize potential return. Use this checklist as a basic structure, and add or subtract the particulars of your own unique plan.

# How to Hire Marketing Talent

Medical practices, especially specialty and subspecialty practices that need to be assertive in their marketing efforts, generally have three resource options for marketing talent. A medical practice will often use all three options, depending on the complexity and goals of the marketing effort, the size of the practice and budget, and other considerations

## Hiring a Staff Marketing Person

The success or failure of hiring an in-house marketing person depends largely on how you define the job and the expectations that apply to that position.

1. *Create a position description that supports clear goals.* Avoid the classic assumption that the "marketing position" is able to deliver a complete spectrum of services and handle virtually anything/everything, from plan administration to creative copywriting to building doctor referrals to "fixing the website."

2. *Hire for the primary skill sets that enable the position.* Hiring for in-house marketing smarts is an excellent strategy, and having an experienced generalist will enable a solid range of support. That said, focus your hiring and performance expectations on the most important tasks and the skill sets needed to achieve them. Professional experience in marketing or communications is more critical than medical office experience.

3. *Marketing communications versus business development.* There are generally two types of "marketing people." The marketing communications category is typically responsible for creating and administering plan items, such as brochures, news releases, social media, Internet content, and brand execution. The second type is business development—an

entirely different skill set—that is a critical sales role responsible for the inbound professional referral system.

4. *Hire or promote only for the right reasons.* Avoid the temptation of filling a position out of convenience. Don't promote someone on staff to fill their time or in the hope they'll "grow into it." Instead, identify and recruit the best talent available, and reward excellent job performance.

## Hiring a Practice Representative

Referral-dependent practices—especially those that do business in increasingly competitive markets—have a continuing need for "feet on the ground" to foster ongoing relationships and oversee an effective system for generating referrals from professional practices.

Every doctor in the practice has a role in supervising and facilitating ongoing relationships with referring doctors as well as in the clinical care of the doctors' mutual patients. But reality dictates that physicians are too busy—highly involved with clinical care and treatment of those patients—to function as the exclusive sales arm of the practice. Additionally, is extensive and exclusive utilization of physician time a good ROI due to the cost of physician time versus revenue generation?

Regardless of the title—physician liaison, physician relations, practice representative—this is a sales role (or, if you prefer, a business development role). The primary responsibility of this position is to grow and protect your most vital asset: referring doctors. And it is a role that can generate hundreds of thousands of dollars in revenue. Many success factors are involved in shaping this task and hiring the right talent. These include the following:

1. *Hire for verified sales talent.* While a clinical background is nice for a candidate to have, sales experience and excellent people skills are essential. Occasionally delivering bagels to the front desk is not the same as having the proven ability to establish and maintain relationships with doctors (and their staffs), convince them to refer, and facilitate a planned support system.

2. *Look for "people skills" and "doctor skills."* A fundamental rule is that people like to do business with people they know, like, and trust. The gold standard for this position is a self-motivated individual with the ability to foster rapport and ongoing relationships with doctors as well as with professional staff members.

3. *Establish measurable performance goals.* Define expectations and accomplishments—at least in part—in specific, quantifiable numbers. This might be as a percentage increase over a baseline, for example, but use a gauge that is available in near-term (monthly or quarterly),

as well as long-term, time periods. It also may be an increase in case numbers from particular referral sources.

4. *Provide supervision and training.* Someone with a strong business development competency will be hungry to absorb clinical and process details. Real-world training furthers the practice representative's sales ability, equips him or her in the art of generating referrals tastefully, and protects your reputation. These representatives must have an understanding of your practice to be able to appropriately sell the importance of your services. Usage of time in training will be a wise investment in this key marketing employee.

5. *Provide appropriate compensation.* Devise an ethical and motivating compensation plan that rewards achievement of monthly or quarterly targets.

6. *Manage the position and the person.* A representative is an extension of the practice, often the best-known face of your business. Communicate your expectations, and review progress and activities regularly. And in addition to "the numbers," there may be more subtle cultural and personality considerations in the medical environment.

7. *Have a clear tracking and reporting system.* Like most employees, salespeople like to know how they're doing in the context of specific objectives. Install a tracking system that accurately reflects the new business attributable to the representative's efforts. Beyond any initial learning curve, you should expect early results.

8. *Don't expect a representative to stay in the office all day.* A productive representative will routinely do much of his work outside the office in direct contact with decision-makers and referring practices.

9. *Expect to endure a learning curve.* Few doctors are experts at identifying, recruiting, training, compensating, and managing sales talent. The process is distinctly different from filling a nine-to-five office staff position, but the potential return is well worth the effort.

## Traits of a Successful/Effective Practice Representative

The job title will vary and the specific tasks will vary, but some of the most important traits to look for when hiring a practice representative include the following:

1. *An extremely motivated, self-starting attitude.* The representative gets the job done, largely on her own.

2. *Excellent communications skills.* Verbal and written skills are vital.

3. *Relationship-building skills.* The representative establishes, cultivates, and maintains positive rapport.

4. *Professional appearance.* This is a reflection of the brand and reputation he represents.

5. *Friendliness and personableness.* No surprise here.

6. *High level of organization.* Customer-relations software helps; this is a detail-driven job.

## Hiring a Health-Care Advertising Agency

By definition, your health-care advertising agency is a partnership arrangement to be chosen and retained with special care. Unlike an ordinary vendor or supplier, an advertising agency is made up of trusted professional colleagues who understand your business, goals, and objectives. A well-qualified agency is a rich resource that brings industry experience, specialized talent, and unique capabilities to the partnership.

A true working relationship with a full-service medical advertising agency is not measured by individual deliverables, such as a brochure or website. Instead, it is where the agency puts itself on the line to produce—and be judged by—tangible and measurable results.

## Why a Specialist Is a Critical Consideration

Advertising agencies quite often have a varied base of experience—technical, retail, business-to-business, entertainment, industrial—because they have captured new clients in divergent industry sectors. Some agency businesses are successful at being generalists, though they would rarely—if ever—use that label.

But the health-care industry is unique in many respects. Finding and hiring marketing talent demands that the agency has specialized (not generalized) experience and talent. Some of the reasons for this include the following:

- Clients expect tangible results, even when resources are limited.
- Health care isn't "sold" the way groceries or auto repairs are sold.
- Health care has a unique culture and mix of patients, providers, payers, and others.
- There are regulations, laws, ethical considerations, and other influences.

With generalist agencies, you might be underwriting their on-the-job training. Are they learning about your profession, specialty, and competition on your budget—and experimenting to find what works?

## Twelve Challenge Questions to Ask before Hiring a Health-Care Agency

After making a candid assessment of your internal capabilities, while understanding your short- and long-term goals, it may be appropriate to partner with a qualified health-care agency. Because this is a vital business relationship, you may become more effectively organized by asking yourself the following questions prior to approaching a prospective agency.

1) "Am I looking for episodic help or long-term support?" Updating a website? Need help with hiring and training a practice rep or continuing strategic and tactical support? The appropriate course will be determined by your objectives or needs. Confirm that you and your agency are on the same page.

2) "What kind of service company are you?" Much like modern medicine and other professionals, marketing is a collective world of specialized skills. It includes writers, graphic designers, search engine optimization experts, and so on. What's more, these firms' business structures can range from an individual consultant model to a full-service enterprise with dozens of employees. Because "agency" businesses differ greatly, get a clear picture of the organization and the resources that may, or may not, support your needs.

3) "Tell me about your experience in health care." Broad experience in marketing, advertising, and PR is good, but go deeper. Drill down on the specifics, and ask for examples regarding the agency's depth and breadth of industry experience as well as specific and documented results for health-care clients.

4) "What sort of strategies are most appropriate to my goals?" Listen closely. The best answer isn't in what they do; it is in what results they expect. An answer shaped around clever execution and winning ad-business awards misses what's important: producing results for the client. Instead, listen for an answer that has a direct connection to achieving your new patient or revenue objectives.

5) "Tell me about your input process." Companies or individuals who are ready with a "treatment plan" before a thorough "diagnosis" may be intent on selling a ready-made solution. Look for a business partner with a comprehensive system for gathering client input and due-diligence details.

6) "Will this marketing partner deliver added value?" A reliable and resourceful marketing partner will not merely be an order taker and ask what it is you want. The partner will add value in strategic thinking, help identify what's needed, help you avoid mistakes, recommend appropriate solutions, and then make it happen.

7) "Are the fees competitive and reasonable given the value added?" Money matters, and comparing fees—and the tangible and intangible deliverables among various resources—is

especially difficult. The answer isn't solely cost. It is cost plus value added. Ultimately, find people you like and trust; it's a big part of what you are buying.

8) "Whom will I be dealing with?" A solid working relationship comes down to people working with people. As discussed, fees are one consideration, and the organization's credentials are another. But also get to know the personality, credentials, and experience of the day-to-day contact person. The best formula for success will include the chemistry of the relationship.

9) "Precisely how will activities be documented and quantifiable results be reported?" Avoid fuzzy and vague references to growing "awareness," "exposure," or "number of impressions." Assuming that you expect tangible results, the answer will be in tracking measurable results, having meaningful metrics, and doing regular reporting of dollars-and-cents ROI.

10) "Will the marketing emphasis be on name awareness or direct response?" Name awareness or general advertising relies on message repetition over a long time period. Conversely, the purpose of a direct-response approach is to inspire immediate action by the target audience. Each method has a valid place and purpose, but be clear about the intended path. With rare exceptions, the nature of health-care advertising—finding a doctor, answering a medical need, and the like—tends to be better served by a firm with a direct-response background.

11) "What about creating a differentiating brand?" Competition is increasingly intense as health-care providers of all types—solo practitioners, group practices, hospital-based practices—demand attention and awareness in the consumer's mind. A well-qualified agency has experience in creating a clear, compelling, and memorable brand message that differentiates the practice from the competition.

12) "Is the firm skilled and experienced in Internet marketing?" Many, if not most, patients begin the purchase-decision process online. Internet-based marketing is an essential component of a well-rounded, effective marketing plan and is one of the best opportunities for an early connection with prospective patients. Beyond creating a professional website, does the agency have strength in search engine optimization, pay-per-click advertising, social media, e-mail marketing, and the like?

**When Outsourcing Makes Sense**

Hiring a full-service health-care advertising agency (or alternatively, short-term creative help) makes sense when the need for marketing services exceeds in-house strengths and capabilities. Use internal resources when core competencies can be leveraged. Outsourcing marketing services usually makes sense when the assignment requires specialized skills, knowledge, or equipment, or when capacity is strained.

The decision to work with an experienced and qualified agency—as opposed to a project-defined vendor—will also be guided by the sophistication of the marketing plan, the strategies and tactics to be employed, the work involved, and the goals to be achieved. If working with an agency appears to be the proper course, in addition to the foregoing challenge questions, you need to answer three fundamental questions:

1) Are you willing to make a partnership-level commitment? To be effective, a marketing company will want a mutually trusting, shoulder-to-shoulder relationship. Everyone is aware of the good and the not-so-good issues, and there is a willingness to hear, understand, and accept recommendations and hard decisions in which the agency is the authority.

2) What is your tolerance for risk? Success is never guaranteed, and there is no absolute assurance of success. Marketing and advertising always involve some element of risk. As with the practice of medicine, however, drawing on experience and applying best practices will reduce the degree of risk and enhance the likelihood of success.

3) Do you have a means to quantify and measure results? The most realistic way to qualify success in marketing is in the tangible, hard results, in dollars and cents. A competent and successful marketing effort will be predicated on clearly defined goals and by determining specific ROI metrics. It's about your bottom line.

# 16

## Contract Negotiations for MFM Subspecialists 101

### Arnold W. Cohen, MD

Maternal-fetal medicine (MFM) practices are unique, varied, and different from general obstetrical practices. Because of this, it is important for MFM subspecialists to understand how to negotiate as a subspecialist, and not just as a general obstetrician-gynecologist (ob-gyn). Over the last several years, negotiation strategies may not have changed, but the people you are negotiating with may have. In the past, the fee-for-service (FFS) model of reimbursement was the predominant model of payment for services. A fee for each CPT and E&M code ("Current Procedural Terminology" and "evaluation and management," respectively) was negotiated with the insurer. This model has been shown to (1) misalign incentives by encouraging increased utilization of services, (2) be the highest-cost and lowest-quality system in the world among developed nations, and (3) disengage patient services from evidence-based best practices.

With the advent of the Affordable Care Act (ACA) in 2010, which was designed to expand coverage, improve quality, and reduce costs, new models of payment are emerging. These models will, if successful, replace the relative value unit–based (RVU-based) FFS payment system that has been used for the past half century. The ACA attempts to promote payment based on what are known as "quality outcomes". Payment will initially be based on the RVU system or capitation of services with quality incentives but will then progress to bundled payments. Bundled payments will include all services for what is known as an episode of care and will require the providers to distribute portions of the payments to each provider of care. The insurer will no longer be the managing payment. Providers will then be forced to be concerned with unit cost, appropriate utilization, and quality outcomes.

The next phase of payment will place the entire burden of payment on an organization responsible for the population. These accountable-care organizations (ACOs) could be a hospital system or a physician network. They will be responsible for the payment to the physicians, the hospital, and all other parts of the health-care system required for the entire population it serves. Therefore, in the future you will be more likely to negotiate with your hospital administrator or the CEO of the ACO rather than with representatives from the insurance companies.

To adequately understand the negotiation process and the information you need to know *before* you go into any negotiating session, it is imperative that you

- Are able to clearly explain why you as an MFM subspecialist should be treated differently from a general obstetrician;
- Understand the payment methodology of the organization you are negotiating with; and

- Clearly know the outcome "quality measures" that will result in incentives in the payment system.

MFM subspecialists must be able to negotiate contracts that are equitable for not only their own practices but also for the insurers or organizations they are negotiating with. If negotiations are done appropriately, the signed agreement will result in appropriate reimbursement for the MFM subspecialist, a better interaction with the organization, and, hopefully, improved quality with reduced health-care costs.

# Sixteen Steps to Follow for Successful Contract Negotiations

To have successful negotiations, the following sixteen steps need to be taken in sequence.

**Step One: You Should Be Actively Involved in the Contracting Process**

Nobody knows what an MFM subspecialist does better than an MFM practitioner. Therefore, it is absolutely necessary for you to be involved in the contracting process. Contracting with an insurer or ACO is one of the most important parts of your practice. It not only results in fair reimbursement for your practice, but it also allows you to establish a positive relationship with the organization.

One practitioner of the MFM subspecialist practice should be actively involved. This will ensure that the information you feel to be important is appropriately relayed to the contracting entity. The insurer or ACO will also realize that you take pride in being an MFM subspecialist and in providing care to your patients. They will realize that you are committed to quality outcomes for the pregnancy as well as reducing cost without sacrificing quality. This message cannot be adequately delivered by an office manager or billing person. Many aspects of the contracting process can be delegated, but it is important that one MFM subspecialist from the practice be actively involved in all discussions that involve medicine, quality of care, outcome measurements, and the differentiation of MFM subspecialists from other obstetrical providers.

More and more, MFM subspecialists are employed rather than being in private practice. Employed physicians will have difficulty becoming actively involved in the contracting process. Contracts with hospitals, academic medical centers (AMCs), or large physician multispecialty groups are usually negotiated at a very high level and generally do not involve specific physicians or department chairs. The negotiators for these large entities may not even know how an MFM subspecialist differs from a general obstetrician.

Because perinatal services based on percent of billed charges for these organizations are very low (less than 1 percent), all obstetrical care providers are included under the umbrella of the obstetrician. This frequently results in MFM subspecialists being given the same reimbursement as the general obstetricians or radiologists who happen to do the same CPT-coded services. In some cases, the professional component of ultrasounds and testing for inpatients may actually be included in a global reimbursement to the hospital or capitated reimbursement to the radiologist. This will result in the insurer actually denying your claims as being "included in hospital care."

If the reimbursement for the professional component of ultrasound is included in the radiology contract, it will be necessary for the MFM subspecialist to negotiate with the radiology department, not the insurer, for reimbursement. This at times is more difficult than dealing with the insurer. These specific issues should be discussed with the system negotiator prior to any contract being signed so that the issues can be resolved and equitably dealt with during the negotiation process. It is vital that the interests of the MFM subspecialists are known prior to negotiations. If this is not done, the MFM subspecialist will have inadequate reimbursement, which will be very difficult to rectify once the practice discovers that bills are being rejected.

**Step Two: Know How You Will Get Paid**

In the past, negotiations were based on CPT and E&M codes. These services were based on the RVU assigned to each code. This FFS contracting will continue for some time, but the future in contracting will be value based, with incentives for quality and cost savings. These contracts may be based on RVUs, bundled payments, or capitation. Understanding these methods of payment is essential before going into any negotiation.

Value-based pay for performance contracts will provide rewards for the top performers, for those who improve the most, or for those who meet predetermined benchmarks. Those who are the bottom performers, who don't improve, or fail to meet benchmarks will suffer from reduced reimbursement. Incentives will be determined on reduced costs for health care or for achieving outcomes thought to result in cost reduction. Therefore, as an MFM subspecialist, it is necessary to understand how your practice will be judged and to know up front that many of the initial quality measures may not be ones where MFM subspecialists can make a significant impact.

If preventing early deliveries is a quality measure for the insurer or ACO in the hopes of decreasing NICU (neonatal intensive care unit) days and saving costs, then the MFM subspecialist may promote appropriate care, but the decision as to when the patient delivers may be that of the general obstetrician. The adjudication of adulation or blame may not be attributed appropriately. Hence, the MFM subspecialist may be judged on care rendered by others and not that provided by the MFM subspecialist. Therefore, the MFM subspecialist must be sure that the value-based contract applies only to care provided by the practice and is not influenced by others. As of 2018, the Society for Maternal-Fetal Medicine (SMFM) is actively working to establish outcome and process quality measures specific to MFM practices.

Obstetricians have traditionally been reimbursed by the bundled-payment methodology. The CPT codes for delivery include prenatal, intrapartum, and postpartum care. Bundled payments in the future will include not only all the obstetrical care a patient receives from a specific provider but also all tests and care required during the pregnancy, including the following: (Figure 16.1).

> **Figure 16.1. Tests and care required during pregnancy**
>
> - Laboratory services
> - Social services
> - Smoking cessation
> - Drug dependence care
> - Home care
> - Medications
> - Nutrition services
> - Perinatal services
>   - Ultrasound
>   - Antepartum testing (BPP, NST/AFI)
>   - Consults
>   - Genetic counseling
> - Ancillary devices
> - Antepartum admissions
> - Hospital delivery care
> - Incremental cost of cesarean sections
> - Normal newborn care
> - NICU care
> - Long-term care of injured infant

A comprehensive bundled payment will be paid to one main provider or institution, who will then be responsible for payment for the remainder of services for the patient, possibly including MFM services. The provider who is being paid could be the provider who is providing prenatal care or the one who does the delivery.

In Tennessee, where bundled payments have been adopted among a Medicaid population, the payment is made to the delivering provider. This could be an obstetrician, family practitioner, midwife, or MFM subspecialist. Complicated formulas are being developed and utilized to adjust bundled payments based on risk. MFM subspecialists routinely provide services for patients who are transferred because of high-risk situations or because of the need to deliver at a tertiary-care facility for neonatal concerns. As a result, the MFM subspecialist who does the delivery and receives the payment will be responsible for distributing funds for all the services provided throughout the pregnancy.

The other possibility is that a high-risk patient who requires co-management and frequent testing would be delivered by a practitioner who has had no contact with the patient prior to the delivery. This practitioner would then be responsible for reimbursing the MFM subspecialist. This type of experiment in payment has yet to be proven equitable. The Affordable Care Act also proposes the formation of ACOs to be responsible in the care of a set population of patients. The ACO is paid a fixed amount, along with additional incentives based on quality of care and cost savings, which then will be distributed to all providers in the system. This promotes bundled payments or payment for episodes of care, as noted earlier. Providers will be paid on a FFS basis with adjustments (paybacks or reduced future payments) to meet the goals of the organizations. The ACOs will need an adequate network of providers. MFM subspecialists will certainly be part of this network. The MFM subspecialists may be employed or reimbursed on a FFS basis, with adjustments being done at the end of a payment period based on the ACO's budget for MFM services.

The ACO will require advanced IT support and interconnectivity with hospitals, providers, laboratories, and imaging centers as well as dedicated data specialists to analyze the data accumulated for the population. The ACO may be formed from physician organizations, hospital networks, or a combination of both entities. The ACO will be responsible, not the insurer (payer), for distributing funds to each type of provider. The payment to MFM subspecialists will be based on all services rendered (figure 16.2), and payment will be independent of the utilization of resources.

This situation may significantly alter the number and types of tests that are done during pregnancy unless those tests are proven to improve outcomes for the mother or newborn. The implementation of this strategy will put the burden of care *and* financial viability of the ACO directly in the lap of the physicians and hospitals. This scenario has the potential to dramatically change our specialty.

**Figure 16.2. MFM services rendered**

- Ultrasounds scans / pregnancy
  - First trimester
  - Cervical length scans
  - Anatomy scans
  - Follow-up scans
  - Fetal echocardiograms
  - Dopplers
- Consults
- Preterm labor prevention programs
- Follow-up visits
- NSTs
- BPPs
- Invasive procedures

**Step Three: Know Who You Are Contracting With**

Insurers or ACOs usually utilize a recruiter or contract negotiator as the initial person involved with a practice in negotiating the contract. This person may not know what an MFM subspecialist is or how an MFM practice may enhance the physician network, improve patient care, or possibly reduce costs. In fact, the negotiator may consider the MFM subspecialist to be another specialist who will increase the cost of medical care, which will result in a greater loss to the entity's profit margin. Therefore, the negotiator may not have the positive perception of how an MFM subspecialist can positively affect a network.

Negotiators may get paid after the contract is signed, and they will not receive a bonus if the contract is not beneficial to the company. They usually will not service the practice or follow-up after the contract is signed. Because of these factors, it is best to initiate contract negotiations with somebody who understands and values your practice. You must stress how valuable an MFM subspecialist is to the community and the high quality of obstetrical care the members of the plan receive. You should have a discussion about how ineffective high-risk care has downstream effects on NICU costs. You must make the negotiator aware of the fact that you provide services to not only high-risk patients but also to normal patients as well (through routine first-trimester screening and anatomy scans). You must make sure that these services are recognized and reimbursed fairly if you are in a capitated contract or bundled-payment arrangement. You also must be willing to discuss the possible negative effects the contract negotiator's network of physicians would experience if you did not participate with the plan.

If possible, it is best if you can negotiate the contract with a physician who understands all these factors. Unfortunately, in most cases, even physician medical directors may not understand the importance of MFM providers, and even if they are involved in the negotiating process, they, too, must be informed about the importance of your services. Therefore, if you are negotiating with a specific recruiter or contractor, you need to educate that person about the type of practice you have and how your special expertise is valuable and absolutely necessary to ensure that their members receive high-quality care.

**Step Four: Understand the Effect of Plan Participation on Your Practice**

If you are in private practice, you must take the time before entering negotiations to determine the percentage of patients in your practice who are insured by the company or in the ACO that you are negotiating with. You also must consider that the company may have different products (i.e., HMO and non-HMO products). Participation with a company does not mean that you have to participate in all the products. It is possible to negotiate a contract with an insurer in which you participate in non-HMO products but do not participate in HMO products. You should search your billing system and determine not only the percentage of your practice that this company represents, but also what percentage of the patients in that company are in each type of plan that the insurer offers.

You may determine that participation in the HMO product, which requires referrals and utilizes a restricted network, does not represent a significant proportion of your practice and pays less than other plan types. If this is true, consider contracting for select plan types rather than all plans available. Remember, many patients may have an HMO plan that allows them to use out-of-network physicians at a higher rate and that many of your patients may actually stay with your practice and use an out-of-network option. This could result in higher overall reimbursement for your group. The contract negotiator will try to have you participate in all products, however, as this will result in a greater payment to the negotiator.

You may find that your perceived willingness to not participate in all plan types will allow you to negotiate a better contract overall, since if you do decide in the end to participate in all plan types, your participation could result in more commission for the negotiator. During this negotiation process, you may consider trying to get the company to alter the referral or authorization process for your practice. Use the negotiation process to simplify your office processes as much as possible.

If you are an employed physician in a multispecialty group, the leverage you have to get a better contract will depend on your ability to explain to the contractor for your group what you do and how important your services are in assuring quality and possibly decreasing overall costs (e.g., NICU days) to the network. Your negotiating ability, though, is significantly reduced compared to that of a private practitioner.

## Step Five: Know Your Competition

MFM providers usually do not consider themselves to be in competition with other MFM subspecialists or other types of providers. This assumption is untrue. Competition exists not only among other MFM subspecialists in the community but also between radiologists, general obstetricians, and medical subspecialists. If there are other MFM groups within your hospital or hospital system, realize that your competition may be willing to accept lower rates in order to get the increased volume from the specific insurer or to be the sole provider in an ACO.

If there are no other MFM subspecialists within the hospital system or community, and that hospital system or community is an important one for this particular insurer, then your ability to contract for increased rates will be greatly improved. When you have no competition, you may consider not participating in the plan and providing services as an out-of-network, nonparticipating physician. This may result in increased reimbursement to the practice, even if it sees a decrease in the volume of patients.

Because many plans will have radiology sites that will do all levels of ultrasound but are not able to provide MFM consultative services, it is important for you to understand how the radiologist is paid. Ask yourself, "Are they paid on a fee-for-service" basis, or in a capitated (per member per month) basis?" If the radiologist is paid on an FFS basis, then the negotiator will not want to pay the MFM subspecialist more than the radiologist for a specific CPT code. You must convince the negotiator that your services, including the ability to provide consultations, collaborative care, and high-quality ultrasound scans, are important and worth the increased payment for your services.

If the obstetrical ultrasound is in a capitated payment program for the radiologist, it presents more difficult situation—the company will not want to essentially pay "twice" (i.e., once to the radiologist in the capitated payment and then to you in a FFS payment for obstetrical ultrasounds). In this situation, you may want to contract to only perform high-risk ultrasounds (i.e., detailed ultrasound evaluations for anatomy [76811] and ultrasounds on patients with medical or obstetrical conditions). This will allow the contractor to justify the increased reimbursement to the MFM subspecialist over the radiologist.

You may also want to solicit the support of your referring obstetricians and have them indicate to the plan that obstetrical ultrasounds need to be done not by a radiologist, but by an MFM subspecialist. They can stress that the quality of care will be compromised if the scan is done by a general radiologist. Making the contractor understand the importance of your collaboration with the predominant obstetrical providers in their network will sometimes be the factor that allows the negotiator to increase reimbursement to your practice. It is therefore important for you to understand whether there is competition and, when there is competition, to be able to clearly explain to the negotiator why a contract with your group would benefit the plan.

If you are negotiating with an ACO, the ACO may want only one MFM group in the network. If multiple hospitals are in the ACO, this may not be possible and will weaken the negotiating stance of the ACO. Therefore, the MFM provider must evaluate the competition and network in the same fashion as a provider in private practice. Once again, if you are employed by a hospital or network, negotiations specifically for MFM subspecialists may be very difficult to alter.

## Step Six: Understand the Special Expertise You Bring to the Network

As an MFM subspecialist, you have unique expertise that other providers in the network cannot provide. It is important that you leverage this special expertise, realizing that the insurer and ACOs cannot assure quality obstetrical care within a community without the appropriate MFM subspecialist providers in the network. The obstetricians in the network must make the contract negotiator or recruiter understand the special expertise that you as an MFM provider bring to the network. This is true whether you are in private practice or if you are employed. If you can do this appropriately, you will have a much better chance of being able to get a favorable contract or be reimbursed (via salary plus incentives) appropriately.

During this contracting process, emphasize the number of general obstetricians who respect you and refer patients to you, and how they will be adversely affected if you are not in the network. When your practice is well respected in the community and if there are high-profile patients whom you have cared for in that community, it is helpful to remind the contractor of this so that your position in the community becomes an asset to you in the contracting process. This type of conversation sometimes proves to be more powerful in the contracting process than you, for example, emphasizing special expertise in an invasive procedure that you only perform infrequently.

Different MFM subspecialist groups may also have an advantage over their competition, both because they do quality perinatal care and because they may also have unique characteristics within their practices. These could be based on location, gender, race, language skills, heritage, or religion. These factors may or may not enter into the quality of care, but they certainly may enter into the desirability of your practice among certain patients. If you have special properties that make your practice unique from the competitors, make sure you stress this during the negotiation process.

## Step Seven: Know What You Bill For

MFM practices should evaluate what percentage of their revenue comes from specific services and what the profit margin is for each service. The services that usually provide the most revenue for MFM subspecialists are ultrasound studies and antenatal testing; consultations and office visits usually provide less revenue. For some practices, acute obstetrical care and total obstetrical care provide only a small portion of their revenue but are very labor intensive. As a general rule, approximately 80 percent of an MFM consultative practice is generated via outpatient services, versus 20 percent from inpatient services. In addition, the provision of inpatient services is more labor intensive and pertains to patients at much higher risk. Negotiate strongly with the insurer or ACO only for those services that are profitable and provide significant revenue. Some insurers or ACOs may only want to contract with you for consultative and collaborative obstetrical care as well as antepartum testing. They may not want the MFM subspecialist to provide routine ultrasounds or global obstetrical care, because they have an adequate network of radiologists and general obstetricians whom they feel can provide the routine obstetric care and delivery services.

Insurers and ACOs will not want the MFM subspecialist to provide total obstetrical care to low-risk patients, but they will need you to care for those complicated patients whom general obstetricians do not want to provide care for (or who may do so with lower quality and higher eventual cost). It may be to your advantage to not provide any global obstetrical care. Then, if you do see a high-risk patient, you will be able to bill on an FFS basis for each visit, test, and delivery for which you are consulted. This may be very advantageous to your practice.

You should understand these issues before you go into the negotiation process. Discuss them precisely so that you do not end up providing demanding, high-risk care for a large volume of patients at a reimbursement level that results in a minimal gain or eventual loss to your practice. Once again, determine if you should provide specific care to patients with particular plan types. You may find that being a nonparticipating provider for total obstetrical care will result in greater profitability for your practice, because most PPO or POS plans allow members to seek care out of network at a higher copay or coinsurance cost. Using a strategy of being on all plans may result in lower margins and profitability, with increased workloads. Using in-hospital care by out-of-network providers may be profitable to your practice, since once a patient is hospitalized, you may be consulted because the hospital has limited MFM provider choice. Unfortunately, the patient is then subject to increased out-of-pocket costs.

Conversely, when you are contracted as a subspecialist with higher copays and coinsurance, you may suffer from reduced patient satisfaction due to the patient-shouldered costs, which may decrease your reimbursement for in-network patients when contracts have bonuses for patient satisfaction. Be sure to discuss this issue before you sign any contracts.

**Step Eight: Understand Practice Profitability**

In any negotiation you have to realize that you should negotiate with specific quantitative, not just qualitative, information. Every practice has three to five insurers that account for about 80 percent of the practice's patients. Therefore, negotiating with those insurers that provide the greatest number of patients to your practice may be different from negotiating with insurers that provide relatively few patients and little revenue. This information may lead you to the decision not to have contracts with those insurers that provide you with less than 5 percent of your patient population; the negotiator would understand this reasoning.

When negotiating contracts with insurers that provide a significant number of patients to your practice, it is best to understand the practice's profitability. This can be calculated by evaluating the RVUs associated with performing specific CPT or E&M services. You should be able to calculate the cost per RVU for each ultrasound, CPT-coded service, nonstress test, biophysical profile, consultation, and office visit as well as for total obstetrical care. Evaluate your practice's operating costs per RVU, including expenses such as salaries, benefits, rent, malpractice, and office equipment. You must also include expenses that will be incurred with the purchase of future ultrasound machines. It is also important to evaluate your sources of revenue, including revenue from office care, antenatal testing, and deliveries. Revenue from any outside contracts related to teaching or caring for patients in clinics will not have the same overhead as patient care and should be evaluated in this process.

By determining your practice's cost per RVU and plan-specific reimbursement based on RVUs for each service you provide, it is possible to determine your specific margins for each CPT service. Having this information will allow you to make decisions such as whether an individual insurer's reimbursements provide profit to the practice or whether certain services, such as deliveries, can be a loss for the practice. MFM medicine subspecialists often will work at multiple sites where reimbursement arrangements may differ. You may have to do this type of RVU-based calculation for each site, based on the various sites' specific reimbursement mechanisms.

When these RVU-based numbers are known, you can determine what services should be contracted for and if a particular insurer's contract will be profitable for your practice. This calculation will also allow you to determine a capitated payment rate. If you know (1) the total cost of providing care to patients in a particular plan or group, (2) the total cost to you of providing care to a patient, (3) the number of pregnancies per one thousand plan members, and (4) the number of members in the plan in the reproductive age group, then you can calculate an advantageous capitated rate. This rate will result in you being able to provide appropriate services to the entire population in the group and to being favorably reimbursed. If you negotiate with this data in hand, the contractor will better understand your needs and may negotiate a contract that is more favorable to your practice.

## Step Nine: Know Your Insurer's Coverage, Grievance, and Appeal Processes

It is imperative that you understand what the company or ACO pays for as well as the process for appealing payment denials. During the contracting process, you should establish a specific contact person with whom you can discuss any denials of payment. It is best if you know who the medical director in your area is and establish a working relationship with him or her. By forming this relationship, you will have a higher likelihood of convincing the company to reimburse your services to patients when unique circumstances arise. You should consider setting up meetings every six months with those medical directors who make up a large portion of your revenue in order to foster and maintain mutually beneficial working relationships. These meetings should not be based solely on contracting but instead should be centered on new practice quality programs, cost-saving advances or protocols, new accreditations and educational initiatives, and other general issues of importance to patient care. Certain insurers may have a greater number of denials than others. These insurers may not be the ones with whom you want to contract or maintain contracts. Reducing problem insurers will improve the state of your accounts receivable and decrease your administrative costs.

If you enter into a capitated contract, you should not see any denials. You will be able to perform any and all tests that you deem to be necessary. This will eliminate denials, but it means that the cost of doing all testing you deem appropriate for all patients has to be calculated as part of the capitated contract. Using preestablished protocols will help you understand the cost of caring for patients with specific diagnoses. These protocols should be followed by all practitioners in the practice. If increased utilization by certain providers causes variability of care, your practice may not survive in a capitated environment.

For example, if one practitioner does not do any antenatal testing on patients with diet controlled gestational diabetes, but another practitioner starts NSTs weekly, with growth scans every four weeks at twenty-eight weeks, then the second practitioner will be introducing added uncompensated costs to the practice and will adversely affect your profits. In most capitated agreements, you will have an increase in utilization because referring providers will realize that your care does not add costs to the patient. Hence, it is important to have care protocols in place not only for continuation of care but possibly for entry into the practice. Placing too many barriers on patient entry, however, may frustrate referring providers and initiate complaints with an insurer. Communication is critical; you must inform referring providers of the reasons for certain care protocols and entry to care within your practice. The overutilization of care under a capitated arrangement can become problematic. The placement of "risk corridors" into a contract for utilization may assist your practice in these instances. Risk corridors are "kickers" placed within a contract that come into play when utilization is elevated (see sample calculation later in this chapter). This may be secondary to increased overall RVU or increased volume of a CPT code.

Any contract should specify how the accounts receivable should be handled and what the time for payment lag should be. Make sure your practice establishes processes that can resolve outstanding issues so that receivables remain at the lowest possible level. Capitated contracts eliminate accounts receivable as well as the authorization of procedures and consultations, thus resulting in reduced administrative overhead for your practice.

**Step Ten: Get Professional Help**

Many contracts with insurers will have specific mentions of payment methodology, gag clauses, financial incentives for payment, hold-harmless clauses, termination clauses, and renewal clauses that may require renegotiation or "evergreening" of the present contract. It is important that you understand all these contract provisions clearly. In order to guarantee that you clearly understand the contract, you may find it useful to enlist a contract lawyer with experience in medical contracting to review the contract before acceptance.

**Step Eleven: Provide Outcome Data**

Contract negotiations are based on the insurer's or ACO's need for the particular type of provider in the network. When multiple providers provide the same services within the community, there is no quantitative way for the insurer to know which provider is best. Large insurers are used to evaluating financial- and quality-based outcome data. ACOs will obtain outcome data and financial data, either from new internal systems trying to collate data from multiple systems or from large insurers that sell this data to them. You must understand the outcome or process data that the company will be collecting to use for incentives. If you have this data going into the negotiation, then you will be in a better position to negotiate a better contract. You must also understand whether the incentive is guaranteed if you meet the goals or if it will only be paid based on company savings.

As an MFM subspecialist, the outcome data in question—related to maternal and perinatal morbidity and mortality and utilization of NICUs—is dependent on not only the care you provide but also the care provided by the general obstetrician or advanced practitioner. You are therefore subject, in many cases, to the measurement of outcomes that you do not fully control. This outcome-based incentivization for MFM providers has not yet been tested particularly well, since there is no consensus on which outcomes or processes should be specific for MFM subspecialists. As of 2018, the SMFM has been working diligently on developing these quality criteria.

In the face of untested outcome measures, patient satisfaction and data (e.g., how long a patient has to wait for an appointment, ease of scheduling an appointment, amount of time spent in the office, and referring doctors' satisfaction) may be the only data that you can use in order to convince the contractor that the quality of care you provide warrants increased reimbursement. Unfortunately, comparative outcome data is also lacking; this data would establish MFM subspecialists' outcomes as being better than those of other providers of obstetrical care who are working in collaboration with MFM subspecialists. Despite this lack of data, the perception is that MFM subspecialists will add worth to the network. While negotiating, capitalize on this perception.

**Step Twelve: Make the First Offer**

Once the contract negotiations have proceeded to the point where you are negotiating reimbursement for specific CPT codes or bundled payments, don't wait for contract negotiators to tell you how much they will pay you for these services. Take the opportunity to tell the contractor how much you want to be paid for these services based on your costs. This will allow you to negotiate the reimbursement from your first offer, as opposed to you trying to negotiate an increased reimbursement based on a low offer that the insurance company or ACO may make. The contract negotiator may have to go back to others in the company to negotiate a much higher reimbursement than they had previously considered. Do not be upset if the contractor cannot meet your demands during the first negotiation session. It may take several sessions before all reimbursement rates will be suitable to both parties. This usually means that you have done a good job and have gotten a better contract than the company was originally willing to give you.

With capitated contracts, it may be more difficult to establish the appropriate rate per member per month (PMPM), since this figure depends on the total number of pregnancies and the number of high-risk pregnancies, which require more intensive testing and care. As stated previously, the contract should thus have risk corridors where the contract will provide additional reimbursement or be renegotiated if the volume of work or the mix of patients significantly changes during the term of the contract.

One possible example is to pay an FFS rate for any service that is over (or that is 110 percent of) the expected RVU of the previous year on which the contract is calculated. In addition, in this instance, the PMPM should then be recalculated for the next year based on the RVU utilization of the previous year when it is beyond the risk corridor. This should also apply to payers so that they realize you will not be dramatically restricting services, which may increase their eventual cost through NICU utilization or increased general obstetric services that are paid on a FFS basis. An example of a risk-corridor calculation is shown in table 16.1.

**Table 16.1. Risk-corridor calculation example**

| | Contract based year | Current year | Additional FFS payment | Next year change to contract |
|---|---|---|---|---|
| **Example of contract with a risk corridor of 10% with a 25% increase in utilization** | | | | |
| RVU | 10,000 | 12,500 | 1500 | 12,500 |
| Per member per month payment | $1.00 | $1.00 + 15% above risk corridor of 10% | | $1.25 |
| **Example of contract with a risk corridor of 10% with a 5% increase in utilization** | | | | |
| RVU | 10,000 | 10,500 | 0 | 10,000 |
| Per member per month payment | $1.00 | $1.00 | | $1.00 |

### Step Thirteen: Be Prepared to Walk Away

When you enter into contract negotiations, your goal is to improve your practice's financial and operating status. If the proposed contract does not provide your practice with an appropriate profit—either through increased volume or margin on specific or overall codes, bundled care, and decreased administrative workload—be prepared to walk away from the contract. Sometimes a contract may not provide profit but does provide for access to increased numbers of patients, improves your ability to negotiate with hospitals, or allows you to acquire a new practitioner with special expertise. If these special situations do occur, then even a nonprofitable or neutral contract may be worthwhile to the practice. If you realize this, then sign the contract. If these situations do not exist, though, and the contract does not make sense to you, then don't sign it. A bad contract will not get better with time. Understand, however, that if you are not able to walk away, then you really have a poor bargaining hand in the negotiation process.

### Step Fourteen: Walk Away as Friends

When you decide not to sign a contract, remember that it is best to maintain a positive relationship with the company. Part ways as friends. You can be assured that things will change and that you will then need to negotiate another contract with the same entity in the future. Don't close the door. Medicine is changing rapidly. What doesn't seem to be good now may be great in the future. If you maintain good relationships, then taking advantage of changing future situations will be easier.

### Step Fifteen: Ask about Issues besides Payment

Payment is an important but narrow issue of any contract. Many issues need to be considered to achieve a successful contracting outcome. You don't get what you don't ask for.
- If your practice has a good relationship with a plan and a track record of responsible utilization, then you may be able to ask for the elimination of authorization of some or all codes or procedures.

- The time before claims are "stale-dated" should be as long as possible to avoid issues with delayed billing, or billing the wrong insurer due to patients providing old insurance information.
- The requirements for appealing claims should be outlined.
- Delayed payment and the possibility of added interest for clean claims after thirty days may be a possible consideration.
- The addition of a cost-of-living adjustment may be entered into the agreement, especially for contracts with evergreening clauses or of an extended length.
- The requirement for the exit from the contract should be equal for both parties.
- The addition of a possible gain share agreement for savings on NICU days or decreasing a preterm delivery rate may be a possible approach that helps both parties, especially in capitated contracts. Gain sharing agreements are contractual terms between a payer and provider that reward productivity, innovation, and profitability outside of the terms of the usual contracted terms and rewards the provider for financial savings to the payer. Gain share agreements also commonly have downside risk penalties. Of course, you should attempt to minimize or eliminate downside risk while increasing the upside. Usually in gain-share agreements, the gain shared is 50 percent of the cost-savings split between provider and payer. Downside risks are usually much lower.

The more issues you negotiate on, the harder it will be for the insurer not to bend on all the possible terms. Doing so also allows you to give in on a few contract points in order to win on areas that are more important to your practice.

**Step Sixteen: The Contract Is Only the Beginning of a Process**

The final point is that when you sign a contract, it is only the beginning of a relationship with the company or ACO. In order to enhance your relationships, it is important that you make yourself a resource for quality care. Let the medical director know that you are willing to advise him or her when difficult cases arise, to participate in quality-assessment committees, and to assist in the development of policy and clinical pathways for the plan. Knowing the people within the plan by having regular contact in a positive fashion will make you an important resource for the plan. This will help in any future contract negotiations.

## Conclusion

Negotiation should be a process that is good for both sides, both of which need to feel as if they are winners. By following these sixteen simple steps, not only can MFM subspecialists get paid fairly, but they can also positively influence the care processes within the health plans or ACO and thus improve the quality of care all pregnant patients in the community receive. This should be the desired outcome for any negotiation process.

# 17

## Accounts Receivable Management / Accounts Collections

### Dirk Feinblatt, BS

In theory, getting paid for medical services should be an easy process. You provide medical care for the patient and send a claim to the patient's insurance company, and the insurance company then sends you a payment. As we all know, this isn't always how it works out. Payers always seem to come up with more ways to complicate the process, delay payment, and in general make it difficult for medical practices to collect the money they deserve. Private insurance plans can also be complex, with varying deductibles, coinsurances, and the like, which often can be confusing to patients and difficult for providers to navigate. While the billing process is complicated, you can take a few simple steps to enable effective revenue-cycle management that will work toward continuous improvement and the achievement of practice goals.

### Measure, Measure, Measure

If you can't measure it, you can't manage it—especially when it comes to medical billing. Metrics are a crucial element to gaining control over clinic operations and profitability. Without having clearly defined performance indicators, it is difficult to measure the performance of your practice revenue cycle today and over the long haul. The following are essential reporting metrics that should become a mainstay for revenue-cycle management within your organization.

*Net Collection Rate*

The net (or adjusted) collection rate is a measure of a practice's effectiveness in collecting contracted reimbursement. It represents the reimbursement percentage achieved from the possible reimbursement allowed based on contractual obligations. Simplified, this is the percentage collected on what you are supposed to be paid; it is not the percentage collected on what was billed. Practices utilize their net collection rate to see how much revenue is lost from factors such as untimely filing, uncollectable (bad) debt, and other similar noncontractual adjustments. Along with other measures, such as days in accounts receivable (A/R) and denial rates, the net collection rate is vital to developing a clearer understanding of your revenue cycle. To calculate your practice's net collection rate, utilize this formula:

**(Payments − Credits) / (Charges − Contractual Adjustments)**
Otherwise stated as:
**(Payment / Amount supposed to be paid) X 100 = Net collection rate in percent**

In order for this calculation to work properly, the payments need to correspond to their originating charges, so it is best to retrieve your data for this metric based on "date of service" rather than "date of post." As with any metrics, it is important to keep your reporting consistent. In this case, it is generally recommended to see data by utilizing a trailing twelve-month schedule to be able to identify trends and/or eliminate fluctuations in the data.

*Days in A/R*

This is a calculation of the average number of days that it takes for your claims to be paid. This metric is one of the most useful barometers of your practice's financial health, as a low number days in A/R means that it takes fewer days to collect your money owed on patient accounts, while a high number of days in A/R indicates that it takes longer to collect. The days in A/R is typically calculated monthly, as this helps facilitate spotting any fluctuations and trends in your accounts receivable. This formula is commonly used to calculate days in A/R:

**Outstanding Accounts Receivable / Average Gross Charges per Day**

Take the total accounts receivable for the numerator. For the denominator, take your total charges for a given time period (three months, six months, or one year) and divide by the number of days; that will yield the average gross charges per day. This is easiest to do over the last year for charges and divide by 365. If your practice has some fluctuation over the last year, however, such as gain or loss of a provider, then a smaller time period may be preferable. For example, if your accounts receivable is $900,000 and you billed $30,000 in charges per day, then days in A/R would be thirty days. One potential pitfall in this calculation is the improper adjustment of adjusting or writing off a balance at the time of posting, which will provide an inflated number of the monies collected.

*Percentage of A/R over 120 Days*

The percentage of A/R over 120 days is yet another key performance indicator (KPI) that identifies how much of your accounts receivable resides in the older "aging buckets." The aging of accounts receivable is calculated by viewing an aged trial balance (ATB), which usually contains the following categories: 0–30 days, 31–60 days, 61–90 days, 91–120 days, and greater than 120 days. Use this formula to calculate your practice's percentage of A/R over 120 days:

**Accounts Receivable >120 Days / Total Accounts Receivable**

This metric tracked over time can be calculated as an overall aggregate or broken out by specific payer groups. This is yet another method for identifying trends regarding which insurance companies are either slow to pay or are experiencing other issues. While taking a high-level view is necessary, it is also advantageous to be able to produce reporting with more granularity such that you could potentially identify the root causes of an issue (e.g., a credentialing issue with a specific provider or a location-specific concern).

*Clean Claim Rate*

This measure represents the percentage of claims that are processed accurately and completely and reimbursed by the payer the first time the claim was submitted. On average, approximately 95–97 percent of claims should be clean claims. The remaining claims create extra workload, where time is spent inefficiently researching the problem, appealing the claim, sending out multiple statements, and delaying the payment. So the rule of thumb is: Get it right the first time! To calculate the clean claim rate, utilize the following formula:

**(Total number of claims submitted over a time period − number of claims over a time period requiring resubmission) / Total number of claims submitted over a time period**

You can take a few steps to ensure a high clean claim rate. Most practice management systems have edit-management systems or claim-scrubbing software that can automatically flag claims for correction prior to submission based on specific payer rules or requirements. A second layer of security resides at your claims-clearinghouse level, where claim scrubbers can flag claims for payer-specific edits. It is vital to make sure that these edit reports are monitored and managed to submit claims in a timely manner and to identify the root causes that are holding up your claims. You can then make changes to your own processes (or even to your claim-scrubbing software) to allow you to correct any problematic claims prior to initial submission.

*Benchmarking*

The use of benchmarking answers the question, "How are we doing?" This is an integral part of the accounts receivable process, whereby you take your KPIs and compare them with national averages and best-practices performers. Because performance varies greatly, you want to retrieve benchmarking data specific to your specialty and, if possible, specific to your location or state, as regional fluctuations may exist. Benchmarking will likely result in a healthier practice and will facilitate the identification and avoidance of problems.

Once you have your performance data, you will want to find appropriate benchmarking data. The Medical Group Management Association (MGMA) produces an annual cost and revenue report that has long been considered the benchmarking standard among medical groups. MGMA's vast survey data can assist in your benchmarking to help identify your strengths and shortcomings. Typical benchmarks are listed below:

- Net collection rate > 96 percent
- Days in A/R: < 40 days
- A/R > 120 days: < 10–12 percent
- Clean claim rate: 95–97 percent

# Factors That Could Affect Your Billing Performance

The billing and collections process is influenced by several factors, as discussed below.

## Contracts

The first factor is contracts, which can have a variety of elements to consider, as follows.

### *Contract Terms*

- Timely filing limits—understand all payer terms. Many payers have attempted to move this from a past standard of 180 days to 90 days. You should attempt to have a longer timely filing rate to account for any problems or complications with billing processes.
- Pay rates—know what your fee schedule is for every specific procedure code. Please see chapter 16 for more information on contracting strategies.
- Capitation—any procedures that are carved out or paid separately need to be closely monitored. Capitation is a form of payment to a provider for each person assigned to a practice for care, whether or not the person seeks care.
- Payments for injectables (RhoGAM, vaccines, etc.) and supplies. These can vary in cost and need to be reimbursed separately.
- Refund procedures—are they taken directly from checks in the future? What is the appeal process, if any?
- Contracted payment rates for advanced practitioners—usually 80 percent of physician charges for physician assistants (PAs) and nurse practitioners (NPs), but 100 percent for certified nurse midwives (CNMs) (due to the Patient Protection and Affordable Care Act (PPACA).

### *State Laws and Regulations*

- Prompt payment—understand the legal requirements placed on insurance companies.
- Clean claim guidelines—know what insurance companies require.
- Refund guidelines—recognize the maximum amount of time after a claim has been paid in which a payer can request a refund. You should attempt to limit this to one year from time of service.
- Payment guidelines for advanced practitioners (PAs, NPs, and CNMs)—distinguish whether your advanced practitioners bill under their own names, or is incident-to-billing utilized?

## The A/R Process

To effectively manage your revenue cycle, it is vital to have clearly defined billing and collections processes and dedicated teams to ensure that you have all the information required to bill properly. Workloads for your billing team should be monitored to ensure appropriate personnel. An average of 0.5–0.7 billers are needed for each provider, but this of course depends on the workload of each provider, the billing output of the practice, the experience of the billing staff, and the presence of a streamlined workflow. For example, a practice that has spent a large amount of time on reducing the resubmission of claims (unclean claims) will have more time to spend on other parts of the billing process.

In addition, the collection of copayments, coinsurance, and deductibles at the time of service by front-office staff (front-desk, checkout desk, and benefits-checking personnel) will greatly reduce the wasted time of chasing down claims after the patient leaves the office. On average, an office that does not collect these claims at the time of service will lose 40 percent of this money during collection. Having contracts that are capitated will also decrease collection services and will decrease the number of billers required per provider, since collections for service are not paid per CPT code but in a single monthly check based on payer membership numbers.

## Benefits and Eligibility

If possible, before you even schedule a patient for a visit, you should verify the patient's eligibility and benefits with her insurance company. The purpose of this is twofold. First, before any services are rendered, you have verified that the insurance information you have received is correct. If the inquiry results in the patient being ineligible, you then have the opportunity to retrieve the correct or updated insurance information from the patient. Second, during the insurance eligibility verification process, you should obtain other vital benefits information. Namely, specific to the services to be provided on the patient's upcoming visit, you will want to obtain all pertinent coverage service information: copayment/coinsurance amounts and any plan deductible that is due. After the visit is scheduled, the patient should be notified by phone of the financial obligation due at the time of service. This should be done at least two business days prior to the date of service and needs to happen each and every time so that the cost is not a shock to the patient and that the proper copay and deductible amount will be collected at the time of service. This setup also allows patients to make arrangements for payment; enables patients to cancel if necessary, which decreases no-show rates and allows scheduling of other patients; and lessens the possibility of consternation and front-office distractions caused by angry patients who were unaware of their financial responsibility until arriving on the day of service. Most insurance companies *require* the patient to pay her copay at the time of service. The collection of coinsurance and deductibles at time of service is allowed for most plans and is recommended for practices. It is also important that providers within your practice do not write off copays, coinsurance, or deductibles, as doing so may be considered to be an illegal inducement to the patient.

## The Billing Process

Data entry of the procedure codes and diagnoses for services provided is best performed by a clerk with highly accurate keying skills and knowledge of CPT (Current Procedural Terminology) as well as ICD (International Classification of Diseases) coding. It is important to have a process in place to ensure that charges have been entered for all encounters that occurred on any date of service. It is a generally accepted process to batch all "superbill" encounters for a given day, either by physician or specific location; once charge entry has been completed, a system report should be run to reconcile and verify that all charges have been billed.

Most practice management systems also have the ability to provide a missing ticket report, which easily identifies the fact that charges have not been entered. These encounters should then be researched to determine if charges were truly missed, or if the patient canceled or did not show for the appointment. This is also an important means of spotting embezzlement from office personnel who may collect cash from a patient and discard the charge sheet or superbill to hide the fact that the patient had any procedures performed. Many electronic health records (EHR) now have direct entry of charges by the provider, and some institutions demand this be done by the provider. Nonetheless, this is usually a waste of time by the provider, who can more easily circle codes and diagnoses on a superbill (such as one produced by the SMFM coding committee) and have the charges input more quickly by staff members who can then also ensure a clean claim. Charges should be entered daily so as not to adversely affect key performance metrics and to maintain consistent cash flow throughout the month. If hospital charges are provided, then these charges should be entered every two to three days at a minimum.

## Claims Submission

Whether your claims are submitted electronically or by paper, file submission should occur on a daily basis. Paper claims should not be utilized unless a payer is not set up to receive electronic claims or the practice has a contractual obligation to attach medical records that cannot be electronically submitted or other documents as part of the claim-submission process. The clear majority of your claims should be submitted electronically; if not, work with your payers and clearinghouse, as it is much more efficient and timely to submit and process electronic claims. Clearinghouse payer rejections and edits should be closely monitored and worked daily to prevent delayed claim submissions.

## Payment Posting

The cash-posting process also needs to be closely examined and reconciled to guarantee that all payments received are properly posted and credited to the correct invoice or charge. In addition, any contractual adjustments or credits need to be entered properly so that any patient balance is accurately reflected in your accounts receivable. To help facilitate the posting process, most forms of insurance recommend (or require) that practices sign up to receive electronic remittance advices (ERAs) to allow the practice to electronically post the majority of payments associated with a particular bulk explanation of benefits (EOB). The payment-posting process should include the following:

- *Line item payments.* Payments should be posted to the specific procedure code level per the EOB. This will allow you the ability to easily identify if payments received correspond to the contracted rate.
- *Capitation payments.* If you have a contract(s) whereby you receive a bulk payment based on a per member per month (PMPM) calculation, you should have a mechanism to post these payments so that this revenue is accurately reflected in your cash posting. If applicable, any procedures that are carved out and paid separately from the bulk payment should be posted as part of the process.
- *Patient payments.* These should be posted in a timely manner so that the patient does not receive a statement unnecessarily.
- *Lockbox.* Provided by banks, an efficient and sophisticated lockbox service can assist greatly in managing your incoming payments. Under this service, payments from patients or insurance are directed to a post office box, rather than going directly to an office address. The bank then processes the payments received and deposits the funds directly into the bank account for the practice. EOBs are then sent to your office (electronically or by mail) for posting/reconciliation to a patient's individual account.
- *Reconciliation.* This is a vital part of the process to safeguard that all payments received and deposited are posted in the billed system and are reconciled on a daily basis.

## Understanding the Importance of Payer Mix

Having a thorough understanding of your payer mix is vital when it comes to managing your operations. Different payer requirements, referral/authorization mechanisms, and payment methodologies can have a big influence on staffing and operational decisions. Keeping track of patient-mix trends and contractual changes is crucial, as they can have an impact on all areas of your practice. For a financially healthy practice, it is wise to have a balanced payer mix and to not be reliant on only a handful of payers. Generally, if greater than one-third of your practice revenue is dependent on a single payer, your practice may have increased risk of financial harm, as that provider may have the ability to make more contractual demands on your practice. Your payer mix should then also be checked for the RVU production versus the revenue portion a payer might possess. You should strive for a higher revenue-to-RVU production and strive to increase the levels of patients from high-revenue/RVU payers as an organizational strategy. In addition, if your contracts are not based on RVU for reimbursement, then you should evaluate the reimbursement of specific services (such as your top five to ten CPT codes) to evaluate these services for their revenue from your larger payers.

Understanding the payer mix and the payer requirements for patient visits (such as for referrals and authorizations) will help with making staffing determinations. In addition, once you know your payer mix and revenue/RVU ratio, another evaluation can be the determination of "practice employee time" for a specific payer. Practice employee time increases with items such as authorization, declined authorizations requiring appeals, late payments necessitating employee follow-up, and payer records requests. Ideally, RVU production as a percentage of the practice should be equivalent to the revenue percentage and the overall employee workload required. For example, if a practice is 10 percent of the RVU production but 5 percent of the revenue and 20 percent of the employee workload within your practice, then the managing principals within your practice should consider dropping the payer or seeking contractual changes to decrease and realign billing work or improve reimbursement for that plan.

Contractual changes may not only be financial in nature; they could also include the elimination of employee work via the elimination of authorization or reduction in coinsurance or copays (both of which increase office collection efforts) for these payers. In contrast, if the revenue percentage is favorable in comparison to your RVU production and employee workload, then you should consider means of increasing the patient load with this payer.

Comparing your payer mix to the overall mix for your geographic area will show how your practice is positioned in the market. A practice payer mix that mirrors the region shows a healthy distribution of patients. An increase of payers from low-paying insurances, of course, is less desirable. Practice managers and managing physicians should strive to increase the percentage of patients from high-paying providers.

**Payer Types**

Payer types come in a variety of styles, as noted below.

- *PPO*. Preferred provider organizations are health plans that provide flexibility for the patient to see a specialist without seeing a primary-care physician first. Premiums tend to be higher, and these plans usually have a deductible. Utilizing an in-network provider is encouraged, as higher costs (coinsurance and/or copays) are associated with seeing an out-of-network provider.

- *HMO*. Health maintenance organization plans usually require that you see a provider within the HMO network. While premiums are generally lower and they usually have lower deductibles, these plans typically have more restrictions for coverage than other plans. Some requirements may include selecting a primary-care provider (PCP) and getting a PCP referral to see a specialist, or paying the entire cost of medical services for an out-of-network provider.

- *POS*. Point of service is a managed care plan that provides different benefits depending on whether the patient uses an in-network or an out-of-network provider. As such, POS plans combine various features of HMO and PPO plans.

- *EPO*. Exclusive provider organization plans require you to utilize providers and hospitals in the network, as they have no out-of-network benefits. Plans of this type allow you to see an in-network specialist without a PCP referral.

- *Medicare.* Medicare is a federally funded insurance program for patients who are sixty-five years or older or have end-stage renal disease (ESRD) or certain disabilities. Payments under Medicare vary by region and cover hospital services, outpatient services, and prescription drugs. Due to its patient-eligibility requirements, Medicare is a rare payer for pregnancy services.

- *Medicaid.* Medicaid is a joint federal and state program that provides care for low-income families or individuals. Coverage varies by state, and recipients are required to qualify for the program.

- *Capitation.* Capitation is a payment agreement between a health-insurance company whereby the provider agrees to accept a prearranged monthly per-patient payment amount based on the number of patients enrolled in the health plan. The providers within a capitation agreement are the effective insurers for physician services for patients.

- *Indemnity.* Indemnity plans, also referred to as fee-for-service (FFS) plans, allow patients the flexibility to direct their own health care by visiting nearly any provider or hospital they choose. The insurance company pays for a set portion of the total charges based on the usual, customary, and reasonable rate for the service, typically once a patient's annual deductible has been met.

**Payer Mix and Billing and Collections**

It is important to monitor billing and collections to be able to

- Identify potential opportunities to increase reimbursement;
- Recognize any rate changes from payers;
- Compare reimbursements and identify opportunities to negotiate better contractual rates;
- Determine if plan reimbursements are below acceptable rates and to make decisions about whether to accept certain insurances; and
- Work with insurance companies to reduce rejections and increase clean claims based on plan requirements.

Obviously, the payment process is important to the financial well-being of a practice. Having comprehensive plans in place to monitor details, ensure adequate follow-up, and constantly make appropriate changes is key to collection success.

# 18

## Coding and Auditing Your Practice

Fadi Bsat (MD) and Pamela K. Kostantenaco (LPN, CPC, CMC)

As in other medical specialties, having solid coding and auditing processes in place is an imperative part of a successful maternal-fetal medicine (MFM) practice. This process starts with the physicians/providers, followed by employing highly trained support staff (billers, coders, and the like). This chapter emphasizes the importance of coding and auditing your practice to ensure that the physicians' practice standards are current and accurate, that the staff members responsible for any aspect of the practice are properly carrying out their responsibilities, and that claims are submitted appropriately.

## Coding

The Society for Maternal-Fetal Medicine (SMFM) provides a comprehensive coding manual (kit) that covers the common Current Procedural Terminology (CPT) procedures, diagnoses codes, and modifiers. In addition, there is now a separate manual, called ICD-10-CM for MFM. ICD-10-CM is the mandated replacement of the ICD-9 code sets used by physicians, medical coders, and billers to report health-care diagnoses. ICD-10-CM has radically changed the way documentation and coding is done and requires a significant effort to implement. You should obtain copies of these manuals for your practice through the SMFM website.[183]

The Society for Maternal-Fetal Medicine also organizes semiannual coding conferences specifically targeted for MFM specialists and practices, including outpatient and inpatient coding. More information on these and all coding resources can also be found at the SMFM website.

### Who Is Responsible

It is ultimately the provider's responsibility and liability, not the office staff's, to select the appropriate CPT and ICD codes based on the service provided and supporting documentation. In some practices, often the ancillary staff initially assigns the appropriate ICD and/or CPT codes for the particular visit or procedure. From a compliance and coding perspective, the provider should always confirm that the right codes were chosen and correct them as needed, because the charges are reported under the provider's name and ID number. The physicians/providers should have a keen knowledge of the proper coding guidelines, be aware of the need for supporting documentation, understand the medical necessity of all services, and keep up to date with the ongoing changes in the coding world.

---

[183] Please visit www.smfm.org/products for these manuals.

## Documentation

Having supporting documentation of the encounter is a crucial piece of the coding process. This documentation provides the who, what, and why. In addition, the documentation should substantiate the level of care provided and the medical necessity for the services rendered. Remember, the medical record is the legal record for the practice, so having the necessary supporting documentation is key. A common statement in the medical field is that if something wasn't documented, then it didn't happen.

## Superbill/Charge Ticket

With the implementation of electronic medical records (EMR) or electronic health records (EHR) over the last several years, some practices have decided not to utilize "superbills" or "charge tickets." Some practices, however, still use these documents. The purpose of utilizing these documents is to relay the information from the medical record into the corresponding alphanumeric coding language. These forms are available as well on the SMFM website.

The procedural services (i.e., the CPT codes) and all applicable diagnosis codes (ICD-10) should be selected on the form. The "linkage/sequencing" of the diagnosis codes should also ideally be performed by the physicians/providers. The terms linking or sequencing signify that the clinical indication (diagnosis) for each procedure (CPT) be matched. More and more payers have lists of clinically indicated diagnosis codes for procedures. The coding staff will then review this information accuracy prior to entering it into a billing system and transmitting it to the appropriate insurance carrier. It is helpful to share these approved diagnoses codes, since they correspond to procedure codes, based on national standards and payers' guidelines. Doing so will help streamline the billing submission and avoid denials and/or further processing correspondence and efforts. For example, Aetna, in conjunction with SMFM, has provided the codes that indicate certain ultrasound procedures; this information can be found online by searching for "Aetna, SMFM, and the CPT code." It may be helpful to download this information and place it in a guide within your office for billing staff and providers.

## Coding Personnel

Large institutions typically have a compliance officer in charge of all compliance activities for the individual practices under the institutional umbrella. This position usually includes coding personnel. Independent and smaller practices should employ one or more qualified persons ("coders") who have an overall understanding of coding in order to have an effective coding process in place. The staff who are directly involved in the coding, however, must have specific qualifications, including proficiency with documentation guidelines, billing/coding guidelines, payer requirements, and an auditing background. The responsibilities of a qualified coder typically include (but are not limited to):

- Coding and abstracting of all professional services (outpatient and inpatient), as would be provided by the MFM division based on the current CPT manual or American Medical Association (AMA), SMFM, and Medicare coding guidelines;

- Linking the CPT and ICD codes to support clinical necessity;
- Providing ongoing education to the physician(s) and staff;
- Acting as a liaison between your office and the payers;
- Reviewing charge tickets for changes that occur during the year;
- Working in tandem with the entire billing organization to ensure accurate billing and minimal claim denial rates.

The coder should be responsible for reviewing the charges for any discrepancies and for bringing any issues to the provider's attention. If the coder does not feel that the level of service is appropriate, then the coder would typically meet with the provider to discuss any concerns. Coders are strongly recommended to have or obtain a certification through the Academy of Professional Coders (Certified Professional Coder, or CPC) or the American Health Information Management Association (Certified Coding Specialist—Physician-based, or CCS-P). It is paramount for coders to stay updated on coding changes, maintain their certification, and keep their educational background up to date.

The physician practice may work with its third-party billing company. If one is used, then that company should utilize at least one certified coder and commit to working closely with the practice to ensure that billing practices and documentation are appropriate for submission on behalf of the providers.

**Educational Tools**

The practice should ensure that staff members who are directly involved with billing and coding receive the necessary extensive education specific to their responsibilities. A few examples of items that could be covered in coding and billing training include the following:

- Coding requirements
- Claim development and submission processes
- Proper documentation of services rendered
- Proper billing standards and procedures
- The legal sanctions for submitting deliberately false or reckless billings

The training may be done internally with in-service sessions or at outside seminars. SMFM organizes semiannual coding meetings specifically targeted to MFM practices. More information can be found on the SMFM website.

## Auditing Your Practice

The Office of Inspector General (OIG) Compliance Program Guidance Audit Protocol recommends that an organization maintain an ongoing evaluation process that not only examines whether a provider practice's standards are current and accurate, but also determines whether staff members are properly carrying out their responsibilities and that claims are submitted appropriately. In addition to the standards and procedures themselves, bills and medical records should be reviewed for compliance with applicable coding, billing, and documentation requirements.

The development of this type of compliance program will allow health-care providers to use internal controls to more efficiently monitor adherence to applicable statutes, regulations, and program requirements. Many MFM practices are solo or small practices, or are hospital based. For hospital-based practices, MFM providers should follow the compliance programs of their respective institutions.

A compliance program for individual and small-group practices contains seven components that provide a solid and effective basis for the program. Due to resource constraints, the program is best implemented in a step-by-step fashion. The program includes (1) implementing compliance and practice standards, (2) designating a compliance officer or contact, (3) conducting appropriate training and education, (4) conducting internal monitoring and auditing, (5) responding appropriately to detected offenses and developing corrective action, (6) developing open lines of communication, and (7) enforcing disciplinary standards.

## Who Will Audit?

Large institutions typically have a compliance officer in charge of all compliance activities for the individual practices under the institutional umbrella. For smaller or private practices, an audit officer or team should be established with the responsibility of developing and implementing a compliance plan. A physician "champion" is essential, but the team may also include the office or billing manager, nursing staff, and coder(s). Their responsibilities will include establishing the compliance plan, evaluating its effectiveness, defining and monitoring measuring tools, proposing training and educational activities, and setting the budget for the compliance activities.

## Why Audit?

Providers should view compliance programs as analogous to practicing preventive medicine for their practice. By implementing a compliance program, practices can realize numerous benefits, including

1. Increased the accuracy of documentation that may lead to patient care benefits;
2. Speed and optimized proper payment of claims;
3. Minimized billing mistakes;
4. The prevention of erroneous or fraudulent claims;
5. Reduction of the chances that an audit will be conducted by the Centers for Medicare and Medicaid Services (CMS) or the OIG; and
6. Avoidance of conflicts with self-referral and anti-kickback statutes.

Although innocent erroneous claims may happen, these should be minimized, because they are a significant drain on public and private health programs. On the other hand, fraudulent claims (intentionally or recklessly false claims) are governed by the civil False Claims Act and may lead to civil penalties, limitations of practice, or even jail. You should be aware of the following four potential risk areas.

*Coding and Billing*

This risk area includes

- Billing for items or services not rendered or not provided as claimed;
- Submitting claims for equipment, medical supplies, and services that are not reasonable and necessary;
- Double billing, resulting in duplicate payments;
- Billing for non-covered services as if they are covered;
- Knowingly misusing provider identification numbers, which results in improper billing;
- Unbundling (billing for each component of the service instead of billing or using an all-inclusive code);
- Failing to properly use coding modifiers;
- Upcoding the level of service.

*Reasonable and Necessary Services*

You can avoid this risk area by making sure that (1) claims are to be submitted only for services that the practice finds to be reasonable and necessary in the particular case and (2) the practice should be able to provide documentation (such as a patient's medical records and orders) that support the appropriateness of the service.

*Documentation*

Providing timely, accurate, and complete documentation is important to clinical patient care. Documentation serves a second function: when a bill is submitted for payment, documentation serves as verification that the bill is accurate as submitted. Documentation may also be used to validate the site of service, the appropriateness of the services provided, the accuracy of the billing, and the identity of the caregiver.

*Improper Inducements, Kickbacks, and Self-Referrals*

This risk is eliminated by having standards and procedures in place that encourage compliance with the anti-kickback statute and the physician self-referral law. Arrangements with hospitals, hospices, nursing facilities, home-health agencies, durable medical equipment suppliers, pharmaceutical manufacturers, and vendors are all areas of potential concern. Physicians should avoid offering inappropriate inducements to patients. Examples of this include routinely waiving coinsurance or deductible amounts, either without a good-faith determination that the patient is in financial need or by failing to make reasonable efforts to collect the cost-sharing amount.

**Educational Tools**

For providers and managers, educational activities and resources may be found on the SMFM website. For coders, these tools are available at the SMFM website and at their respective coder-certification websites, such as the Academy of Professional Coders or the American Health Information Management Association.

The compliance team or officer has the responsibility of determining what training is required. Essential elements of that will include (1) defining the importance of the compliance program and the consequences of violating the standards and procedures set forth in the program (i.e., compliance is a condition of continued employment), (2) defining the role of each member in the program, and (3) determining what training is necessary for which staff members in the practice.

**Self-Audit**

A self-audit will primarily focus on the following components:

- Bills are accurately coded and accurately reflect the services provided as documented.
- Documentation is being completed correctly.
- Services or items provided are reasonable and necessary.
- Proper supervision is provided for all patient services.
- Appropriate adherence to supervision and billing requirements for all "incident to" services is provided.
- Copays and deductibles are collected in accordance with any third-party, federal, and state guidelines.

The OIG recommends that a baseline audit be used to enable a practice to evaluate its progress in reducing or eliminating potential vulnerability over time. The baseline audit will establish a consistent methodology for selecting and examining records, and this methodology will then serve as the basis for future audits. Following the baseline audit, periodic audits should be conducted at least once each year. Optimally, a randomly selected number of medical records should be reviewed in order to ensure that the coding was performed accurately. Although there is no set formula as to how many records should be reviewed, here is a basic guide. Categories should include (but not be limited to):

- Outpatient evaluation and management services (e.g., new/established office visits, outpatient consultation, observation care);
- Inpatient evaluation and management services (admissions, subsequent care, consultations, critical care, prolonged services, etc.);

- Diagnostic/fetal assessments and procedures (ultrasounds, biophysical profiles, nonstress testing, Dopplers, echoes, nuchal translucency, etc.); and
- Surgical procedures (cerclage, in-utero fetal shunts, catheterization, amniocentesis, chorionic villus sampling [CVS], multifetal reductions, deliveries, etc.).

One of the most important components of a successful quality assurance/auditing program is having an appropriate response when the physician practice identifies a problem. While no boilerplate solutions on how to handle problems when identified are available, the response should incorporate the following: (1) take action as soon as possible after the date the problem is identified, (2) preserve information that tracks the physician practice's reaction to and solution for the issue, and (3) develop a method for dealing with those risk areas identified by the audit through the practice's standards and procedures.

**Sample Size**

The audit should review ten to twenty patient records (per provider) annually or semiannually; ten to twenty medical records per federal payer (Medicare or Medicaid) should also be examined. The sample size can be smaller if audits are more frequent; a larger sample size allows the coder/auditor the ability to select from a broader range of dates. If problems surface, a focused review should be conducted more frequently.

**Record Keeping**

The length of time that a practice's records are to be retained can be specified in the physician practice's standards and procedures. (Federal and state statutes should be consulted for specific time frames, if applicable.) Medical records, if in the possession of the physician practice, need to be secured against loss, destruction, unauthorized access, unauthorized reproduction, corruption, or damage. Standards and procedures can stipulate the disposition of medical records in the event that the practice is sold or closed.

**Record Retrieval**

If the audit is performed by an external auditor, then we strongly encourage that the auditor have the necessary expertise in the field of MFM and not just a general coding/auditing background. If it is an on-site audit (recommended on most initial audits), that allows easy access to patient charts and corresponding charge ticket availability. An off-site audit (not recommended for most initial audits) can possibly cause (1) incomplete documentation to be sent, which can cause delays; (2) a high volume of photocopies to be produced; and (3) concerns about HIPAA (Health Insurance Portability and Accountability Act) patient confidentially, which would require a HIPAA business partnership agreement.

## Types of Audits

Several different types of audits may be conducted. In a *prospective review*, the auditor looks at charges before billing. The advantages of this type of audit are that claims can be fixed prior to submission and that the auditor is not required to report findings. The disadvantages include billing delays, lack of access to payment information, and a lack of availability of records. In the commonly performed *retrospective review*, the auditor charges after billing/payment. The advantages of this style of audit include larger sample sizes, no billing delays, access to payment data, and easy availability of records. The main disadvantage is that the auditor is required to report and refund overpayments. In a *focused review*, the audit is performed once after the initial review has taken place for problem areas; this is usually performed after educational courses have been taken and is subsequently performed three months after the educational session.

## Corrective Actions

In developing its compliance program, the practice should develop its own set of monitors and warning indicators. These may include:

- Significant changes in the number and/or types of claim rejections and/or reductions;
- Correspondence from insurers challenging the medical necessity or validity of claims;
- Illogical patterns or unusual changes in the pattern of CPT, HCPCS (Healthcare Common Procedure Coding System), or ICD–10 code utilization; and
- High volumes of unusual charge or payment-adjustment transactions.

For potential criminal violations, the compliance program should include steps for prompt referral or disclosure to the appropriate governmental authority. For overpayment, the practice should take appropriate corrective action, including prompt identification and repayment of any overpayment to the affected payer. Violations of the compliance program should be reviewed with the responsible provider and staff and then documented in writing. The compliance program standards and procedures should include provisions to ensure that a violation is not compounded once discovered. In instances that involve individual misconduct, the standards and procedures might also advise as to whether the people involved in the violation be retrained, disciplined, or, if appropriate, terminated.

# Conclusion

Keeping open channels of communication between all the providers and staff involved with coding and auditing is paramount for the success of any such program. In particular, the staff should be comfortable discussing coding and compliance concerns with the providers in general, and the compliance officer or team in particular. To achieve meaningful and open communication, a compliance program can include the following:

- The creation of a user-friendly process (such as by using Dropbox);

- The requirement that employees report conduct that a reasonable person would, in good faith, believe to be erroneous or fraudulent;
- Provisions in the standards and procedures that state that a failure to report erroneous or fraudulent conduct is a violation of the compliance program;
- The use of a process that maintains the anonymity of the reporting person; and
- Provisions in the standards and procedures that no retribution will occur for reporting conduct that a reasonable person who is acting in good faith would believe to be erroneous or fraudulent.

The compliance plan should be communicated in writing to all providers and staff, with details as to the content and frequency of audits, educational expectations, and remedial plan details. Any communication that results in a finding of noncompliant conduct should be documented in the compliance files by including the date of the incident, the name of the reporting party, the name of the person responsible for taking action, and the follow-up action taken.

Finally, a compliance program does not need to be time or resource intensive and may be implemented progressively in an ongoing fashion. It should be regularly reviewed and revised as necessary to adhere to coding and auditing requirement changes. When it comes to the coding and documentation, a team effort is necessary between the physicians/providers and support staff.

# 19

## Benchmarking Provider Work and Coding

Brian K. Iriye, MD

Benchmarking is an often discussed but insufficiently employed tool in the modern medical practice. Physicians and administrators often request benchmarks for relative value unit (RVU) production, daily sonographer production, median office space, or a myriad of other topics in a maternal-fetal medicine (MFM) practice. In this way, a benchmark is used to compare performance to a recognized standard and to provide a metric for one practice to another within an industry.

Nonetheless, comparisons like these are often shortsighted and fail to assist with the true role of benchmark utilization, which is to spur improvement and change. Comparisons from benchmarking exercises should seek to understand and utilize practices from other organizations, and sometimes even different industries, in order to enforce regulations that already exist within a practice, to drive internal process improvement, and to initiate and stimulate personal provider and employee motivation. Using benchmarks as standards helps to give a practice clues on how to identify and reward successes as well as how to correct problems when falling below specific goals. Essentially, benchmarking should be used as a form of comparative analysis to gauge performance; a practice can then seek alternatives to its present processes if necessary. Since all practices should strive for continued process improvement, benchmarking should be a key recurring function of the premier medical practice.

Benchmarking should follow a specific plan for instruction and correction. Examining a practice against unrealistic standards will result in a process that is destructive rather than instructive. Initially a practice should decide who and what to benchmark, visualize how the process will allow an analysis of the activities within the practice, and then commit to evaluation and possible change based on the results. An initial analysis should be performed to determine if the data desired could be collected, to assess the probable accuracy of information, and to address the time and work needed to collect and analyze the data. After this information is collected, any gaps in benchmarks and performance, or the lack thereof, can be identified. If needed, an action plan can then be devised and implemented. After a reasonable amount of time has elapsed, the data can then be re-collected and examined to see if the action plan has created meaningful change.

Benchmarking can be done at both the internal and external levels. Internal benchmarking is done within a practice, while external benchmarking compares the practice to other practice types in MFM (university, hospital owned, or private practice) or even to other practice specialties or industries. The more the comparisons are made externally to different specialties or other industries, the higher the chance for error in comparisons. When benchmarking is done internally within a practice, however, sufficient variation may not exist to make a valid or worthwhile comparison, as a practice dynamic or culture may not have enough significant differences to estimate the true benchmark value.

The Association for Maternal Fetal Medicine Management (AMFMM) RVU study of 2015 was a collection of data from over 150 MFM physicians from across the United States; the study included coding data from the different types of MFM subspecialist practices in order to examine billing and utilization. The information from this study is invaluable for possible benchmarking efforts.[184] The data from the AMFMM benchmarking survey of 2011 looked at other issues such as ancillary worker employment and production, exam time, and office characteristics; it was previously published in the book commemorating the fortieth anniversary of the Society for Maternal-Fetal Medicine (SMFM) called *40 Years of Leading Maternal and Fetal Care*.

# Benchmarking Your Practice Coding

As noted above, benchmarking can be conducted at both the internal and external levels, both of which are described below.

**Internal Benchmarking**

An excellent example of internal benchmarking of a practice is the examination of coding by providers. There are many reasons to evaluate provider and practice coding, including:

- Elimination of variation in coding
- Enhancement of correct coding
- Prevention of overcoding
- Elimination of undercoding or noncoding
- Assessment of workloads and production per patient or day
- Assurance that protocols of certain consultations or procedures are being performed for specific diagnoses or office visits

The following example illustrates a hypothetical internal benchmarking and evaluation of a possible coding analysis of a practice (see figure 19.1). Eight physicians are utilized in this practice example for evaluation. An analysis of possible scenarios for variance of the data is provided after each example. Attempt to evaluate each example as if it were your practice, and study each scenario. Produce reasons to explain the variation prior to reading the possible causes. The explanations involved are not complete but do provide a few alternatives to assist you. Providing reasons for the variation will facilitate your examination of deviation that involves benchmarking factors in the future.

---

[184] See www.smfm.org.

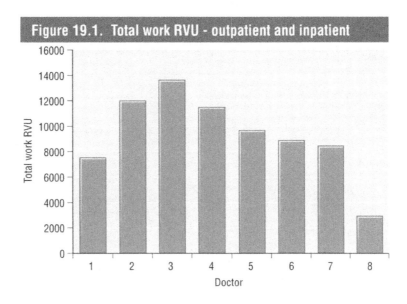

As figure 19.1 shows, the numbers 1–8, which represent the eight doctors, show extensive variation. What are some of the possibilities for the variation present? First, why is number 8 so low? Possible reasons are that:

- Physician 8 is newer to the practice, does not have his own patient population, and is being started slowly to learn practice processes and thus was not present during the whole time of evaluation.
- The decrease is due to part-time work status.
- The physician is more frequently at a site with fewer patients due to being at a newer office or having fewer relationships with referring providers.
- The RVU is dependent on technical and professional components, and physician 8 works at a site that does not allow attribution of technical components (this should be eliminated by using only work RVU).

Next, why do physicians 2, 3, and 4 have much higher RVU numbers?

- Maybe physicians 2, 3, and 4 work more clinical days per week than other physicians.
- The physicians work at different offices, where the number of patients may be different.
- The higher numbers may possibly be attributed to the inclusion of technical-component RVU.

To look at these issues, you must drill down in the data further to find out the real story.

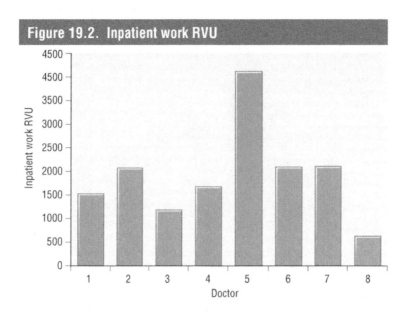

Figure 19.2. Inpatient work RVU

In this case, why is the RVU of physician 5 so high in figure 19.2? Here are a few possible reasons:
- The inpatient RVU can also vary by amount of days in the hospital versus days in the office. Does physician 5 work more days in the hospital?
- Is she a popular doctor for consultation?
- Does physician 5 bill more consultations and higher-level consultations for inpatient work?
- Does physician 5 do most of the antepartum testing and hospital ultrasound?
- Alternatively, do all the other physicians undercode within the inpatient realm?

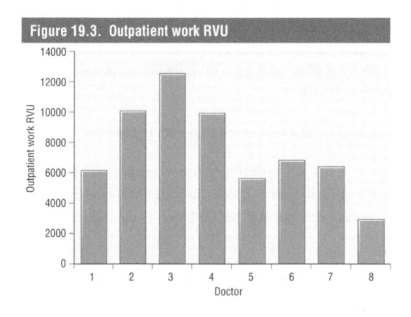

Figure 19.3. Outpatient work RVU

Why the extreme variation in outpatient RVU shown in figure 19.3?
- Again, the variation could possibly be from the amount of clinic days versus inpatient days.

- Are there multiple clinics with differences in workloads?
- It also could possibly be due to coding variation between doctors as well (or both).

Are there any possible ways of examining this further?

By analyzing outpatient RVU by clinic day and looking only at work RVU, as shown in figure 19.4, we start to find further clarity. By examining data per clinic day and work RVU, variables are eliminated so that we can scrutinize production in the outpatient setting. One must be responsible enough to actually count the days worked in clinic, thus eliminating vacation days and partial clinic days worked. In this data, you can see as much as 31 percent variation between the highest and the lowest physician in regard to RVU production.

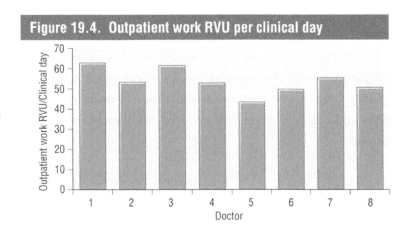

Why the 31 percent variation in production? Multiple reasons could explain this scenario, including (1) coding irregularity (both high and low), (2) variation in the performance of consultations, (3) patient volumes, or (4) types of ultrasound procedures that are performed. There is a way to delve further and examine these possibilities. Can you guess what this approach might be?

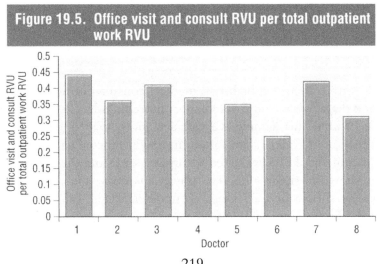

One can look further at whether the previous outpatient RVU per clinic day discrepancy is ultrasound-based or consultation- and office visit–based by looking at the RVU generated by office visits and consultations as a percentage of the total RVU per day (see figure 19.5). Using this method, large discrepancies in consultation percentages appear. Again, what are some of the reasons for the variation?

- Are differences in consultation and office visits secondary to a compensation plan based on production?

- Are consultations not being performed because there is no production bonus? When there is no production bonus, the bonus to the provider comes from time not spent in dictating or typing the consultation—hence, the provider may leave work earlier. In these instances the physician may write recommendations within an ultrasound report to pass on to a referring provider but not bill the patient.

- Is a provider not providing the consultation for another reason? Though it is surprising, you may find that a provider may not perform office visits or will downcode to reduce the patient's copays and coinsurance in order to increase patient satisfaction by decreasing the cost to the patient.

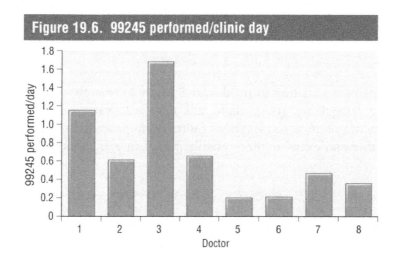

Within a practice with a focus on high-risk medical consultation in pregnancy versus a group focused on ultrasound diagnostics, you would expect more high-level consultations (level 4- 99244 and level 5- 99245). Within this sample we can see more than a tenfold variation in level 5 consultations. Examination of coding is important in this instance. Development and adherence to protocols for consultation should be evaluated to support or refute the individual physician coding levels and variations shown in figure 19.6. The physicians doing the coding should be examined, and individual providers should be questioned to understand the causes of the noted variability. Possible reasons for the findings are as follows:

- Physicians who code by time instead of by systems is the first possible reason. Coding by time instead of systems will often underestimate the consultation level. If a complete exam, history, and review of systems is performed, then most offices could charge level 4 or 5 visit codes, which would be supported by the documented information and problem complexity in an MFM subspecialist practice. Furthermore, most maternal medical conditions necessitate examination and documentation of medical history.

- Again, lower numbers may be secondary to billing lower-level consultations or not billing consultations to decrease patient copays and coinsurance and increase satisfaction.

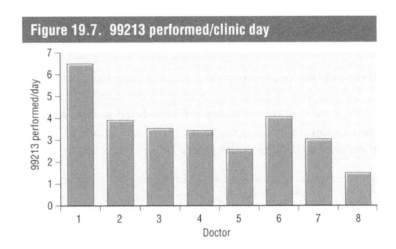

Similarly to initial consultations, follow-up for consultation may be performed more frequently in a practice with a focus on high-risk medical problems. The 99213 code may also be used in high-risk patients for obstetric care outside of a global obstetric (OB) charge for care. The differences here are also somewhat illuminating. Are medical issues being examined and documented at visits appropriately? What are some of the possible reasons for the variances shown in figure 19.7?

- Physician 1 sees more high-risk OB care patients than the other providers.
- Physician 1 sees more maternal medical problems in pregnancy.
- Physician 1 is paid by production and is overbilling.
- Physician 1 bills all visits as 99213 despite some being more likely 99212, 99214, or 99215.
- Physicians 5 and 8 are not billing due to copayments or coinsurance problems for patients and to improve patient satisfaction.
- Physicians 2–8 are not following practice protocols to document visits (if protocols exist).
- Physicians are performing fewer office visits and are not paid by RVU production.

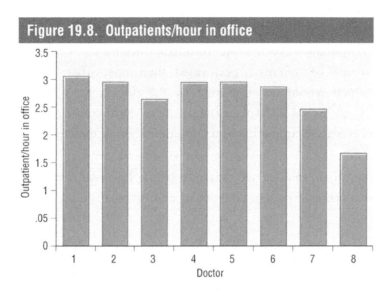

Figure 19.8. Outpatients/hour in office

To examine if part of the total outpatient RVU variance has occurred due to the number of patients who are seen, the number of patients per hour or day can be examined, as shown in figure 19.8. In this way, a practice can analyze whether the scheduled patient loads are equivalent, which is an important consideration to most providers. Any difference in number would make an eventual difference in outpatient RVU if coding were otherwise comparable.

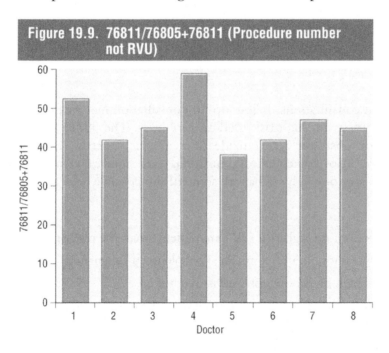

Figure 19.9. 76811/76805+76811 (Procedure number not RVU)

As a matter of ultrasound utilization, every MFM practice should evaluate the ratio shown in figure 19.9. When the patient presents initially for a second- or third-trimester ultrasound and anatomy is evaluated, the provider will code a 76805 or 76811. Hence, the provider will choose between these codes; the frequency of choice (as expressed via the above ratio) may be examined as one general means of assessing appropriate coding. Although the 76811 code has specific indications, many providers (including radiologists and general obstetric providers) have overutilized the code. Clearly, not every patient has an indication for this exam, and it should be rare that two instances of 76811 occur in a single pregnancy.

Of note, the SMFM and Aetna have worked together to form indications for the major types of obstetrical ultrasound (for example 76811, 76805, 76825, and 76820), which may be found online with a simple Google search with the terms "Aetna guidelines obstetric ultrasound." Within a high-risk practice, one would expect a higher level of 76811 utilization as compared to a general obstetrics practice. Some MFM providers may overcode for this procedure, however, as they feel they do the work involved in this code despite the lack of indication—an inadequate reason to perform this test, and 76805 should usually occur in this instance—or the provider may underutilize this code to avoid responsibility for missing something on the ultrasound or because of the cost to the patient.

**External Subspecialty-Specific Benchmarking**

At other times, when comparing your own practice providers to one another, the evaluation can become myopic. Institutions often utilize external specialty-specific benchmarks to acquire further information to evaluate their physicians. Unfortunately, until recently the problem was that little information existed. The AMFMM RVU study of 2015 assisted in providing some RVU-related information based on coding data.[185] You can use the data from this benchmarking study to further investigate the working and efficiency of your practice.

| Table 19.1. 76811/76805+76811 exam ratio (%) | | | | | | | |
|---|---|---|---|---|---|---|---|
| Practice type | Number docs | Average | Median | 10th | 25th | 75th | 90th |
| Company owned | 11 | 71.0 | 81.7 | 50.5 | 54.1 | 86.6 | 91.5 |
| Hospital | 46 | 60.7 | 60.6 | 39.8 | 53.6 | 68.9 | 86.7 |
| Private | 33 | 55.5 | 56.3 | 38.1 | 43.6 | 67.5 | 81.6 |
| University | 57 | 54.3 | 57.8 | 18.3 | 40.8 | 80.7 | 86.1 |
| Total | 147 | 57.9 | 58.9 | 35.4 | 46.3 | 78.1 | 87.3 |

The AMFMM RVU study median and average for 147 physicians performing ultrasound was 58.9 percent and 57.9 percent, respectively. Data that falls outside the 25th percentile and 75th percentile (46.3 percent to 78.1 percent) should be examined for proper coding utilization. Now, if we compare the data shown in figure 19.9 (a single practice's data) to the single-subspecialty MFM data (from a national sample) shown in table 19.1, we will see that this practice's overall utilization of the 76811 code is less than the median. Can you think of possible reasons for this and other findings? Here are a few possibilities:

- The practice does a significant number of low-risk examinations.

---

[185] See the SMFM website (www.smfm.org) to examine the results of the 2015 AMFMM RVU study.

- The practice is undercoding.
- Again, physician 5 is lower in this realm as well. Is some assistance needed here in overall indications for coding?

| Table 19.2. Percent of scans as repeated scans 76816/76816 +76805+76811 | | | | | | | |
|---|---|---|---|---|---|---|---|
| Practice type | Number docs | Average | Median | 10th | 25th | 75th | 90th |
| Company owned | 11 | 49.1 | 48.7 | 41.6 | 42.7 | 53.2 | 59.9 |
| Hospital | 46 | 47.6 | 42.1 | 21.3 | 31.9 | 53.8 | 63.6 |
| Private | 33 | 46.8 | 44.1 | 18.8 | 25.9 | 60.3 | 66.5 |
| University | 65 | 46.3 | 53.6 | 6.1 | 42.1 | 57.4 | 100.0 |
| Total | 155 | 47.1 | 48.1 | 18.1 | 35.5 | 57.1 | 66.5 |

Another code that is often utilized within MFM practices is the repeat ultrasound code, 76816. The repeat ultrasound code should be utilized when a patient is seen for the same diagnosis as on a subsequent visit. This code can be observed in benchmarking studies to assess whether follow-ups are being done too frequently or to evaluate over- or undercoding, which are important metrics within a value-based medicine practice. The best means of determining this is by creating a ratio of the repeat ultrasound code as a fraction of all second and third trimester scans (76816 / [76816 + 76805 + 76811]), see table 19.2.

The bar graph above (figure 19.10) is again from the 2014 AMFMM RVU study. The shaded areas show the 10th–90th percentiles. We can see significant variation in ultrasound coding in the survey of providers from the study (as described in this graph) as compared to national benchmarks as seen in table 19.2, which is somewhat worrisome, as the averages and medians are relatively close among all practice types (university, private, hospital, or company owned) for MFM subspecialists. For your practice, the 25th and 75th percentiles should give most leaders and managers cause to investigate the reasoning for the coding deviance.

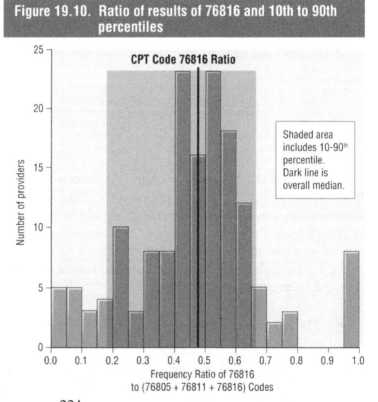

Figure 19.10. Ratio of results of 76816 and 10th to 90th percentiles

Shaded area includes 10-90th percentile. Dark line is overall median.

Umbilical artery Doppler is another CPT code that is often overutilized. Nonetheless, this code has specific indications derived from SMFM recommendations. This code is often used as an adjunct to the codes 76805, 76811, or 76816. Hence within the AMFMM RVU study, a ratio was again created to assess utilization [76820 / (76805 + 76811 + 76816)]. The AMFMM RVU study showed that the average and median rate of 76820 RVU as a percentage of total ultrasound percentage was 17.0 and 10.8 percent, respectively (table 19.3).

| Table 19.3. 76820/(76805+76811+76816) expressed from the total number of ultrasound exams in percent | | | | | | | |
|---|---|---|---|---|---|---|---|
| Practice type | Number docs | Average | Median | 10th | 25th | 75th | 90th |
| Company owned | 11 | 18.0 | 12.5 | 9.6 | 10.9 | 24.0 | 31.2 |
| Hospital | 45 | 27.7 | 10.8 | 5.2 | 7.9 | 45.6 | 60.1 |
| Private | 33 | 9.1 | 7.9 | 3.5 | 5.4 | 12.7 | 19.1 |
| University | 64 | 13.1 | 11.5 | 6.4 | 9.0 | 15.5 | 19.3 |
| Total | 153 | 17.0 | 10.8 | 5.0 | 7.7 | 15.9 | 30.5 |

The median of 10.8 percent is probably much more indicative of a normal number, as the median appears to be inflated. Results of less than 5.0 percent and greater than 15.9 percent (25th–75th percentile) should merit observation. Utilizing this ratio is important to reduce variation and waste within your practice. The AMFMM RVU study displayed large variation between providers for umbilical artery Doppler (figure 19.11) and this is likely to be a future target for payers to examine provider and practice variation.

Figure 19.11. Ratio of results of 76820 and 10th to 90th percentiles

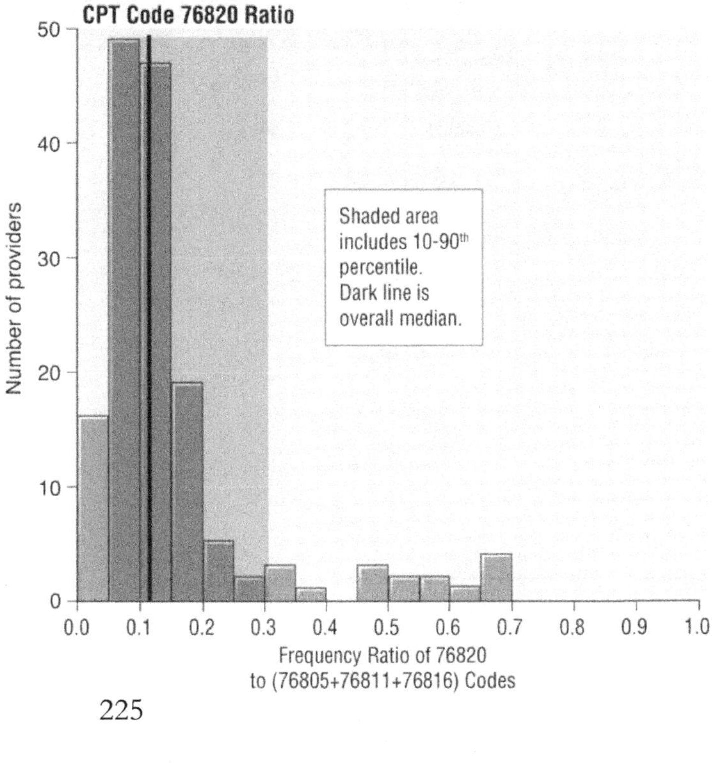

## Common Practice Benchmarks

Other common benchmarks within a practice can be found via different organizations. The Medical Group Management Association (MGMA) and the American Association of Medical Colleges (AAMC) put out yearly data on RVU and salaries for MFM providers. Although both of these organizations' data are considered gold standards, their data do have a few problems. First, the MGMA and the AAMC data are self-reported from providers or their surrogates. This creates the possibility that some practices may have included incorrect data for RVU, such as including technical components in some RVU information. Second, the MGMA study has large variation in the number of participants who are surveyed annually, with occasional years of woefully inadequate numbers of respondents. In contrast, AAMC data includes only university institutions, which make up only approximately 40 percent of practices, and also may have misreporting of data for the same reasons in the MGMA benchmark. Both the AAMC and MGMA ask for the final calculations of work RVU, which may not be possible for lower-performing practices to calculate, especially practices without EMR; those with smaller, less intensive systems; and those without the personnel to access and provide the data.

The AMFMM RVU study attempted to fix these shortcomings by instead asking for coding data[186]. This allowed the study researchers to more accurately calculate the work RVU. Asking for coding data also allowed this author's group of researchers to look on a more granular level at CPT coding and actual billing within an MFM practice. The study from data collected in 2014-2015, was performed for over 150 physicians in the United States and from a wide variety of practice types. The overall blend was 43 percent university based and 57 percent community based, which is very close to the ratio in practice across the United States.

**AMFMM RVU Study Data**

If we look at the data shown in table 19.4, of interest is that the RVU generation from the AMFMM RVU study is 13 percent greater than the MGMA data. University physicians appear to have the lowest RVU generation, which makes sense because of the additional duties of education and research in combination with other institutional challenges and responsibilities.

**Table 19.4. MFM work RVU generation**

| Practice type | Number docs | Average | Median | 10th | 25th | 75th | 90th |
|---|---|---|---|---|---|---|---|
| Company owned | 11 | 8497 | 8601 | 6250 | 6463 | 10284 | 11329 |
| Hospital | 47 | 8460 | 8538 | 3183 | 4837 | 10249 | 14350 |
| Private | 34 | 9704 | 9567 | 3699 | 7338 | 12400 | 14896 |
| University | 71 | 6112 | 5298 | 1769 | 3672 | 7455 | 11646 |
| Total | 163 | 7699 +/- 4564 | 6976 | 2834 | 4361 | 9921 | 14387 |

---

[186] Iriye B, Hancock L, Hancock J, Ghamsary M. An accurate assessment of MFM provider productivity: results of the AMFMM RVU Survey. Am J Obstet Gynecol. Jan 2016; S283.

| Table 19.5. Work RVU per clinical day worked ||||||||
|---|---|---|---|---|---|---|---|
| Practice type | Number docs | Average | Median | 10th | 25th | 75th | 90th |
| Company owned | 11 | 45.7 | 43.7 | 34.6 | 38.6 | 52.7 | 61.6 |
| Hospital | 47 | 63.1 | 41.9 | 17.5 | 28.4 | 70.2 | 130.0 |
| Private | 34 | 54.8 | 56.1 | 26.3 | 43.2 | 66.4 | 73.0 |
| University | 71 | 47.7 | 40.0 | 22.6 | 31.0 | 63.1 | 83.0 |
| Total | 163 | 53.5 | 45.2 | 19.7 | 31.7 | 64.2 | 85.6 |

Within the AMFMM RVU data, respondents were asked the number of clinical days they worked; this information was used with the overall work RVU to calculate RVU per clinical day (see Table 19.5). Private practitioners had a median amount of 11–16 more work RVU generated per clinical day. Nonetheless, this information is important in order to analyze individual work production within different office environments. The data shown in table 19.5 may be slightly skewed, as all ultrasound within the AMFMM study was attributed to outpatient services.

Within practices I have seen that have financial difficulty, the lack of performing and billing of consultations by providers is often a problem, which leads to underperformance. Examination of office visit and consult RVU as a percentage of total outpatient work allows a practice to examine its overall performance of office visits and consultation as a contribution to the total outpatient RVU production (table 19.6).

| Table 19.6. Office visits+consult RVU as a percentage of total outpatient work RVU and ultrasound ||||||||
|---|---|---|---|---|---|---|---|
| Practice type | Number docs | Average | Median | 10th | 25th | 75th | 90th |
| Company owned | 11 | 27.1 | 28.2 | 11.6 | 18.6 | 34.0 | 44.1 |
| Hospital | 47 | 21.6 | 16.9 | 9.3 | 10.5 | 28.6 | 36.8 |
| Private | 34 | 21.8 | 18.3 | 7.8 | 12.4 | 27.0 | 38.4 |
| University | 71 | 33.0 | 27.5 | 5.0 | 10.7 | 43.1 | 67.9 |
| Total | 163 | 27.0 | 20.9 | 7.4 | 11.3 | 33.2 | 48.6 |

Further examination, as in table 19.7, shows the spread of consultation types charged by respondent subspecialists as a percentage of total consultations. Managers and practices should look at the above data to find instances of over- and undercoding. Practices should also note that differences in level of consultation may differ because of time-based versus component-based billing.

Table 19.7. Average overall percentage of type of consult

| Practice type | Number | 99241% | 99242% | 99243% | 99244% | 99245% |
|---|---|---|---|---|---|---|
| Company owned | 10 | 7.1 | 11.8 | 42.8 | 24.0 | 14.4 |
| Hospital | 42 | 16.5 | 29.8 | 42.6 | 10.0 | 1.2 |
| Private | 32 | 38.9 | 24.3 | 16.3 | 15.6 | 5.0 |
| University | 58 | 21.0 | 28.7 | 29.2 | 15.8 | 5.3 |
| Total | 142 | 22.7 | 26.8 | 31.2 | 14.6 | 4.6 |

As of 2018, most MFM practices perform inpatient and outpatient services. It is important to realize that practice types differ in their production of work RVU in these different environments (table 19.8). Most outpatient services are easier and require less manpower and effort to produce. Recognizing the source of your work RVU production is important in realizing if efforts are needed to expand outreach and broaden services in either the inpatient or outpatient realm.

Table 19.8. Average inpatient work RVU/ total work RVU per doctor (%)

| Practice type | Number docs | Average | Median | 10th | 25th | 75th | 90th |
|---|---|---|---|---|---|---|---|
| Company owned | 11 | 20 | 11 | 5 | 8 | 23 | 30 |
| Hospital | 47 | 34 | 26 | 4 | 9 | 37 | 46 |
| Private | 37 | 35 | 12 | 0 | 1 | 23 | 41 |
| University | 71 | 54.3 | 21 | 0 | 6 | 42 | 83 |
| Total | 166 | 29 | 20 | 0 | 6 | 37 | 58 |

**Other Important AMFMM Survey Data**

Salary and Compensation

Presented in table 19.9 are the data regarding total physician compensation in 2014-2015 for the MFM subspecialist. When taking the work RVU data and dividing it by total compensation, we can present the compensation per work RVU (table 19.10), which is helpful for providers working with production based contracts.

### Table 19.9. Total compensation

| Practice type | Number docs | Average | Median | 10th | 25th | 75th | 90th |
|---|---|---|---|---|---|---|---|
| Company owned | 11 | 457,521 | 480,000 | 322,738 | 385,000 | 542,500 | 610,000 |
| Hospital | 47 | 593,187 | 536,043 | 296,414 | 475,921 | 764,156 | 949,804 |
| Private | 37 | 478,704 | 400,000 | 171,503 | 350,000 | 469,976 | 994,069 |
| University | 71 | 335,497 | 327,508 | 210,324 | 264,333 | 426,803 | 460,000 |
| Total | 166 | 448,463 | 402,859 | 206,576 | 309,375 | 525,000 | 774,912 |

### Table 19.10. Total compensation (US Dollars) per work RVU

| Practice type | Number docs | Average | Median | 10th | 25th | 75th | 90th |
|---|---|---|---|---|---|---|---|
| Company owned | 11 | 88.30 | 74.28 | 48.17 | 53.56 | 120.58 | 159.06 |
| Hospital | 47 | 134.00 | 108.24 | 60.64 | 81.79 | 145.28 | 193.98 |
| Private | 37 | 83.45 | 70.88 | 45.70 | 63.00 | 104.11 | 118.93 |
| University | 71 | 106.64 | 79.65 | 38.00 | 56.34 | 108.31 | 162.47 |
| Total | 166 | 108.00 | 84.48 | 43.69 | 64.09 | 119.73 | 162.47 |

Many providers believe that performing more deliveries increases compensation. However, this benefit is only seen when performing 25-49 deliveries and there does not appear to be increasing compensation when performing over 50 deliveries per provider per year (table 19.11). One possible reason for this may be that increasing deliveries requires the MFM provider to spend more time out of the outpatient office limiting outpatient revenue production. Alternatively, MFM providers performing more deliveries may be seen as a threat to general obstetric providers which may reduce referrals.

### Table 19.11. Salary based on number of deliveries

| Delivery number | Corp | Hospital | Private | University | Total |
|---|---|---|---|---|---|
| Less than 25 | 455,274 | 585,039 | 466,880 | 246,736 | 433,609 |
| Greater or equal to 25 | 480,000 | 597,392 | 576,250 | 370,306 | 461,951 |
| Less than 50 | 455,273 | 571,443 | 478,148 | 312,422 | 450,421 |
| Greater or equal to 50 | 480,000 | 650,055 | 485,000 | 360,609 | 444,047 |

Miscellaneous

Practices should look at the coding of office visits as a means of tackling variation between providers and one means of looking for adequate billing and coding (table 19.12). A similar approach may also be done for consult coding.

| Table 19.12. Average overall percentage of type of new visit | | | | | | |
|---|---|---|---|---|---|---|
| Practice type | Number | 99201% | 99202% | 99203% | 99204% | 99205% |
| Corporate | 9 | 24.8 | 6.6 | 34.5 | 16.8 | 17.4 |
| Hospital owned | 38 | 11.3 | 22.1 | 45.1 | 14.5 | 7.0 |
| Privately owned | 34 | 26.5 | 12.4 | 24.2 | 17.3 | 19.7 |
| University owned | 66 | 12.2 | 14.4 | 34.2 | 23.9 | 15.3 |
| Total | 147 | 16.1 | 15.4 | 34.7 | 19.5 | 14.3 |

Table 19.13 presents data on MFM C-section rates. This figure only includes physicians who perform deliveries.

| Table 19.13. Cesarean delivery rate (%) excluding multiple gestations | | | | | | | |
|---|---|---|---|---|---|---|---|
| Practice type | Number docs | Average | Median | 10th | 25th | 75th | 90th |
| Company owned | 4 | 42 | 100 | 68 | 68 | 100 | 100 |
| Hospital | 35 | 69 | 65 | 44 | 58 | 74 | 87 |
| Private | 19 | 46 | 50 | 0 | 25 | 78 | 94 |
| University | 59 | 38 | 40 | 16 | 26 | 48 | 70 |
| Total | 117 | 49 | 48 | 20 | 33 | 70 | 88 |

Conclusion

One of the key roles of AMFMM, now the SMFM Practice Management Division, has been to survey practices to obtain vital benchmarking information for MFM practices. In the future, this role will be assumed by a new benchmarking group within the SMFM. Physicians and managers should be part of the solution in the future by answering similar surveys to provide information that can be utilized as a standard for future practice evaluation and improvement. Utilizing benchmarking data should be tailored toward improving the practice and setting standards rather than administering arbitrary punishments or rewards. Results should be interpreted to look for valid reasons for variation, similar to the risk adjustment of data in medical research. Only then can numbers be trusted and appropriate modifications be accomplished.

This approach to examining the results of a benchmarking process requires thorough analysis. As previously shown, any performance gap should be examined for reasonable explanations of data variance from a benchmark. Managers and decision-makers should also search if a best practice is evident. This last step will accelerate change by avoiding untested techniques and helping skeptics join in with a solution. Having a proper benchmarking plan in place will overcome possible resistance and complacency and will propel a practice forward with a functioning plan of action.

Any strategy should involve the affected parties to make implementation more likely and to assist the affected parties in problem recognition. Thereafter, a forecast of future performance should be set and monitored for any improvements. Recalibration and reassessment of benchmarking goals should then be done, and the plan for improvement or the goal itself should be evaluated from the new performance data. Benchmarking efforts often lead to a positive influence when done correctly, as they promote a culture of continuous improvement, learning, and competitiveness.

# 20

## Planning Your Office Space

### Wilbert Fortson Jr., MD

Planning to open or relocating to a new office space requires careful planning, given the limited resources available in today's medical and economic climate. This chapter assumes that your practice has found it reasonable to open a new office space. Whether you are in private practice, are in a community office setting, or are at a university center, the approach to opening a new office space is similar despite the varied practice types. Carefully evaluating the many factors involved will help enable you to meet your goals. The initial steps in planning your office space are listed below:

- Identify the needs of the community.
- Identify the needs of the practice.
- Decide whether to open the office in a facility or nonfacility location. An office space located within a hospital is known as a facility location, while a nonfacility location is an office space located in a freestanding building outside the confines of a hospital.
- Evaluate several geographic variables to aid in finding the ideal location for your practice.
- Choose the ideal space.
- Decide whether to use an existing footprint or to proceed with a new build-out.
- Design the layout.
- Identify equipment needs.

This list is provided again in checklist 1 at the end of the chapter.

## Location Considerations

The Center for Medicare and Medicaid Services (CMS) provides a few examples of facility locations, including hospitals, surgery centers, skilled nursing facilities, and nursing homes.[187] A freestanding office space that is not located within the confines of one of the above examples would be considered a nonfacility location. Both types of location have their pros and cons. One of the definite positive features of a facility location is the immediate proximity to the desired hospital. This allows the provider a significant level of comfort in timely management of high-risk pregnancies. For example, antepartum testing units are often located in close proximity to or

---

[187] Centers for Medicare and Medicaid Services, *How to Use the Searchable Medicare Physicians Fee Schedule (MPFS) Medicare Learning Network Booklet*. April 2014. http://www.cms.gov/Outreach-and-Education/Medicare-Learning-Network-MLN/MLNProducts/downloads/How_to_MPFS_Booklet_ICN901344.pdf.

within a labor delivery unit in the event that an expedited delivery is indicated. In addition, the facility itself then staffs many of these units and provides the equipment rather than the provider's practice, which may be a means of lowering overhead for the practice, although CMS accounts for these costs during the billing and reimbursement process.

If the office space is located within the hospital and the hospital owns the equipment, then the provider can only bill for the "professional component" of the care rendered. For most procedural codes used by maternal-fetal medicine (MFM) subspecialists, the professional component of the billing is approximately 25–35 percent of the "technical component," which is the portion of an exam that is due to costs of equipment, supplies, nonprovider personnel, and office space. In most cases, facility reimbursement when billed by hospital systems is higher than that of the nonfacility reimbursement, because typically hospital facilities have increased overhead. This differential in payments is known as the "site of service payment differential."[188] Leasing office space within a facility often includes payment for utilities, cleaning services, tenant upgrades, and maintenance costs within the lease price. Conversely, in this arrangement the practice may have limited options when choosing utility services and tenant upgrades. In addition, the responsibility of cleaning services, security, and other services are a tenant obligation but are the duty of the facility itself.

Nonfacility locations also have advantages and disadvantages. Typically, in a nonfacility location, the practice has the complete decision-making authority to choose how the office space is to be set up and maintained (e.g., cleaning services, tenant upgrades, staffing, and choice of equipment). While having this authority lends itself to enjoying more autonomy, it also requires careful resource management, further contracting and negotiation with multiple entities, and additional responsibilities in supervision.

Both facility types also offer different advantages with regard to your strategic objectives. For example, you may choose to place an office within a hospital because of its high volume of complicated patients and because its surrounding population is expected to increase over the next few years. In contrast, you may choose a nonfacility location equidistant between two hospitals that both have very busy labor and delivery units to provide equal coverage to both facilities.

In most cases, the type of practice will determine whether a facility or nonfacility location is best. For example, if your practice type is one that provides total obstetrical care including deliveries, then a facility location might be your best option. Consultative-only models may find it beneficial to be in a nonfacility location. Employed physicians often work in facility locations. These locations are advantageous to their employers for multiple reasons: existing IT infrastructure, proximity to the labor and antepartum units they want their providers to utilize, simpler oversight by administrative personnel, and (most important) increased facility billing charges and collections.

---

[188] Centers for Medicare and Medicaid Services, "Physicians/Nonphysician Practitioners," chapter 12 in *Medicare Claims Processing Manual*. October 17, 2014. http://www.cms.gov/Regulations-and-Guidance/Guidance/Manuals/downloads/clm104c12.pdf.

## How to Choose a Location

One of the most important aspects in choosing where to place your office is to consider the needs of the community. There are certain demographics to consider. In a 2012 article for the *American Journal of Perinatology*, William Rayburn and his coauthors suggested that for MFM specialists, there should be approximately one MFM subspecialist to support 3,100 deliveries annually in a particular "catchment area," or one MFM subspecialist for every twenty-four ob-gyns.[189] The catchment area is defined as the area in which a city attracts a population for the utilization of services within that city. The article is informative but only counted MFM subspecialists who were members of the American College of Obstetricians and Gynecologists (ACOG). The SMFM had approximately 1,650 members at the time of the article's publication and hence underestimates the current (2017) MFM provider population by approximately 20 percent. Utilizing this additional information, the number of deliveries to support a single MFM subspecialist is approximately 2,600. When evaluating hospitals in your area, if may be beneficial to create a list similar to the one shown in table 20.1.

**Table 20.1. List of hospitals and respective delivery volumes in a particular geographic area**

| Hospitals | Number of Deliveries |
|---|---|
| Hospital 1 | 8,000 |
| Hospital 2 | 5,500 |
| Hospital 3 | 3,000 |
| Hospital 4 | 1,500 |
| Total | 18,000 |

Let's say that 18,000 deliveries take place within a given community. When we perform the calculation (18,000/2,600), we find that approximately seven MFM subspecialists would be needed in a community with 18,000 deliveries. This would be an immediate need. You also have to consider the potential of an increase in the volume of deliveries over the next three to five years.

However, delivery volume is only one of many demographic factors to consider. You should also evaluate whether the overall population in the catchment is expected to increase. For example, Hospital X attracts reproductive-aged women from a seventy-five-mile radius who utilize its labor and delivery units. It may be of strategic advantage to place an office between two or more hospitals that have a wide catchment area for MFM services. Is there expected to be an increase in the number of reproductive-aged women (15–44 years old) in the community over the next three to five years? Rayburn's data, collected in 2010, showed at least 1 MFM subspecialist for every 47,000 reproductive-aged women,[190] but that number would decrease to 1 in 37,600 with the underestimation in providers of approximately 20 percent.

It is also important to point out that the age range of reproductive women is increasing with the utilization of assisted reproductive technologies. Therefore, a community with high utilization of such technologies may require additional MFM support. Data on deliveries in a

---

[189] W. F. Rayburn et al., "Maternal-Fetal Medicine Workforce in the United States," *American Journal of Perinatology* 29 (2012): 741–46.
[190] W. F. Rayburn et al., "Maternal-Fetal Medicine Workforce in the United States," 741–76.

community can often be obtained from hospital administrators who utilize sources such as Intellimed to obtain information.[191]

The location of your referring provider's offices may be of particular importance when determining the physical location of your office. Referring providers will appreciate that your services are within close proximity when they need them. As of this writing, ob-gyn specialists are performing an increasing number of ultrasound exams. As a result, some ob-gyns are identifying a higher number of suspected abnormalities and often desire same-day consultations due to high patient anxiety. Locating your office within close proximity to as many referring providers as possible will thus expedite the referral process. This may also require an additional office space if the referring ob-gyns are spread across a large geographic region.

As MFM subspecialists, our overall goal should be to provide the highest quality of care to an expecting mother with increased risk. MFM subspecialists have differing opinions about how to provide the highest quality of care. As a result, there is a competitive side to running a medical practice. The importance of your competitors' office locations can't be underestimated. For example, if your main competitor is located in a large facility that has a large catchment area to draw from, it would be of great benefit to you to place one or more satellite nonfacility locations distant from your competitor and in close proximity to one or more referring providers in that catchment area. These decisions will be improved by having knowledge of the delivery volume of individual physicians and groups, which can be obtained from Intellimed.

**Geographic Variables**

Again, knowing the catchment area for hospitals where you have privileges is an important aspect when deciding where to place an office (see table 20.2).

Table 20.2. Distance to Hospitals in Catchment Area

| Hospitals | Distance (miles) |
|---|---|
| Hospital A | 100 |
| Hospital B | 50 |
| Hospital C | 25 |

Table 20.2 shows three hospitals that have varying distances in their respective catchment areas. Let's say that Hospital A has a catchment area of one hundred miles, but the bulk of the reproductive-aged patients are traveling between forty and fifty miles for health-care services. Placing a satellite office so that patients would only have to drive twenty-five miles for outpatient care would be beneficial to you, as this may increase patient volume as well as patient compliance and satisfaction by reducing their travel times. In a 2012 article, Rayburn, Richards, and Ewell found that approximately 1.3 million reproductive-aged women needed to drive at least sixty minutes to reach a level III facility at that time[192] (see below for a discussion of the different levels). It also may be possible in some instances to establish a telemedicine presence instead of having providers travel to practice sites, which would affect the setup of both existing and satellite facilities.

---

[191] Resources are available at https://www.intellimed.com.
[192] W. F. Rayburn, M. E. Richards, and E. C. Ewell, "Drive Times to Hospitals with Perinatal Care in the United States," *Obstetrics & Gynecology* 119 (2012): 611–16.

Of equal importance is having access to facilities that can provide a high level of ancillary support. Higher-level neonatal intensive care units (NICUs) are an integral part of the health-care delivery system for MFM subspecialists. NICU care standards are defined as follows:[193]

**Level I.** Provides basic level of care to low-risk neonates and possesses the capability of stabilizing and providing care for infants born at thirty-five to thirty-seven weeks of gestation until transfer can be accomplished.

**Level II.** Should have the capabilities of a level I facility plus provide care for infants born at thirty-two weeks of gestation or later and weigh 1,500 g at birth, with problems expected to resolve rapidly without the need for urgent subspecialty pediatric care.

**Level III.** Should have the capabilities of level I and II facilities plus provide sustained life support. Should provide comprehensive care for infants born before thirty-two weeks of gestation and who weigh less than 1,500 g. Further, a level III facility should be able to provide prompt access to a range of pediatric medical and surgical subspecialists. Level III facilities should also ideally have neonatology and MFM services.

**Level IV.** Includes the capabilities of level III nurseries, with additional capabilities and experience with the most complex and critically ill newborns; pediatric medical and surgery subspecialists are available twenty-four hours a day.

It is important to have your main office located in close proximity to a level III or IV facility. Having privileges at a level III/IV facility will enable you to provide complete care for all expectant mothers at all gestational ages; 98 percent of all MFM subspecialists are located in a county with one or more level III perinatal centers.[194]

As mentioned earlier, the local population growth and the population's demand for MFM services is another factor to consider when deciding where to place an office space. The housing market, particularly new subdivision construction, can be an indicator of an increasing local population. The building of new schools, markets, and large shopping malls are positive indicators of population growth as well. Your local city's planning department and the US Census Bureau are good sources for population data. You can also find data on the most common ICD-10 codes (from the International Classification of Diseases) in a given area or zip code; the association of a high number of pregnancy-related codes would be a good sign of a region that is in need of services.

---

[193] Committee on Fetus and Newborn, "Levels of Neonatal Care Committee on Fetus and Newborn," *Pediatrics* 130, no. 3 (2012): 587–97.
[194] Rayburn, Richards, and Ewell, "Drive Times to Hospitals with Perinatal Care in the United States," 611–16.

Finally, growth in local industry plays an important role in growing a population and therefore should be considered in your planning. Job growth is critical to a community's financial stability. For example, plans for a new factory or plant to be built in the community, new companies moving to the area, and an increase in the growth of new businesses in the area over the last three years are all signs of economic growth and stability. An area with strong housing and job growth will invariably lead to a higher population of reproductive-aged women and consequently a higher volume of referrals. This information can be obtained from your city's planning and development department.

## Space Considerations

Now that you've decided on the location of your office, it's time to create your office work space. The decision to buy or lease depends on your financial situation and goals. The financial implications of buying versus leasing are beyond the scope of this chapter and should be discussed with a financial consultant or accountant to maximize financial advantages. Whether leasing or buying, the options are to move into an existing office space or perform a complete build-out from a shell.

The major advantage to moving into an existing office space is the lower-cost construction, while the major disadvantage is that most existing offices spaces are not designed for pregnant patients. Because most standard exam rooms are not large enough to accommodate an exam table as well as large ultrasound systems, most existing office spaces will need to undergo some sort of redesign or upgrade before they can be used. Costs associated with redesigns and upgrades are typically cheaper than complete build-outs. Limiting the amount of plumbing changes to the existing footprint will keep costs down. More important, if leasing, minor redesigns and upgrades may be included in the tenant-improvement portion of the lease. If it is not a part of the lease, then you should negotiate to have it added.

The major advantage to performing a complete build-out is that the result will be a brand-new space specifically designed for you and your office's workflow. As stated above, however, build-outs can be costly. When leasing, this could have a substantial impact on the monthly rent amount as well as the term of the lease. Obviously, the property owner plans to recoup any cost associated with build-out, which is typically done by charging a higher rent amount or longer lease terms. Construction times are typically longer for a complete build-out than a redesign, which should also be kept in mind with office development.

## Space Layout

The primary focus of your office should be to provide high-quality health care in the most efficient manner. As MFM subspecialists, we spend a great deal of time reading about the newest advancements in medical interventions and therapies, but we often fail to spend enough time evaluating the efficiency with which our office operates. As we continue to face the pressures of operating an office in the face of declining reimbursements, the efficient management of patient volume has become imperative. We have to treat many more patients to meet our ever-increasing overhead expenditures. Patient wait times are increasing, which may contribute to lost work hours for the patient. As a result, patient compliance with follow-up visits may be in jeopardy, given the reluctance of patients to use paid time off from work for doctor visits.

Operational efficiency is critical to any business, and the medical business is no different. Incorporate ideas into your office design to reduce the amount of walking your providers and employees have to do to travel through areas of the office. A sample office plan is included in this chapter to exhibit flow patterns that may be beneficial to office design (fig. 20.1). Office design should be implemented based on provider patterns of care in regard to ultrasound and consultation. A complete evaluation of operational efficiency should be done annually. You can use relative value unit (RVU) production to objectively evaluate your practice's efficiency. (Please see chapter 19 on benchmarking provider work and coding.) The office layout should therefore be done with efficiency in mind.

## Waiting Area and Registration

The waiting room delivers the first impression of the physical office. The office layout should be designed to have different entry/exit doors for patients and staff. The color of the waiting area should be warm, calming, and aesthetically pleasing. The registration desk should be easy to access and yet distant enough to allow privacy from the patient sitting area. Another way to protect privacy and promote efficiency can be accomplished by utilizing a registration kiosk or the utilization of a tablet sign-in station. These electronic alternatives to paper can be used as patient portals and integrated directly with the electronic medical record (EMR). Electronic registration also allows a way to track patient wait times from the many EMRs that possess these capabilities.

The patient sitting area of the waiting room should be designed to maintain privacy and promote a sense of calmness. A distance of five to six feet between the registration desk and the start of the sitting area is recommended. The sitting area should have enough seating to accommodate waiting patients and at least one significant other. A general rule is to have two chairs per "active patient encounter." An active patient encounter is an encounter in which the patient has checked in but has not checked out of the office. Therefore, if you typically have at least six to seven active patient encounters at any one time, then your waiting area should have seating for at least twelve to fourteen people. Having a restroom in the waiting room or common area of a larger building may also be desirable to limit unnecessary traffic flow in and out of the patient care areas.

## Patient Intake Area

The patient intake area is the area generally used to obtain vitals, reconcile medications, and take medical histories. Therefore, this area must also be designed to maintain privacy. Having a separate room for patient intake is ideal; alternatively, you could use an area that is separate from the flow of patient traffic.

## Genetic Counselor's Consultation Suite

If you utilize genetic counselors, this room should be included in your plans. The room should be large enough to accommodate the genetic counselor and at least two others and should be approximately ten feet by ten feet. This office should be within close proximity of the ultrasound suites, given that the genetic counselors and sonographers will often need to communicate during a patient encounter. Genetic teaching aids should be available in order to effectively communicate complex genetic concepts to patients. For example, it is important to have sample karyotype reports available, which demonstrate to patients what normal and abnormal karyotypes are. Patient information pamphlets describing the various testing options available (e.g., first trimester screening, serum screening, advanced carrier screening, noninvasive prenatal diagnosis, and invasive diagnostic procedure information pamphlets) should be kept in this area.

## Ultrasound Suites and Exam Rooms

This area is of vital importance to the MFM subspecialist. It should be state of the art, comfortable for the patient, and well maintained at all times. The room should be large enough to accommodate a standard sink area, exam table, ultrasound machine, and two additional chairs. A separate wall or ceiling-mountable viewing monitor for the patient and her significant others to view the exam should be added as well. The rooms should have separate temperature controls in order to maintain the proper operating temperatures for the ultrasound systems and to maintain patient comfort. This may require separate ultrasound heating and cooling systems that are separate from the remaining office system. Adding gel- and towel warmers to your rooms also adds an additional comfort feature. Towel warmers, for example, can be used to keep moist towels warm for patient use after her exam.

Adding a dimmable light switch near the ultrasound machine will aid the sonographer in adjusting the room lights during and after an exam without having to move back and forth throughout the room. Depending on provider preference, a separate sonographer image review and report generation area may be located within or outside of the ultrasound suite. Generally an ultrasound suite needs to be larger than other medical offices due to the ultrasound equipment, the guests the patient may bring to visits, and the need for a sink and storage areas for towels and medical supplies. Rooms smaller than twelve feet by twelve feet are at the lower end of functionality for these areas. These rooms require Internet connectivity for the ultrasound machines so that off-site diagnostics can be performed on ultrasound equipment. This connectivity is also needed for the transmission of images to a PACS (picture archiving communication system) and the transmission of ultrasound data to a reporting system.

## Antepartum Testing

If you choose to perform antepartum testing within your office, the area should be able to accommodate at least two patients at a time. The nonstress test (NST) rooms are typically for patient monitoring only. These rooms may be public or semiprivate, given that patient health information is not typically discussed here. These rooms should be equipped with gel warmers and reclining NST chairs. I recommend computerized NST machines with a paperless function and the ability to monitor the fetal strips remotely. The NST monitors should also have the capability of storing the NST in PDF format and integrating with most EMRs. This allows for long-term paperless storage of the fetal-monitoring tracings.

You may also wish to add a smaller ultrasound room off the area where NSTs are performed. This room can be ten by ten feet and house an ultrasound system of midlevel quality for the more limited functions of biophysical profiles. Again, it is important that this system can connect to a PACS and reporting system.

## Consultation Room

Some providers use a separate office for face-to-face consultation, while other providers prefer to perform consultations in the ultrasound suite. If you as the provider choose to use your office, then your desk should be set up in such a way that there is empty space between you and your patient and so that you are always facing the patient.

Dual computer monitors should be used in the physician consultation room. The monitors should be set up to allow you and patient to view the content on the screens simultaneously. This setup allows you to review and compare multiple exams from the same patient. In addition, this setup allows you to compare and contrast normal and abnormal images for patient education.

## Administration and Business Office Space

If you perform your own billing, then a separate space will be needed for the billing personnel. This space should also be private, given the nature of the position. University and hospital-based practices usually will have this in a separate section. The practice administrator's office should also be private and in close proximity to the billing personnel, as they will frequently need to communicate regarding scheduling, benefits verification, billing, and reimbursement issues. Depending on the volume of your practice, you may need additional space for referral management personnel. The practice administrator and the billing and referral management personnel collectively function as the administrative department of your practice. Administrative personnel may be located in the clinical office or a separate location. Again, the practice volume and space availability will dictate where these offices are located.

## Information Technology (IT) Space

The twenty-first century has seen an explosion in the utilization of IT services in the MFM practice. Due to the increasing use of high-resolution imaging, EMRs, and ultrasound reporting software, practices require larger computer databases, more powerful servers, and redundant backup systems. With the exception of the ultrasound systems, the IT equipment can be some of the most expensive equipment a practice purchases. Given the delicate nature of IT equipment, it should be kept in its own space: a separate temperature-controlled room that is easy to access and remote from patient care areas. Keeping the IT room separate from the clinical area and patient traffic prevents disruptions in patient care in the event that repairs are required during office hours.

Even more important than maintenance access is the need for physical security. Placing vital computer infrastructure assets in secured areas is the first step in preventing unauthorized access.[195] A total of 329 breaches of health-care records (with more than 500 records per episode) occurred in 2016, affecting over 16 million records.[196] Medical information fetches a higher payment on what is known as the dark web, at approximately $0.50 to $1.00 per individual record versus $0.01 to $0.05 cents for other information; this higher payment is due to the plethora of identifying information found in medical records.

Physical access should be controlled to this area via keys, ID card swipes, or keypad systems, with regular access code changes. Removable ceiling tiles should be fastened for at least six to eight feet surrounding the area to help avoid access via ladder and by circumventing other forms of security. For these same reasons, critical network components and phone systems should also be located in the IT room. Your data-transfer needs should be professionally evaluated, given the large amount of data that enters and exits the MFM practice today via the Internet; insufficient bandwidth can cripple your network, causing frustration for staff and patients alike. Higher bandwidth is especially necessary for offices with satellite locations that send diagnostic imagery back to the primary office for storage.

**Employee Break Room and Restrooms**

If space is available, a break room equipped with a refrigerator, microwave, coffee maker, television, table, chairs, and a toaster should be added. This area is important for staff morale. Most of the staff and providers will use this place to reenergize themselves throughout the day. Separate employee restrooms should also be located nearby.

## Equipment Considerations

MFM practices must also maintain space for a variety of different kinds of equipment, as noted below.

**Ultrasound Systems**
The ultrasound system is an essential piece of equipment for the practicing MFM subspecialist. A variety of options are available for such systems, and the ideal system is a matter of personal preference. The ultrasound systems and their associated probes are often the most expensive purchase for your office. The standard purchase options are buying versus leasing, although the pros and cons of buying versus leasing are beyond the scope of this chapter; consider consulting your accountant regarding the tax implications of both options.

---

[195] KISI, "How to Make Your Office Physical Security HIPAA Compliant." November 12, 2015. https://blog.getkisi.com/make-office-physical-security-hipaa-compliant/.
[196] HIPAA Journal, "Largest Heathcare Data Breaches of 2016." Posted January 4, 2017. https://www.hipaajournal.com/largest-healthcare-data-breaches-of-2016-8631/.

Two of the highest-priced options for ultrasound systems are the maintenance and extended warranty contracts, which are typically sold separately. Most systems today typically have a warranty for only the first year after lease or purchase. All maintenance and repairs beyond the first year will be the responsibility of the practice. It is also important to note that documented regular maintenance to your system is required by the American Institute of Ultrasound Medicine (AIUM) if you desire to become an accredited practice. The Society for Maternal-Fetal Medicine recommends that MFM subspecialists perform ultrasounds as part of an accredited practice.[197] If your office is located in an area that is subject to power shortages, then systems should be plugged in to battery backups to prevent the loss of critical information.

**Ultrasound Reporting Software**

MFM practices have used ultrasound report generation software for many years now. Some ultrasound system vendors now offer proprietary reporting software with the lease or purchase of one of their systems. It is imperative that ample time is spent in evaluating the reporting software prior to purchase. Switching from one vendor to another can be expensive and difficult and will result in lost productivity. Sonographer input is an invaluable part of the evaluation process, given that the sonographers are often the primary users of this software. Although this list is not exhaustive, a few key attributes to consider when purchasing ultrasound reporting software include the following. It should have

- A simple user interface;
- Customizable reports;
- The ability to create and modify templates;
- Image capture and image archiving capabilities;
- Remote access capability via the system or other remote software (such as VMware or Citrix);
- Fax and e-mail reporting capability;
- The ability to interface with multiple ultrasound vendors for direct data download;
- The ability to save reports in multiple document formats (PDF, Word document, etc.);
- A searchable database;
- Be HIPAA (Health Insurance Portability and Accountability Act) compliant; and
- Feature possible bidirectional development of/with EMR.

---

[197] Society for Maternal-Fetal Medicine, "SMFM Resolution on Ultrasound Practice Accreditation." https://www.smfm.org/publications/150-smfm-resolution-on-ultrasound-practice-accreditation. Accessed December 22, 2017.

# Electronic Medical Records (EMR) and Practice Management (PM) Software

As of 2018, EMR utilization has become the standard across nearly all medical practices. While EMR implementation can be a laborious process, once fully integrated into the practice, EMR has many important benefits. Some of the advantages include a searchable database, a paperless and readily available documentation system, integrated patient scheduling, practice management capabilities, and the convenience of having all your medical records stored on a server. As with ultrasound reporting software, each provider should spend ample demo time evaluating an EMR prior to purchase. The list below details a few of the most important features of a functional EMR:

- simple user interface
- robust ob-gyn module
- ability to generate consultative reporting
- ability to create and modify templates
- ability to e-mail and fax reports
- a patient portal
- remote access capabilities
- fully functional practice management (PM) components
- lab integration
- electronic prescribing
- searchable database
- automated coding
- automated appointment reminders
- HIPAA compliant

The practice management (PM) component of the EMR refers to the part that contains the patient scheduling, billing, and coding, which are components primarily used by the back-office personnel. This component of the EMR is invaluable, because it should ensure the timely and correct pathways for billing, authorization, benefits checking, and report generation on performance. Reports should be available on the EMR regarding average patient volume (by RVU or exam number), patient wait times, and information on billing performance (see chapter 19 for examples).

The ability to obtain this kind of information with minimal difficulty will aid in resource management. EMR/PM software may be purchased and stored on an internal server maintained by the practice. Alternatively, many EMR/PM vendors offer a cloud-based service where the software is stored on a remote server that is usually maintained by the software vendor. See Chapter 22 on Information Technology for Your Practice.

**Computer Servers**

Given the demands of EMR systems, ultrasound reporting software, and PACS, an office-hosted system should possess a robust office computer network and server for your office space. The server should have large storage and backup capabilities. In addition, servers and other major computer assets should be scalable so that you can easily expand your network to meet the needs of your growing practice. The security of your imaging systems should not be overlooked: the data in your EMR should be encrypted, but your imaging systems also need to encrypt diagnostic imagery to meet HIPAA requirements.

A properly configured business-class firewall will help prevent network intrusions, while antivirus software and regular operating system updates for all computer assets can help prevent or mitigate the effects of emerging malware and virus threats.[198] Arrangements should also be made for copies of the EMR, ultrasound reporting system, and PACS to be regularly and routinely made and secured off-site. A comprehensive and regularly tested disaster-recovery plan can help meet regulatory retention requirements for your patient records. You should consult with a competent and experienced IT professional who has knowledge of medical systems and needs for advice about the specific needs of your practice.

**Other Supplies**

Other standard medical office supplies and recurrent-use items (such as syringes, needles, gauze, plastic speculums, soap and soap dispensers, exam table paper, ultrasound gel, and ultrasound imaging paper) can be purchased in large volumes through medical supply vendors. Some believe that this industry may change in the coming years; the middleman system of health-care supply companies may become obsolete, while online purchasing, such as through Amazon or Walmart, may become a future medical supply option. Until then, joining a group purchasing organization (GPO), an entity that utilizes collective bargaining for a group of medical practices, will assist in obtaining discounts from vendors.

# Conclusion

Opening or relocating to a new office space involves a significant amount of planning and attention to detail. When investigating a new location, be sure to consider the location's strategic placement compared to your competitors as well as its proximity to a level III NICU and your referring providers. The health of the local economy and the population's growth potential should also be included in the decision-making process.

The space layout should be based on your workflow. The design should promote patient comfort, allow for efficient patient traffic flow, and maximize patient privacy. EMR and ultrasound reporting software and PACS are necessary components of the MFM practice. The use

---

[198] James Norvell, vice president of infrastructure, SPINEN (Specialized Information Environments), personal communication with the author, July 22–25, 2015.

of these electronic charting systems, practice management software, and data analysis can provide operational information to help you manage your office more efficiently. While the location, space layout, and equipment utilized will be specific to each individual practice, this chapter has provided a good reference point from which to start. The following checklists can be used to help in the process.

## Checklist 1. Identifying a New Location

- Identify the needs of the community.
- Identify the needs of the practice.
- Decide whether to open the office in a facility or nonfacility location. An office space located within a hospital is known as facility location, while a nonfacility location is an office space located in a freestanding building outside the confines of a hospital.
- Evaluate several geographic variables to aid in finding the ideal location for your practice.
- Choose the ideal space.
- Decide whether to use an existing footprint or proceed with a new build-out.
- Design the layout.
- Identify equipment needs.

## Checklist 2. Office Suites

- waiting and registration
- patient intake
- genetic counselor's consultation
- ultrasound suites and exam rooms
- NST suite
- provider consultation suite
- administration and billing
- information technology (IT)
- break room

# Electronic Health Records / Practice Management Selection—A Guide to Making the Right Choice for Your Practice

Frank Ciafone, MBA

"Find us a good computer system." These are the most dreaded words a consultant can hear from client physicians looking for the first time or seeking to replace their present practice-management office system. To many physicians it seems simple enough: find a good vendor, check out a couple of references, schedule the installation, and within a couple of months the practice will be benefiting from all those capabilities they were shown in the sales demonstration. Check again with that practice a few months after installation, and too frequently one will find frustrated staff, unhappy physicians, and a lawyer looking at the fine points of the contract to make a case for reimbursement.

## Eight Steps for Information-Needs Assessment

What can you do to protect yourself from the myriad of pitfalls the buyer of an office system faces? The answer, most simply, is to do your homework, get good advice, and have reasonable expectations. To assist in this process, you should consider the following as your practice chooses a new solution to your information needs.

### 1. Set a Timeline for the Selection Process

System selection can be a laborious exercise, and without buy-in from everyone concerned in the practice, the process can drag on for months, often to the point of making initial examinations outdated and, worse, possibly useless. No matter the size of the practice, publish a memo detailing the time frame you have in mind for completing the process. The timeline should have five major benchmarks:

- completion of practice requirements
- vendor request for information (RFI) completion
- selection of presenters
- determination of finalists
- vendor selection

The timeline will serve as a statement of commitment for both your practice and interested vendors and will assist in keeping necessary studies on target.

## 2. Examine Your Practice

Look at the way you practice medicine in all aspects, from scheduling to collections to marketing. Ask yourself, "What are the nuances of the practice in the scheduling of physicians, rooms, or procedures that might go beyond a straightforward application?" If you bill for carrier reimbursement, for example, then examine how you post (or would like to post) payments to procedures, what reports you need to track claims and patient responsibility, and what collection support (such as letter writing) you get from your present manual or automated system. If you internally market to your patient base, how you track procedures, create patient recalls, or communicate about new procedures will also be important as you consider system offerings.

This exercise is critical in system selection, and in most cases, the practice should fully engage all staff resources in this examination. First, a physician "champion" needs to take the lead, since eventually a relationship with the selected vendor will be based on this study, and a vested interest should be established in the earliest stages of selection. A committee should be established with representatives from the various departments who will be affected by the future system selection. Ideally, this committee will consist of people from scheduling, billing, and the back office, plus a key provider of the practice, particularly if an EMR (electronic medical records) system is part of the selection process. The committee should set up a timeline for the study and choose a date for the practice study results. At its conclusion, a report should be created and distributed to all staff members who will be affected by a new system to solicit their feedback. It is particularly important, in the case of an EMR, that all providers agree on a common presentation of chart information or at least understand the issues the practice faces in this area.

## 3. Explore the Industry

Unless you are well versed in technology-related issues, you may wish to contract with a system consultant who is familiar with the medical software marketplace and its applications. No hard-and-fast findings are available to definitively point to a particular vendor, but having knowledge of quality players in the marketplace in your area will help narrow your search. It is always an advantage to work with vendors that are in a good financial position, but many quality companies are private, which makes their financial situations difficult to assess. A growing client base may be an indicator of a company's position, but while you are doing this research, avoid the common mistake of looking solely at the largest vendor in your area or the number of installations performed by the company nationally. A large vendor will have the advantage of stability in the marketplace, but a small vendor can be more responsive to any requested software changes. Look instead at vendors that will share their complete client list in your area, and pay particular attention to client comments regarding local support. Ultimately, this attention at the local level will most determine the success of your implementation choice, assuming other factors regarding finalists are approximately equal.

So now you understand your practice's needs, you've prioritized their importance in choosing a system, and you've achieved a comfort level with a number of vendors serving your area with good support. Now it's time to looking at vendor offerings.

### 4. Issue an RFI

A good first step in avoiding sales pressure is the creation of a request for information (RFI) from selected vendors. This document should be concise. Do not waste vendor time asking questions that you can research easily or will not affect your decision. Ask specifics that pertain to important issues for your practice. If you need to block rooms in the scheduler according to provider availability, then ask for this capability specifically. Prioritize your needs into categories, ranging from must-haves at installation to advantageous to a long-term wish. Assigning a numeric ranking to these needs will help you score vendor responses and will allow the vendor to prepare demonstrations to answer your needs.

One of the more difficult tasks in the RFI is to obtain a sense of cost for each offering. The platforms, annual maintenance, and upgrade pricing will differ greatly among vendors, but try to provide input such as number of screens anticipated or remote access needs so that the vendor can provide better details on cost. Remember that the purpose of the RFI is to get you and your potential vendor in the same room, so it's better to know upfront if you can afford what the vendor is offering.

### 5. Invite Vendor Demonstrations

Based on the results of the RFI, develop a short list of no more than three vendors that meet your essential needs. If you have developed a good RFI and identified well-supported systems in your area, then it should not be difficult to rule out inappropriate systems for your office. A short list should be used in determining vendor invitees, as demonstrations can be a draining experience for staff and physicians alike: after you have viewed more than three demonstrations, the individual system features begin to blur, and the sales presentation replaces system capabilities in differentiation.

If possible, delegate a team member to be a scribe for the demonstration, and assign a particular area of interest so that one staff member will become an expert—for example, on the scheduling features for all the systems presented. Structure the demonstration to your wishes as to time and format. Allow perhaps thirty minutes for vendors to present their companies' strengths, support approaches, and any areas of differentiation that they may wish to express. For the remainder of the demonstration, format the meeting based on your "hot button" issues. If scheduling is critical, then ask for perhaps thirty minutes on these topics alone, allowing less time for a less-than-critical topic. Work backward from a total meeting duration to determine subject blocks, with a meeting cap of ninety minutes or less. The vendor can always address additional questions following the demonstration, but a vendor should be able to perform a concise demonstration within that time parameter.

### 6. Conduct a Client Visit

A visit to an installation can be informative, but use it to see how the system operates more than to obtain an endorsement. You wouldn't send a potential patient to see an underperforming physician practice, and neither would a vendor. In a client visit, check for workarounds that the practice may have to perform in response to any software shortcomings. For example, if comment fields are used to input desired data because there is no other place in the program to enter information, then these fields may not be searchable in system reports. System speed, screen presentation, and patient/system interaction are good areas to examine in a live environment.

### 7. Perform a Final Consensus Check

At this point, you should have been able to differentiate among system alternatives to narrow your choice to perhaps two finalists. For practice peace and unity, selection-team members should meet and report to the committee their perspectives on the vendor offerings. The team should then create and disseminate a report to appropriate managers and providers for review and sign-off. This is the chance for everyone in the practice to make their objections known and to discuss them prior to moving into negotiations with the selected vendor. The goal in this step is to create buy-in and appreciation of the process, thereby lessening any "I told you so" frustrations during installation.

### 8. Begin the Contracting Process

Your vendor will present you with a templated standard form contract for your acceptance, with stated pricing for purchase and maintenance. Your ability to negotiate cost changes to this contract will depend on a number of factors:

- the importance of sales closure
- the size of the project
- any established relationship to refer potential sales
- existing vendor market share

Unfortunately, many practices concentrate their contracting energy on pricing, at the cost of performance warranties, and they regret this oversight greatly over the course of the vendor relationship. High-performing practices will incur a far greater cost from not holding their vendors accountable for downtime than the one-time savings of a strongly negotiated sales price. It is critical that you ensure that *all* core service and performance obligations are expressly and specifically stated in your EMR contract.

The following are a few baseline performance requirements that you should expect your vendor contract to address to your satisfaction:

- system-scheduled downtime
- response time to downtime
- backup and data recovery
- accountability (hardware/software performance and maintenance)
- updates and modification request response times
- training (hours of initial and follow-up)
- future costs (licenses, training per hour, updates, maintenance)

- data conversion (cost, delivery)
- installation timeline
- practice sign-off for satisfied implementation

In addition to the practice's consideration of the clinical aspects of delivery, your practice's attorney should also be satisfied about the terms related to clearly defined delivery issues, performance issues, and remedies for nonperformance. Pay particular attention to the contract's definition of breach of contract in terms of vendor failure and the jurisdiction location for any curative legal action.

## Transitioning to a Health System or Hospital-Established EMR

Over the past few years (as of 2018), working within an existing hospital or system-wide EMR has become the major operational challenge to practices that are transitioning from private practice to employed-physician models. The following are system-related issues that can derail the smooth integration of transitioning practices, create daily frustration for staff and physicians, and impede optimal efficiency.

1. **Your Relationship with the Software Developer Is No Longer Direct**

The recommended course of action discussed previously in this chapter for a private practice that is selecting a vendor will establish a relationship between customer and vendor that fosters cooperation and accountability. Operating within the health system's EMR will most often dictate that you will be working with the hospital's IT and information services departments, who in turn maintain the relationship with their vendor.

2. **Your System Will Be Less Customizable**

System-wide EMRs face the challenge of serving a wide variety of specialties, particularly in software design and maintenance. Vendors and internal system support staff understand that any change to a data-input field that benefits your practice may negatively affect the organization as a whole. In addition, the vendor must address any software changes in new revision levels, which will create a nightmare for development and implementation staff.

3. **Response to System and Training Needs Will Be Variable**

Working with two support suppliers (vendor and hospital) creates the challenges of availability and accountability in optimizing the EMR. If your organization is in an aggressive expansion mode, then the support staff will be stretched in implementing and supporting these practices. Requests for service will be prioritized and response times dictated by urgency, real or perceived. Finally, maternal-fetal medicine will most likely be one of the smaller departments within the system and as such will be challenged to effectively lobby for change and service.

So how can your practice succeed in obtaining help for its system needs in this scenario? The following are a few suggestions in optimizing your experience:

- Establish a relationship with key management that will advocate for your practice through the ranks of your organization and to the vendor.
- Become knowledgeable in the basic architecture of your system and its reporting capabilities. Having proficiency in system operations will help tremendously in discussions with all levels of support.
- Be proactive in your relationship with IT and information services. Request quarterly reviews of your practice's application, and be sure to establish timelines on any projects that affect your system.
- Be tenacious in following up on requested training or services. Every conclusion to a service discussion should have an action plan and delivery date in place.

# 22

## Information Technology for Your Practice

Greg Ferrante (MSCE, CCNA) and Megan Ferrante (BS)

One of today's increasingly important elements for any practice is the thorough consideration of the information technology platform that you, your staff, and your patients will utilize and rely on every day. Whether in-house or cloud based, this platform's reliability and availability are important to keep in mind, as they will have a direct impact on the efficiency of your office's daily productivity. Six key areas should be addressed when looking at information technology for your practice:

1. *Understand your practice's needs.* Understanding how your practice utilizes IT equipment will help you better understand your practice's present and future needs, which in turn will help you better consider the recommendations you receive from IT consultants, vendors, or staff.

2. *Choose an in-house or cloud-based system.* Should your practice go in-house or cloud? Based on the size of your practice, the number of imaging devices, and the number of active exam rooms, your answers to these questions will have a direct bearing on what type of IT platform to consider.

3. *Compile a list of necessary equipment.* Make an overview of the many items that go into a comprehensive IT platform for a medical practice, from the workstations and printers down to the long-term data storage of picture archiving communication system (PACS) servers.

4. *Choose IT professionals for your practice.* Choosing the right personnel or professionals to manage the day-to-day operations of the IT department of your practice is critical to the overall efficiency of your IT systems on which the entire practice now depends.

5. *Consider all security issues.* Any implementation of a network, large or small, requires careful consideration of all potential security issues of the infrastructure. Add access and security surrounding the network both inside and out, and keep in mind the ever-changing requirements of HIPAA/HITECH (the Health Insurance Portability and Accountability Act and the Health Information Technology for Economic and Clinical Health Act).

6. *Plan for IT requirements before office construction or remodeling.* IT requirements are often overlooked when constructing a new office or practice, whether it's a complete build-out or simple structural modifications. Understanding those requirements during the planning stages of any construction project will minimize the impact and future costs while keeping security and efficiency in mind.

The IT platform that you and your staff use will have a direct effect on you and your staff's ability to perform efficiently hour to hour of each day.

## Understanding How Maternal-Fetal Medicine (MFM) Utilizes IT

Whether you are starting a new practice or running an existing one, the information systems in an MFM practice will be utilized for similar tasks: appointment scheduling, checking in patients, exam room and office data entry, physician entry of chart notes, and patient checkout and billing. Each of these is discussed below.

### Appointment Scheduling

Usually the first interaction with a patient occurs during appointment scheduling. The staff members required to handle scheduling utilize the practice management system to check the availability of the physician, availability of staff for imaging and/or monitoring, and assessment of availability for any other services performed by the MFM practice.

### Patient Check-In and Intake

Typically the practice management software is used to check in the patient, which requires the interaction of the workstation with the practice management server while the data is being entered into the system. The staff member checking in the patient typically verifies with the billing department and/or interface for any copays if the practice requires the copay be paid before the appointment. Benefits checking will also occur prior to the visit and will require input into the practice management system.

If the patient is a new patient, she will typically fill out the intake forms before arriving; these forms will also need to be entered into the system prior to her being taken to an exam room. Some practice management systems allow the patient to fill out the patient intake information online before arriving at the office, which can streamline the check-in process. This solution does require a web interface for patients to access at their convenience while not compromising the security of the practice's patient data.

### Exam Room and Office Data Entry

The patient is then directed to an exam room to meet with doctors, advanced practitioners, and sonographers, who will conduct exams of various levels. An imaging exam will typically result in a number of ultrasound images, video clips, and measurement data that are then transmitted by the ultrasound machine to the ultrasound reporting system or PACS server. The ultrasound machine transmits quite a bit of imaging data at this time, as the typical exam can range from a few hundred megabytes to upward of five to ten gigabytes of data. This is a key area of the practice's efficiency needs, as this amount of data multiplied by the number of primary exam rooms with imaging devices will give you a good idea of how much data transmitting and storing a practice will do throughout each day. Another factor to keep in mind in this particular area is the number of exam rooms that are remote from your office (i.e., at a satellite office).

The efficient transmission of ultrasound data from the imaging device to the PACS server will depend on the speed of the connection between the ultrasound machine and the PACS server itself. Within the walls of a single office, a standard high-speed, switch-based network will work sufficiently. When you have remote offices, however, you must consider the connection speed and data-connection types that will be required. PACS vendors should also weigh in on this decision or at least offer baseline requirements for WAN (wide area network) connectivity between their equipment and PACS servers.

## Physician Entry of Chart Notes

After the exam comes the doctor's direct interaction with the workstation and the time it takes to complete the exam observations and render the report. The doctor's workstation is a key element in daily efficiency, as the doctor can only work at the pace the computer can perform. This may be done through a hardwired computer terminal or via a laptop or other portable entry device with sufficient secure wireless connectivity.

## Patient Checkout and Billing

While the doctor is wrapping up the exam, typically the patient heads to checkout for another interaction with staff and the practice management system. This part of the interaction will consist of processing the payment (if it was not done at check-in), entering that information into the practice management system for billing, and of course scheduling the next visit. While not as much data is transmitted as in the exam itself, this area is also a key component of the patient interaction.

Meanwhile, the billing department, scheduling department, and various other departments are all working in other areas of the practice management system and PACS, all of which use data speed on the network. All this usage multiplied by the overall number of staff will give you a pretty good idea of just how high a data-transmission speed you will require as well as the amount of data storage required to secure and maintain this network and data activity.

Although practices vary in their patient interactions, a typical patient visit provides a baseline of the impact on your IT equipment and network connections. Key areas to consider when decision-making are the number of exam rooms with ultrasound machines, the number of doctors and staff workstations needed to run the practice, the number of remote or satellite offices, and the number of remote staff members. This information will help you determine whether running a cloud-based or in-house IT platform will be right for you and your practice.

## To Cloud or Not to Cloud

This is a legitimate question in this era of high-speed Internet and the multitude of data-warehousing options available today. Deciding whether to have internal servers host your EMR data or to have the data hosted on the cloud depends on the size, goals, and requirements of the practice.

### Cloud Hosting

When your EMR data is hosted in the cloud, your data essentially resides on a set of servers at a secure location; some providers make sure that copies of the data reside at other locations as well for redundancy purposes. With a cloud-hosted platform, the practice does not have to worry about purchasing extensive server hardware or operating systems, or maintenance or upgrades to the same. Cloud-based solutions are typically hosted in locations with heavy security, including biometrics for access, security cameras, and patrolling guards.

With a cloud-hosted platform, however, the provider tends to face a higher likelihood of hacking attempts, denial-of-service (DoS) attacks, and other potential security problems. In the event of a DoS attack, or even loss of an Internet connection at the provider's office, the staff will not have access to the EMR data. In addition, hosting fees can be expensive, and many cloud providers charge based on the amount of data being stored. So if the practice is a high-volume practice with a lot of providers and patients, the costs for hosting can become quite high. If the practice experiences any billing issues or disagreements, the cloud provider can block access to the software until the billing issue is resolved. If the practice desires to switch practice management solutions, the problem is then retaining access to records from a company you no longer do business with. A move to a new EMR without a contractual predetermined handling of the transition may result in delays in getting your data, or an expensive transfer of data via the development of an interface for reassignment of the information.

The connection speed between the office and the location where the data is stored can also become an issue. For smaller practices that transmit minimal imaging data, hosting on the cloud may not be an issue. For a practice with a large number of images, video, and data, the connection between the cloud and the practice can hinder the speed at which data is stored and retrieved. The more traffic there is, the slower the response times.

Software vendors that offer their services on the cloud are required to be HIPAA and HITECH compliant. Therefore, some security issues that normally have to be addressed by the practice when using in-house servers should already have been resolved by vendors on their cloud services, which may be an advantage that would interest some practices.

### On-Premise Servers

If you keep your EMR data on-site, you will have to ensure that your servers are stored in a secure room within the practice. For this option, the practice will not only have more control over local security and access to the software but to the hardware as well. Unlike with a cloud solution, if the Internet is down, the users will still be able to access the data while at the office.

Depending on the amount of data being handled, the practice may need to purchase and maintain a significant amount of hardware to maintain the system's reliability, redundancy, and backup requirements. This will also entail keeping up with all operating system updates and security releases to maintain the data's security. As the practice and/or patient base grows, more hardware will need to be purchased to store additional data.

On-premise servers can be more susceptible to virus infections, locked systems, and system crashes than a cloud solution, unless systems are in place to prevent and/or contain these issues. Preventing any downtime caused by these issues requires hardware redundancy, a reliable backup method, and intrusion-prevention systems.

**Mixture of In-House and Cloud Services**

Another option is to do a mix of the two and use both in-house servers and cloud services—it doesn't have to be one or the other. A practice may choose to have the practice management system be a cloud-based system while managing the PACS on in-house servers, or vice versa. A practice can use other cloud-based services that assist in day-to-day operations without any significant passing of data between the cloud and the practice's network or interfering in day-to-day operations (e.g., off-site backup and spam filtering).

**Deciding Which Way Is Best**

A cloud solution is most likely better suited for smaller practices that do not have a large provider and ultrasound footprint. Purchasing the hardware for servers, storage space, backup solutions, and networking can be a significant expense. Moving to the cloud can minimize that large expense, but it will have a higher ongoing expense because of the various hosting fees. While having a cloud-based system can seem like a great solution that will minimize hardware purchases and maintenance as well as ongoing maintenance of the system, such a system can have a significant impact on the efficiency of an MFM practice. A physician having quick access to a patient's chart, ultrasound images, and/or video is paramount, and a cloud-based system for a medium-to-large practice can seriously affect the speed at which a physician can access the data. Before investing in a cloud-based system, a practice needs to have knowledge about typical downtime issues, the time spent fixing these instances of limited access, and the speed of information access during times of maximal traffic. Meaningful investigation and due diligence are both required, and a practice should ask current customers of similar size for a review of their experiences.

# Components of the IT Platform

Although this section covers components of the IT platform, it is strongly recommended that you consult with an IT professional who has experience in both data-center build-outs and medical practices and who utilizes PACS and EHR systems.

Whichever direction you decide on when reviewing cloud or in-house IT platforms, you must constantly evaluate and update a number of components as time goes on. Oddly enough, in-house IT platforms are very similar to cloud platforms. Working our way from the staff and their desks, we'll move into the network to the application servers and data-storage systems and then out to the Internet. Figure 22.1 shows a small sample of a basic network.

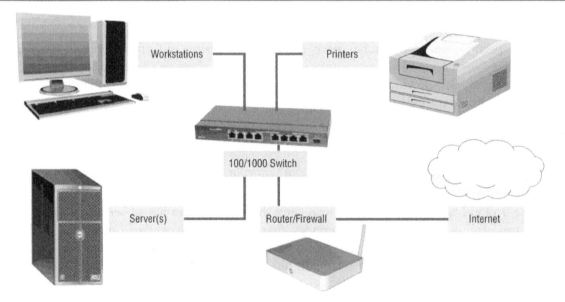

Fig 22.1. Sample network within a medical office

## Workstations

At each desk, you will find a PC or workstation. This is typically a business-grade computer with the "professional" version of the Microsoft operating system, which should have a good balance between cost and speed.

## Switch

Each one of the workstations is then connected via network cables to a central set of switches that tie the workstations, servers, and Internet together. As of the publication of this book (early 2018), standard switch speeds are 1 Gbps or 1,000 Mb per second, with 10 Gbps or 10,000 Mb per second switches just starting to become cost effective.

## Servers

In the "in-house" IT platform scenario, you will have servers in a secure data room in your practice that are also connected to the central switch. Servers should be designed to handle their respective tasks (in some cases more than one) and have ample CPU power, RAM, and hard-disk space to survive the practice's growth rate for three to five years. Application servers are designed to run your software, such as EHR or PACS application software. Other servers may include (1) domain controllers, which handle authentication to your network of computers; (2) e-mail servers;

(3) print servers; and (4) backup servers, which perform routine backup procedures on all the other servers.

For a smaller practice, some of these functions can be combined onto one or two servers (i.e., the authentication, e-mail, and print serving can be handled on one server). As the practice grows, servers will need to be broken up to handle their assigned tasks in order to minimize the load.

### Storage Area Network

Ideally the servers should be connected to a central data repository, also known as a storage area network or SAN. SAN servers should be completely redundant within themselves, meaning that they have two power supplies, two motherboards, two disk controllers, and four or more hard drives. The SAN server or any device that acts as your data repository is, simply put, the most important piece of equipment you will buy and maintain in an in-house system.

### Backup

Although the SAN server or data-storage server should be fully redundant, routine backups of data are an absolute requirement, and an off-site copy of your practice's data should also be maintained. If your office has two or more locations, it could be feasible to copy the backup data out to one of your outside locations, or you could locate a HIPAA-compliant cloud backup provider to send your backups to for a nominal fee.

### Router/Firewall

Beyond the switches is the device known as a router or firewall that connects you to the Internet and potentially to outside offices. Firewalls with unified threat management (UTM) software subscriptions should be used to scan and prevent unwanted viruses, malware, or other undesired content from entering your network. They should also prevent and log any attempted intrusion attempts into the network.

### Remote Office Locations

In a scenario where you have multiple practice locations and an in-house data facility, you will need to incorporate the cost of a wide area network connection (or WAN) back to your primary location that houses your IT platform servers. The transmission-speed requirements and cost of these lines will depend on how many staff, workstations, exam rooms, ultrasound machines, and doctors are set to operate at the given remote location. Private metro-Ethernet or fiber lines between offices should be your first consideration and addition to your budget. Once again, the speed of this connection will have a direct impact on your staff's productivity at the remote location. Keep this in mind when limiting your budget in this area—it could cost you more than you will save by going with service below your true needs.

## Other Services and Requirements

While the above items are the fundamental elements that you will see in an in-house or cloud-based IT platform for your practice, a number of other items will come up as well. Your option to buy or use cloud services is also an option for these services. These other items include spam and virus filtering of e-mail, e-mail encryption, virus scanning of servers and workstations, web-content filtering, server-uptime monitoring, environmental controls, and many more.

## Selecting IT Support Management Staff

When it comes to selecting in-house staff or outsourced professionals to manage your IT platform, it is important to consider a number of elements. You might be asking yourself, "Do I hire full-time staff or contract with a professional team?" Similar in some ways to the "Do I go cloud?" question, your decision process on this element should be founded on your practice's needs, its frequency or demand of IT staff interaction, and the overall self-sustainability of your practice's IT platform.

### Internal IT Support

On the upper side of the budget, a single full-time IT staff member can oversee the IT department and be on premises forty hours per week. In the MFM industry, most likely this person will also need to be available after hours as well. Having an on-site IT person will ensure that the person is present and available for whatever issues arise, whether it be a malfunctioning printer or a server-down situation. Additionally, an internal IT support staff has your practice/institution as his or her primary and only responsibility. But most practices don't have the resources to hire more than one full-time IT staff member, so backup arrangements should be made in case that staff member is unavailable because of vacations, sick days, or any other events.

    A full-time in-house IT person will need to be provided the same benefits provided to the other employees, including desk space, a workstation, ongoing training materials and classes, management software or subscriptions, and of course vacation time, sick days, and benefits. In addition to all the tools and training materials, you have to keep in mind that the IT staff member will come into contact with your staff as well as have some exposure to a certain percentage of your patients. A professional and outgoing personality as well as the ability to clearly communicate with, help, or train staff are necessary prerequisites.

### Contracted Support

Moving down in budget costs, but typically higher in value, is the contracting of IT professionals to maintain and manage your IT department. Most successful IT companies have transitioned into what are known as MSPs, or managed service providers. MSPs typically have a wide array of automated management software systems that can be installed on every computer in your office; they can automatically maintain and monitor those systems as well as conduct service request interactions or act on support tickets between staff and IT support at the click of a button. In most cases, management agreements can be forged with an MSP that will consist of a fixed monthly cost that will cover all support needs, thus giving you a fully staffed IT department in most cases for less cost than from having one in-house IT manager.

One primary difference between in-house staff who only deal with your network and an MSP is the fact that in-house employees are more likely to be sheltered from ongoing cyberattack threats and issues happening in the world that day, unless they happens to get press coverage (which most do not). In contrast, an MSP handles multiple clients and gains a much broader view of the daily events going on in the IT world, even receiving new information on an hour-by-hour basis. For example, if one or more of the other clients of an MSP organization are hit by the same virus on the same day, a typical response by a good MSP company is to roll out a warning and/or a protective measure to its other clients. Likewise, MSPs gain experience in events that occur with other organizations they may handle. Those experiences are then passed on to their other clients in order to reduce future workloads.

On the downside, if you are a smaller entity, then contracted support may not be as responsive as in-house personnel, since they may be responding to other customers' issues—your problems may not be their top priority.

**Last Word—In-House versus Contracted Staff**

Out of all these considerations, one important factor to keep in mind is that the professionals you choose to manage your practice's IT department should have direct experience working with other MFM practices or, at a minimum, extensive experience working with high-volume networks with multiple PACS providers in the medical field. Other good qualities to look for include extensive experience with WAN, IT management and security, and experience with multiple firewall and intrusion prevention systems (IPS) vendors. Experience in working with and training less technically inclined people is another plus.

# IT and Security

Whether you choose to keep your servers in-house or store data on the cloud, whether you have on-site IT staff or decide to outsource, you always need to address the issue of security. The following are some of the factors to consider: (1) how your patients do their intake, (2) how staff access patient data, (3) how patient data is stored and retrieved, and (4) how patient data is kept safe, secure, and reliable.

In addition, regardless of whether the EMR and PACS data is stored on the cloud or locally, the HIPAA security and privacy rules[199] require technical safeguards to be in place:
- access control
    - unique user identification
    - emergency access procedure

---

[199] Centers for Medicare and Medicaid, "HIPAA Security Series," Department of Health and Human Services, vol. 2, paper 4, May 2005, revised March 2007.

- automatic logoff
- encryption and decryption
* audit controls
* integrity
* person or entity authentication
* transmission security
  - integrity controls
  - encryption

As earlier sections of this chapter discussed, security should be interwoven with how MFM practices utilize IT, the components of IT, and IT staff management, whether local or cloud based. While the HIPAA guidelines are fairly generic in nature, an MFM practice should keep a few specific things in mind, no matter how small or large the practice, including the following.

1. All users should have unique log-ins, with the network and practice management software requiring regular password changes and not allowing the repetition of passwords. User accounts should be configured to automatically lock after a few attempts of inputting an incorrect password, and auditing logs should reflect these attempts.

2. Workstations should be configured to be locked when not in use after a certain amount of time, and they should require a password in order to be unlocked.

3. Computer screens that could potentially be seen by patients need to be angled in such a way that they cannot read them.

4. Managed switches that connect the computers to the servers need to be installed and configured to have complex passwords.

5. If using in-house servers, then the servers need to be kept in a locked, air-conditioned room along with all other networking equipment, including switches and routers. The air temperature of this room should be monitored; a monitoring system for any potential problems regarding system status should be utilized as well. Servers also need to be in a "logged off" or "locked" state when not in use, and they should only be accessible to the IT support staff/vendor and practice management. It is not recommended to store the servers in the same room as the janitorial equipment, office supplies, or anything else that would make the room accessible to non-IT or non-management personnel.

6. All Wi-Fi access to the network needs to be assigned complex passwords, and the Wi-Fi should not be discoverable to outside of your office employees.

7. Routers/firewalls should be configured to minimize any potential threats by limiting the number of ports that provide access to the network from the outside. Any required services that require an "open door" on the router should require usernames and passwords, as previously described, and they should be audited on a regular basis for unauthorized access.

These recommended basic guidelines are fairly easy to implement regardless of the practice's size. What's often not considered a part of keeping a practice's patient data secure is how the office is constructed, which is the subject of the next section.

## Office Construction and IT

Something that is commonly overlooked when acquiring space to operate your practice is the construction build-out required to handle your IT platform. When constructing a new building or building out an existing location suitable for your practice, it is crucial to handle all the details of the IT networking, including the location of computers and monitors in relation to patient flows and, for those who elect to run in-house IT platforms, server room facilities with adequate space, power, and cooling.

Beginning in the waiting room, where the patient has the first physical contact with and impression of your practice, it is important that your front desks be designed to accommodate a small workstation; the monitors should face away from the waiting room so they do not expose any patient information. Workstation displays should be low enough to allow your staff to see everything going on in the waiting area and, likewise, to allow the patients to easily see and communicate with your staff. Each desk area should have two to four power outlets for its workstation and any other electronic equipment staff may require, such as credit card machines, calculators, and the like. Each desk area should have a minimum of two but preferably four network jacks, all of which need to be tested and marked to indicate their endpoint on the patch panel in the data room (the patch panel has corresponding numbers to indicate which port it came from). Figure 22.2 shows a simple example of how network jacks can be labeled and how they correspond to the connections in the data room.

These network jacks are also known as network runs or network drops. Each network drop is a physical connection back to your server room or telephone closet, where all network drops in your office come together to connect to a central switch device that connects all your workstations together. The location of these jacks should be under or near each desk area where you plan to place a workstation or network-connected device. This way you avoid running cables over walkways or across long distances, both of which could present a safety hazard for your staff. You should work closely with your IT consultant to determine network locations during the construction phase of your practice or when redesigning existing space.

As we move deeper into the practice and back-office areas where patient flow is expected, we should configure the desks so that displays face away from patient traffic as much as possible. Likewise, for each and every desk and cubicle for the back office, give the same consideration to power and network-jack location in order to reduce the length of cables and power cords required for your IT workstations.

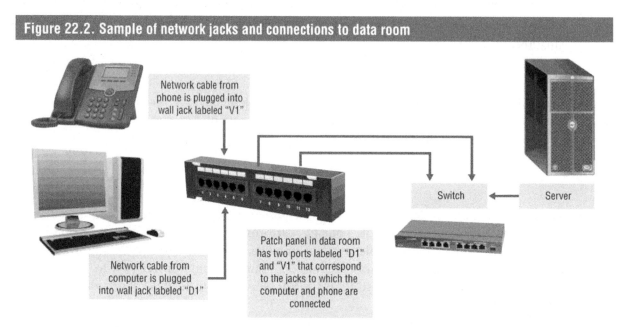

Figure 22.2. Sample of network jacks and connections to data room

For those who have elected to run an in-house IT platform, the server room should be carefully designed as a central data room that will house the application and data-storage servers as well as networking equipment for your practice. The data room should be designed so that it provides ample room for the racks that will hold your servers, switches, data-storage devices, and backup systems along with telephone systems, security, and other electronic equipment. In addition to all this equipment, the network patch panels—where all the network wiring in your practice should come together—will be in your data room as well. Your data room should be large enough to comfortably situate the rack or racks you require to house your servers and other IT equipment in the center of the room, with enough space for technicians to work in front of and behind the equipment. This space also provides the necessary airflow for your servers. If possible, you should also allow yourself at least an additional 25 percent of space to accommodate any growth—for example, in the event that you expect to grow the current location or add outside locations to your practice. Racks should be lined up right to left, and airflow should run from front to back.

Inside the data room, you should have a minimum of two to four dedicated power circuits at twenty amps or above, each. These power jacks should be located so that they easily connect with your uninterruptable power-supply devices without having to run power cords over walkways or work areas. Uninterruptable power supplies (UPS) equipment is generally connected to these circuits, and your IT equipment is plugged into those UPS devices. UPS devices are essentially boxes of batteries and sophisticated circuitry that maintain an even flow of power to the IT equipment located in your data room. Any equipment plugged into these UPS devices will continue to run for a period of time in the event of power failures, spikes, or sags, all of which would otherwise harm or temporarily interrupt your servers and equipment functionality.

Servers, data-storage devices, high-speed switches, and routers tend to put off a modest amount of heat, which is typically rated in British thermal units (BTUs). Most IT equipment will have a BTU rating, so you can easily calculate the amount of cooling capacity your air-conditioning units can achieve. For smaller data rooms, more compact ductless air-conditioning units or even portable air-conditioning units can suffice. For larger operations, it may be best to have two air-conditioning units for redundancy and shared workload in cooling your data room. Air handlers should be kept on dedicated power circuits separately from your other data-room outlets. It is also recommended that the temperature of the data room be maintained below 80°F at all times. Typically, when temperatures rise above 88°F over extended periods of time, data-storage equipment wear and failure become accelerated.

## Conclusion

Many things must be considered and addressed when choosing your practice's information technology platform: from constructing and building out your practice to determining how your staff and patients will interact with your systems to choosing how that data is accessed, stored, and kept secure. Understanding how your practice utilizes IT hardware is key in making decisions in this regard. Information technology is the lifeblood of your operation, and it contains and controls all the information on which you, your staff, and your patients depend. It should be cost effective yet fast, secure, and reliable. Your information systems platform should be treated as an important line item in your budget, because your practice's efficiency will depend on its speed and reliability. It should be secure from both inside and outside threats, and you should have multiple backup sets of your data in the event of data corruption or loss. Imagine, if you will, going for hours or days without access to your electronic medical records and practice management system. This thought should rest firmly within your decision-making process when you consider what will truly serve as the electronic foundation of your practice and give it the ability to function in today's paperless world.

# 23

## Phone Systems and Service

### Brian K. Iriye, MD

An argument can be made that the most important piece of technology in your office is not your ultrasound equipment or computer systems, but your phone system and its proper setup and utilization. A good exercise to perform is to call your own office to assess phone etiquette or to have a friend or family member call, acting as a patient, to assess the service. Does the phone ring endlessly? Are you placed on hold without explanation? Does the call go to voice mail? Does your "patient" have an impersonal experience or a bothersome first impression from staff? An organization that measures patient experience for health-care organizations, Press Ganey, has stated in a 2011 report, "Patients continue to voice frustrations over the ease of scheduling appointments, the helpfulness of telephone staff, and the promptness of return calls."[200] A telephone system with exemplary service gives your practice a true chance to stand out and be remarkable.

Over the course of twenty years, our practice in Las Vegas has grown from a practice of two doctors, one office, and sixty to seventy patients per day to twelve doctors, three offices, 275 patients per day, and over five hundred new referrals per week. But although we increased the number of our phone lines, our front desk answered all phone calls, and one office took the majority of those calls. This created a system where the patient on the phone appeared to be a higher priority than the patients in our office due to the continuous time spent answering and then triaging phone calls. In addition, the calls would initially have to be triaged, as the front office was not the ideal place to receive calls from people attempting to contact different areas of our practice. Some calls would get left on extended hold in the attempt to get them to the right area, which created further issues. We had to admit: the office had a problem. We set out to study our needs, realized that the average cost of losing disgruntled patients was approximately $1,500 each, and attempted to create team awareness and ownership of our phone problems and office attention and dedication to move forward with a large-scale change.

## Prepping for Success

The first step to having an effective phone system is to understand call volume. If you know the number of calls your practice receives per day, then you can calculate the number of phone lines you will need. A proper number of lines in an office can be determined as follows:[201]

---

[200] 2011 Pulse report: Perspectives on American Health Care. Press Ganey. Accessed January 30, 2018. https://helpandtraining.pressganey.com/Documents_secure/Pulse%20Reports/2011_Press_Ganey_Pulse_Report.pdf

[201] S. Peller, *Own the Phone* (Phoenix, MD: Greenbranch Publishing, 2015), 17.

- 1–99 calls/day: 1 main line and 2 rollover lines
- 100–199 calls/day: 1 main line and 3 rollover lines
- 1 extra rollover line for each 100 calls per day

To ensure that your practice is actually providing quality phone service, you should consider a call-recording system, which allows you to assess the service and make remediations and improvements as needed. To record calls in most US states, you may have to state that "your call may be monitored to provide better customer service." To stay compliant with the Health Insurance Portability and Accountability Act (HIPAA) and record phone calls to improve your service, you must maintain several safeguards:

- Store recordings with encryption.
- Access recordings with a username and password.
- Do not e-mail any patient recordings.
- If working with other entities for call recording, they must
  - sign a HIPAA business associate agreement;
  - properly destroy recordings when no longer needed; and
  - outline what steps they will follow in case of data breach.

Larger practices should definitely invest in a private branch exchange (PBX) phone system. These systems allow calls to be switched between office users on local lines while also allowing the office to share a certain number of external phone lines. Voice over Internet protocol (VoIP) systems can be combined with a system with PBX functionality to reduce long-distance charges and converge voice and data capability on a single network. Many modern systems have data-gathering features that can analyze a wealth of data, including dropped calls (patients hanging up), wait times, numbers of calls answered per employee at a desk, total calls per day, calls per hour, and other data that will help you determine staffing numbers and timing as well as analyze employee workloads.

## Have a Core Team

You should have a core team who answers the majority of calls that cannot be triaged by a PBX. This team needs to have enthusiasm for your mission, empathy for callers and concern for their well-being, patience and professionalism even under sometimes difficult circumstances, and the ability to answer or triage questions quickly and confidently. The emotions of your staff are not always manageable, but their attitudes while answering calls can be. Hence, it is important to know your team's skill sets and to place appropriate people in the phone service role of your practice.

Many of us bristle at the thought of integrated voice response (IVR) systems and their options from one to nine and then secondary options after the initial selections. Large industries' misuse of these systems has created widespread loathing of IVR systems. Nonetheless, these systems, when used properly, actually present advantages. When a patient calls, the initial phone message via an IVR system should state the practice name and a short mission statement and then provide three to four options. This entire message should last less than thirty seconds. When utilized in this manner, the call is quickly routed to the best person for the specific patient concern, and staff time is minimized with the caller as well. An appropriate IVR answering system message could be something similar to this: "Welcome to ABC Perinatal Services, helping you to achieve a better pregnancy outcome. For scheduling, press 1. For billing, press 2. For all other questions, please press 3."

From the time the IVR system hands off the call, the goal is to answer in three rings or less. Each ring lasts three to four seconds, and the general rule is to answer calls in ten seconds or less to avoid hang-ups. Hang-ups are costly to your practice because if a patient hangs up, she has a decreased likelihood of calling back. For a new-patient referral, the average revenue generated within a maternal-fetal medicine (MFM) office over the time of the pregnancy is $1,500. If the patient is a returning patient, then her frustration may lead to decreased patient satisfaction, insurance payment penalties, or unpleasant social media reviews that affect your business. In addition, voice mail should not be used as an option for new-patient calls. One informal study has shown that only 10 percent of new patients leave a voice mail when given this option.[202]

Your core team should use hands-free headsets to answer calls. Holding your neck straight when answering calls gives you a clearer voice, and having free hands allows you to input information more rapidly into your computer systems for appointment scheduling or documentation-of-care-by-call conversations. Your call-answering team should also have mirrors at their desks. Approximately seventy-five percent of the message over the phone is communicated in the tone of voice of the person on the call, and this positive energy starts with a smile.[203] It is extremely difficult to say something in a bad manner while smiling. This is a hallmark of call centers, which often use the mantra "Smile and dial."

Keeping written reminders of this at people's desks is also helpful. New callers should never be sent to a voice-mail machine, as this is frustrating from a patient perspective, especially for a patient with increased risk of complications. For people who require further triaging of phone calls, your system should have call parking to avoid accidental hang-ups and also to have repeat rings for calls that have been parked too long. When people are on hold, your practice should use messaging; recorded messages in which you market the services and accolades of your practice and remind the patient of the importance of your services are preferable. These sometimes reassure the patient, reset her mind-set, and remind her of why she is receiving care from your office in the first place.

## Call Scripting

Most scenarios in a practice occur frequently and hence should have a scripted format to ensure compliance with desired office responses. These scripts do not always need to be read verbatim, but having your team use the scripts initially will teach them to follow the pattern these calls should take.

---

[202] Ibid., 33.
[203] Telesales. Dragos Iliescu. Accessed January 30, 2018. http://bookboon.com/en/telesales-ebook

*New Patients*

New patients want to be treated with kindness, feel the practice is qualified and will meet their needs, be treated in a desired period of time, and have the feeling that the charges will be manageable. Initial scripting should provide a warm hello, state the name of the practice and the mission, provide the staff member's name, and request the caller's name and possibly phone number in case of disconnection. Asking the phone number also starts the collection of demographic information, which initiates the process toward the patient booking an appointment.

*Existing Patients*

These patients want to feel special and remembered and to be able to book their desired appointment times. Being able to open their records within the practice's electronic medical record (EMR) and having one to two personal details about the patient is often helpful for the receptionist who answers the call. The opening of records immediately also lets the patient know that her records can be accessed quickly as well as making her wish to handle the matters of her call as quickly as possible.

*Rescheduling Patients*

Patients who reschedule are costly to a practice because, if the rescheduling is done at the last minute, their slots often cannot be filled and become nonrevenue-generating time slots. These patients should be advised that rescheduling should be avoided (1) in order to comply with a prescribed treatment plan for their pregnancy and because (2) the provider is also concerned and invested in the patient care and treatment plan. A possible response may be, "We usually ask for two business days prior to cancellations due to the fact that our calendar is very full, and other patients have been requesting appointments. Is there any way you can still make the appointment?" This type of phrasing notifies the patient that rescheduling is difficult due to the practice being particularly busy. If she still insists that she cannot make the appointment, then a follow-up appointment should be made at the time of cancellation.

An example of scripting for rescheduling at the time of cancellation is, "We understand urgent circumstances can occur, and we really don't want you to lose your progress in your care. If you can't come to your appointment, we might be able to fit you in later this week to make sure we keep going forward with your plan to help your pregnancy. Does Friday at one p.m. fit into your schedule?"

*Upset Patients*

Patients who are angry or upset want to be heard and listened to about their concerns. Making such patients feel that their concerns are being acknowledged may help them to decompress emotionally and act in a more rational manner. Sometimes telling the patient that you will research the matter and call her back will give her a time period to calm herself for future communications. Hence, these patients should be listened to without attempting to argue or interrupt them. Refrain from questioning the correctness of the patient at this time, even if she is obviously incorrect, and instead work to empathize and apologize. Your team members should also keep their composure and request the patient to offer a solution that the practice can provide. Again, it is not important to give in to the request if it is not possible or reasonable, but have the team assure the patient that your practice will research the problem further and will contact the patient again.

## Conclusion

Phone service is an underappreciated means of showcasing your practice and providing a superior customer experience. Obtaining data on your current situation, providing a proper system infrastructure, and choosing a proper team are important factors in providing an improved and efficient means of communication with your patients. Thereafter, preparing your staff with responses to specific common scenarios will decrease the likelihood of experiencing unpleasant interactions at stressful times, which will invariably present themselves on occasion. Building this infrastructure with proper equipment and using a motivated team approach will give your practice an increased likelihood of success.

# Appendix 1

## Miscellaneous Employee Forms and Employee Manual

Note: prior to using any of the forms listed in appendices 1–3, the user should verify if the form meets the legal requirements for the place of utilization (e.g., an MFM practice). The authors and editors take no responsibility for validity and legal usage in the place of utilization. The usage of these forms is done at the user's own and sole discretion.

# Central Business Office

## End-of-Day Reconciliation

1. Put encounter forms in sequential order.
2. Document missing encounter forms.
3. Run tape to include charges and payments.
4. Run system-applicable daily activity summary (worksheets).
5. Compare totals from system report to manual tape totals.

   If totals are the same, then business-day activity has been successfully reconciled.
   If totals do not match, rerun tape.
   If still out of balance, then utilize daily account summary and check for activity from each encounter form.
   Once balanced, print bank deposit off system.
   Print batch posting journal off system.

At end of day, a copy of the day-end balancing worksheet, encounter forms, and copy of system-generated bank deposit should be filed by date. The system-generated batch posting journal is then sent to the central billing office with validated deposit slip attached, along with daily activity sheet.

Bank deposits are to be made daily.

# Disciplinary Action Form

Employee: _____  Date: _____

| Action Taken:<br><br>☐ Verbal warning<br>☐ Written warning<br>☐ Suspension<br>☐ Termination | Type of violation:<br><br>Date(s) of violation: |
|---|---|

Description of event/incident:




Previous related incidents:




Plan of action (to include goals/objectives, measurements to be taken to improve behavior/performance, time frames, etc.):




Supervisor/Manager Signature: _____  Date: _____

I have read this statement and have been given the opportunity to comment. My signature acknowledges only that I have received a copy of this statement.

_____  _____

Employee Signature                Date

_____  _____

Witness Signature (if applicable)  Date

**Employee Confidentiality Statement**

I agree to respect and maintain the confidentiality of all discussions, deliberations, records, and other information generated in connection with the _____. I agree to make no voluntary disclosures of such information, except to persons authorized to receive it in the course of business affairs.

Furthermore, my participation in business operations is in reliance on the belief that every other member of the staff will similarly preserve the confidentiality of these activities. I understand that the _____and staff are entitled to undertake such action as deemed appropriate to ensure that this confidentiality is maintained, including action necessitated by any breach, or threatened breach, of this agreement.

_____          _____
Printed Name                                                                       Date


_____
Signature

# Business Relations

## Nature of Employment

Your relationship with **[Practice Name Here]** is that of an employee-at-will. Your job status does not guarantee employment for any specific length of time. Your employment with **[Practice Name Here]** is entered into voluntarily, and both you and **[Practice Name Here]** are free to end the employment relationship at any time, for any reason, with or without cause or advance notice. Your employment-at-will status with **[Practice Name Here]** may be altered only with specific, written authorization by the Officers. Nothing in this Employee Handbook should be construed as a contractual agreement, right to or promise of any specific employment period, or of any other term, condition, or benefit of employment. All policies and procedures in this handbook may be altered or revoked without prior notice, at the sole discretion of **[Practice Name Here]**, and should not be relied upon by the employee as an entitlement to any substantive or procedural matter.

## Employee Relations

**[Practice Name Here]** believes that the work conditions, wages, and benefits it offers to its employees are competitive with those offered by other employers in the medical community. Should any employee have concerns about work conditions or compensation, the employee is strongly encouraged to voice these concerns openly and directly to management.

Our experience has shown that when employees deal openly and directly with supervisors and management, the work environment can be excellent, communication can be clear, and attitudes can be positive. We believe that **[Practice Name Here]** amply demonstrates its commitment to its employees by responding effectively to employee concerns.

## Employment Categories

Each employee is designated as either hourly or salary for federal and state wage and hour laws. Hourly employees are entitled to overtime pay under the specific provisions of federal and state laws. Salary employees are excluded from specific provisions of federal and state wage and hour laws. An employee's compensation classification may be changed upon written notice by management.

Temporary employees are those who are hired as interim replacements to temporarily supplement the workforce or to assist in the completion of a specific project. Employment assignments in this category are of limited duration. Employment beyond any initially stated period does not in any way imply a change in employment status. Temporary employees retain that status unless and until notified of a change. While temporary employees receive all legally mandated benefits such as workers' compensation insurance and Social Security, they are ineligible for all of **[Practice Name Here]**'s other benefit programs.

Part-time employees are those who are assigned to a position and specific responsibilities. These employees work continuously for a specified number of hours per week, which is less than a regular schedule of thirty hours per week. All part-time employees receive all legally mandated benefits such as Social Security along with all of **[Practice Name Here]**'s other benefit programs.

Full-time employees are those who are not in a temporary status and who are regularly scheduled to work at **[Practice Name Here]** for a minimum of thirty hours per week. Generally, full-time employees are eligible for **[Practice Name Here]**'s benefit package, subject to the terms, conditions, and limitations of each benefit program after a minimum ninety-day on-the-job training program.

**Equal Employment Opportunity**

In order to provide equal employment and advancement opportunities to all individuals, employment decisions at **[Practice Name Here]** will be based on merit, qualifications, and abilities. **[Practice Name Here]** is an equal opportunity employer and does not discriminate against any person because of race, color, creed, religion, sex, national origin, disability, age, or any other characteristic protected by law, to the extent required by applicable law. This nondiscrimination policy extends to all terms, conditions, and privileges of employment as well as to the use of all company facilities, participation in all company-sponsored activities, and all employment actions such as promotions, compensation, benefits, and termination of employment.

**[Practice Name Here]** will make reasonable accommodations for qualified individuals with known disabilities unless doing so would result in undue hardship. This policy governs all aspects of employment, including selection, job assignment, compensation, discipline, termination, and access to benefits and training.

Any employee with questions or concerns about any type of discrimination or other personnel issue in the workplace is encouraged to bring these issues to the immediate attention of his or her supervisor, office manager, or chief physician. Employees can raise concerns and make reports without fear of reprisal. Anyone found to be engaging in any type of unlawful discrimination will be subject to disciplinary action, up to and including termination of employment.

## Compliance and Conduct

**Business Ethics and Conduct**

The successful business operation and reputation of [**Practice Name Here**] is built upon the principles of fair dealing and ethical conduct of our employees. Our reputation for integrity and excellence requires careful observance of the spirit and letter of all applicable laws and regulations, as well as a scrupulous regard for the highest standards of conduct and personal integrity.

The continued success of [**Practice Name Here**] is dependent upon our patients' trust, and we are dedicated to preserving that trust. Employees owe a duty to [**Practice Name Here**] and its patients and shareholders to act in a way that merits the continued trust and confidence of the public.

[**Practice Name Here**] will comply with all applicable laws and regulations and expects its directors, officers, and employees to conduct business in accordance with the letter, spirit, and intent of all relevant laws and to refrain from any illegal, dishonest, or unethical conduct.

In general, the use of good judgment, based on high ethical principles, will guide you with respect to lines of acceptable conduct. If a situation arises where it is difficult to determine the proper course of action, the matter should be discussed openly with your immediate supervisor for advice and consultation.

All employees are expected to perform their assigned responsibilities during normal business hours. [**Practice Name Here**] expects each employee to cooperate with other employees and treat other employees with respect. Any employee having a conflict with another employee is required to address the matter directly and professionally to the other employee. [**Practice Name Here**] will not tolerate gossip of any sort among coworkers, as this causes distractions and affects morale. If an issue arises and cannot be resolved among the parties involved, then the matter shall immediately be brought to the attention of the immediate supervisor.

Compliance with this policy of business ethics and conduct is the responsibility of every [**Practice Name Here**] employee. Disregarding or failing to comply with this standard of business ethics and conduct could lead to disciplinary action, up to and including possible termination of employment.

**Employee Conduct and Work Rules**

To ensure orderly operations and provide the best possible work environment, [**Practice Name Here**] expects employees to follow rules of conduct that will protect the interests and safety of all employees and the organization.

It is not possible to list all the forms of behavior that are considered unacceptable in the workplace. The following are examples of infractions of rules of conduct that may result in disciplinary action, up to and including termination of employment:

- Supplying false or misleading information when applying for employment or during employment
- Personal use of company credit card or extension of terms and credit
- Theft or inappropriate removal or possession of property
- Falsification of timekeeping records
- Working under the influence of alcohol or illegal drugs
- Possession, distribution, sale, transfer, or use of alcohol or illegal drugs or abuse of prescription drugs in the workplace while on duty or while operating company-owned equipment
- Failure or refusal to submit or consent to a required alcohol or drug test
- Fighting or threatening behavior in the workplace
- Boisterous or disruptive activity in the workplace

- Negligence or improper conduct leading to damage of company property or any other property on company premises
- Insubordination or other disrespectful conduct
- Engaging in unethical or illegal conduct
- Having a conflict of interest
- Violation of safety rules, health rules, and HIPAA (Health Insurance Portability and Accountability Act) policies
- Smoking in prohibited areas
- Sexual or other unlawful or unwelcome harassment
- Possession of dangerous or unauthorized materials, such as explosives or firearms, in the workplace
- Excessive absenteeism or tardiness or any absence without notice
- Unauthorized use of telephones, mail system, or other equipment
- Conduct that reflects adversely upon you or [**Practice Name Here**]
- Making or publishing a false or malicious statement concerning a physician, employee, patient, supplier, contract laborer, or [**Practice Name Here's**] violation-of-personnel policies
- Unsatisfactory performance or conduct that does not meet the requirements of the position
- Other circumstances that warrant discipline

Nothing in this policy requires [**Practice Name Here**] to follow any certain type or number of steps in the disciplining or termination of its employees. Each situation must be considered on its own facts and circumstances in order for [**Practice Name Here**] to determine the appropriate measures to be taken, including termination without prior warning, disciplinary action, or notice. Either [**Practice Name Here**] or the employee may terminate the relationship at any time with or without advance notice.

## Use of Phone and Mail Systems

Personal use of the telephone for long-distance and toll calls is not permitted. Employees are required to practice discretion when making local personal calls. Employee cell phones must be silenced within the office during office hours, and calls must be taken out of sight of the patients. The use of [**Practice Name Here's**] paid postage for personal correspondence is not permitted.

## Computer and E-Mail Usage

Computers, computer files, the e-mail system, and software furnished to the employees are property of [**Practice Name Here**] and are intended for business use only. Employees should not use a password, access a file, or retrieve any stored communication without authorization. While computer and e-mail use are intended for job-related activities, incidental and occasional brief personal use is permitted within reasonable limits, as determined by the sole discretion of [**Practice Name Here**]. To ensure compliance with this policy, computer and e-mail usage may be monitored by [**Practice Name Here**] without prior notice or consent. Employees have no right or expectation of privacy in any computer or e-mail usage occurring through or on [**Practice Name Here**] computers or e-mail systems or accounts, even if it is the employee's own personal e-mail or other account being accessed.

[**Practice Name Here**] strives to maintain a workplace free of harassment and is sensitive to the diversity of its employees. Therefore, [**Practice Name Here**] prohibits the use of computers and e-mail in ways that are disruptive, offensive to others, or harmful to morale. For example, the display or transmission of sexually explicit images, messages, and/or cartoons is not allowed. Other such misuse includes, but is not limited to, ethnic slurs, racial comments, off-color jokes, or anything else that may be construed as harassment or as showing disrespect to others.

E-mail may not be used to solicit others for commercial ventures, religious or political causes, outside organizations, or other nonbusiness matters.

[**Practice Name Here**] purchases and licenses the use of various types of computer software for business purposes and does not own the copyrights to this software or related documentation. Unless authorized by the software developer, [**Practice Name Here**] does not have the right to reproduce such software for use on more than one computer.

Employees may only use software on local area networks (LANs) or on multiple machines according to the software license agreement. [**Practice Name Here**] prohibits the illegal duplication of software and its related documentation.

Employees should notify management immediately upon learning of any violations of this policy. Employees who violate this policy will be subject to disciplinary action, up to and including termination of employment.

**Internet and Other Communications/Electronic Devices Usage**

Internet access to global electronic information resources is provided by [**Practice Name Here**] to assist employees in obtaining work-related data and claims filing. The following guidelines have been established to help ensure responsible and productive Internet usage. While Internet and other company-provided communications/electronic devices are intended for job-related activities, incidental and occasional brief personal use is permitted within reasonable limits, as determined by the sole discretion of [**Practice Name Here**]. To the extent that the Internet is accessed through computers, computer files, e-mail systems, and software furnished to the employees—all of which are property of [**Practice Name Here**] and are intended for business use—employees should be aware that their Internet usage may be monitored by [**Practice Name Here**] without prior notice or consent. Employees have no right to or expectation of privacy in any Internet usage occurring through or on [**Practice Name Here**] computers or e-mail systems or accounts, even if it is the employee's own personal e-mail or other account being accessed. To the extent that [**Practice Name Here**] provides employees with any electronic or communications devices, or pays for any portion of the use of such devices (including pagers or cell phones), this policy applies to the company's monitoring of and the employee's use of such devices.

All Internet data that is composed, transmitted, or received via our computer communications systems is considered to be part of the official records of [**Practice Name Here**] and, as such, is subject to disclosure of law enforcement or other third parties. Consequently, employees should always ensure that the business information contained in Internet e-mail messages, and other transmissions is accurate, appropriate, ethical, and lawful.

The equipment, services, and technology provided to access the Internet remain at all times the property of [**Practice Name Here**]. As such, [**Practice Name Here**] reserves the right to monitor Internet traffic and to retrieve and read any data composed, sent, or received through our online connections and stored in our computer systems.

Data that is composed, transmitted, accessed, or received via the Internet must not contain content that could be considered discriminatory, offensive, obscene, threatening, harassing, intimidating, or disruptive to any employee or other person. Examples of unacceptable content may include, but are not limited to, sexual comments or images, racial slurs, gender-specific comments, or any other comments or images that could reasonably offend someone on the basis of race, age, sex, religious or political beliefs, national origin, disability, sexual orientation, or any other characteristic protected by law.

Abuse of the Internet access provided by [**Practice Name Here**] in violation of law or [**Practice Name Here's**] policies will result in disciplinary action, up to and including termination of employment. Employees may also be held personally liable for any violations of this policy. The following behaviors are examples of previously stated or additional actions and activities that are prohibited and can result in disciplinary action:

- Sending and posting disciplinary, harassing, or threatening messages or images
- Using the organization's time and resources for personal gain
- Stealing, using, or disclosing someone else's code or password without authorization
- Copying, pirating, or downloading software and electronic files without permission

- Sending and posting confidential material, trade secrets, or proprietary information outside of the organization
- Violating copyright law
- Failing to observe licensing agreements
- Engaging in unauthorized transactions that may incur a cost to the organization or initiate unwanted Internet services and transmissions
- Sending or posting messages or material that could result in damage to the organization's image or reputation
- Participating in the viewing or exchange of pornography or other obscene materials
- Sending or posting messages that defame or slander other individuals
- Attempting to break into the computer system of another organization or person
- Refusing to coordinate with a security investigation
- Sending or posting chain letters, solicitations, or advertisements not related to business purposes or activities
- Using the Internet for political causes or activities, religious activities, or any sort of gambling
- Jeopardizing the security of the organization's electronic communications systems
- Sending and posting messages that disparage another organization's products or services
- Sending anonymous e-mail messages
- Engaging in any other illegal activities

## Workplace Monitoring

Workplace monitoring may be conducted by [**Practice Name Here**] to ensure quality control, employee safety, general security, and customer satisfaction.

While on [**Practice Name Here**]'s premises, employees have no expectation of privacy in their belongings or in the nonprivate workplace areas, which include, but are not limited to, offices, work locations, company-provided designated parking areas, desks, computers, rest and eating areas, and any other belongings on or in any of the above.

Employees who regularly communicate via the telephone may have their conversations monitored or recorded. Telephone monitoring is used to identify and correct performance problems through targeted training. Improved job performance enhances our customers' image of [**Practice Name Here**] as well as their satisfaction with our services.

Computers furnished to employees are the property of [**Practice Name Here**]. As such, computer usage and files, including e-mail usage and related files, are also the property of [**Practice Name Here**] and may be monitored or accessed at any time with or without acknowledgment from the employee.

[**Practice Name Here**] may conduct video surveillance of any nonprivate workplace areas. Video monitoring is used to identify safety concerns, maintain quality control, detect theft and misconduct, and discourage or prevent acts of harassment and workplace violence.

Because [**Practice Name Here**] is sensitive to the legitimate privacy rights of employees, every effort will be made to conduct workplace monitoring in an ethical and respectful manner.

## Immigration Law Compliance

[**Practice Name Here**] is committed to employing only US citizens as well as aliens who are authorized to work in the United States, and we do not unlawfully discriminate on the basis of citizenship or national origin.

In compliance with the Immigration Reform and Control Act of 1986, each new employee, as a condition of employment, must complete the Employment Eligibility Verification Form I-9 and present documentation establishing identity and employment eligibility. Former employees who are rehired must also complete the form.

**Disability Accommodations**

**[Practice Name Here]** is committed to complying fully with the Americans with Disabilities Act (ADA) and applicable state law as well as to ensuring equal opportunity in employment for qualified persons with disabilities, to the extent required by law. All employment practices and activities are conducted on a nondiscriminatory basis.

Hiring procedures are designed to provide persons with disabilities meaningful employment opportunities. Preemployment inquiries are made only regarding an applicant's ability to perform the duties of the position.

Reasonable accommodations for qualified individuals with known disabilities will be made unless to do so would be an undue hardship. All employment decisions are based on the merits of the situation in accordance with defined criteria, not the disability of the individual.

# Confidentiality

**Nondisclosure**

The protection of confidential business and personal information is vital to the interests and the success of [**Practice Name Here**]. All employees of [**Practice Name Here**] must respect the confidences placed upon them. The relationship between [**Practice Name Here**] and each patient demands that no disclosure of information occur without proper authorization.

Under no circumstances will confidential matters concerning patients, employees/coworkers, physicians, or other business matters be discussed with outsiders or friends. Such confidential information includes, but is not limited to, the following examples:

- Patient names and medical and financial information
- Patient lists
- Company/employee financial information
- Proprietary processes
- Personal employee/physician information
- Financial information
- Marketing materials
- Business forms

No employee will be allowed or knowingly allow others to deliberately falsify, alter, destroy, or remove company reports or records without prior approval of the relevant authorized official. Each employee shall immediately report to a supervisor any unauthorized disclosure or publication of such information by another employee.

All employees are required to sign a nondisclosure agreement (NDA) as a condition of employment. Employees who improperly use and disclose of confidential business information will be subject to disciplinary action, up to and including termination of employment, even if they do not actually benefit from the disclosed information.

**Access to Personnel Files**

[**Practice Name Here**] maintains a personnel file on each employee. The personnel file includes such information as the employee's résumé, data sheet, records of training, documentation of performance, compensation information, and any other information pertaining to the employee.

Personnel files are the property of [**Practice Name Here**], and access to the information they contain is restricted. Only management and physician partners will have access to this information.

**Personnel Data Changes**

It is the responsibility of each employee to properly notify [**Practice Name Here**] of any changes in personnel data. It is required by law that personal information—including mailing address (no PO boxes are allowed), telephone numbers, names of dependents, emergency contacts, educational accomplishments, and any other such changes—are to be accurate and current at all times. If any personnel data has changed, notify management in writing as soon as possible.

## HIPAA

**[Practice Name Here]** intends to fully comply with the requirements of the Health Insurance Portability and Accountability Act (HIPAA) and any amendments or related provisions. All employees are expected to become familiar with the policies and procedures adopted to comply with these requirements as well as to safeguard the privacy of patient and employee information. Sensitive or confidential information should not be discussed, disclosed, or used except as necessary to perform the functions of the employee's job, as permissible under HIPAA. If an employee is in doubt as to measures to be taken to comply with HIPAA or believes that a breach of HIPAA has occurred (or may occur), the employee should immediately contact the office manager.

# Employment

## Introductory Period

The introductory period is intended to give new employees the opportunity to demonstrate their ability to achieve a satisfactory level of performance and to determine whether the new position meets their expectations. **[Practice Name Here]** uses this time period to evaluate employee capabilities, work habits, personal character, and overall performance. Either the employee or **[Practice Name Here]** may end the employment relationship at will at any time during or after the introductory period, with or without cause or advance notice.

All new and rehired employees begin on a ninety-calendar-day trial period. All benefits are effective on the first day of the month following the completion of the introductory period. If **[Practice Name Here]** determines that the designated introductory period does not allow sufficient time to thoroughly evaluate the employee's performance, the introductory period may be extended for a specified period.

## Performance Evaluations

A formal written performance evaluation may be conducted at the end of the ninety days of employment. Additional formal performance evaluations will be conducted to provide both management and employees the opportunity to discuss job tasks, identify and correct weaknesses, encourage and recognize strengths, and discuss positive, purposeful approaches for meeting goals.

Performance evaluations are scheduled approximately every twelve months, coinciding generally with the anniversary of the employee's date of hire. **[Practice Name Here]** may amend this schedule at its discretion.

Merit-based pay adjustments may be awarded by **[Practice Name Here]** in an effort to recognize truly superior employee performance. The decision to award such an adjustment is dependent upon numerous factors, including the information documented by this formal performance evaluation process.

## Work Schedules

Work schedules for employees vary throughout our organization. Management will advise employees of their individual work schedules. Staffing needs and operational demands may necessitate variations in starting and ending times, as well as variations in the total hours that may be scheduled each day and week.

Company policy mandates that employees will be prepared and ready to work at their required start times. Chronic variations in an individual's required start and stop times will result in disciplinary action and may result in a reduction of benefits.

## Attendance and Punctuality

To maintain a safe and productive work environment, **[Practice Name Here]** expects employees to be reliable and to be punctual in reporting for scheduled work. Employees are also expected to take their lunch/mealtimes within the time limits previously set. Absenteeism and tardiness place a burden on other employees and on **[Practice Name Here]**. In the rare instances when employees cannot avoid being late to work or are unable to work as scheduled, they should notify their team members and management as soon as possible in advance of the anticipated tardiness or absence.

Poor attendance and excessive tardiness are disruptive. Either may lead to disciplinary action, up to and including termination of employment.

## Timekeeping

Accurately recording time worked is the responsibility of every employee. Federal and state laws require [**Practice Name Here**] to keep an accurate record of time worked in order to calculate employee pay and benefits. Time worked is all the time actually spent on the job performing one's assigned duties.

Employees are required to accurately record the time they begin and end their work, as well as the beginning and ending time of each meal period, by utilizing the time clock. Employees must also record, by use of the time clock, any split shifts or departures from work for personal reasons. Time records must accurately reflect all absences, late arrivals, early departures, meal breaks, and regular and overtime hours worked. Employees are prohibited from performing any off-the-clock work, which refers to work they may perform but fail to report. Overtime work must always be approved in writing by management **before** it is performed, except in an emergency situation.

Any employee who fails to report or inaccurately reports any hours worked is in violation of company policy. Altering, falsifying, or tampering with time records or recording time on another employee's time record will also result in disciplinary action, up to and including termination of employment. It is the employee's responsibility to sign his or her time records to certify the accuracy of all time recorded.

If an employee is required to travel from the office to another facility in order to perform work duties, that travel time will be counted as work time to the extent required by law. Any lunch period provided to the employee during the time away from the office will be counted as nonworking time, and the employee will be allowed to use that time as he or she wishes, as provided in the Meal Periods policy discussed below.

## Meal Periods

All full-time employees are provided with a one-hour meal period each workday. Management will determine meal periods to best accommodate operating requirements. Employees will be relieved of all active responsibilities and restrictions during meal periods and will not be compensated for that time.

## Overtime

When operating requirements or other needs cannot be met during regular working hours, employees may be scheduled to work overtime hours. When possible, advance notification of these assignments will be provided. All overtime work must receive **prior** written approval from management, except in an emergency situation. Overtime assignments will be distributed as equitably as is practical to all employees who are qualified to perform the required work.

## Paydays

All employees are paid biweekly on Fridays. Each paycheck will include earnings for the prior payroll period. The timeliness of payroll processing begins three business days prior to the actual pay date. If any unforeseen changes in compensation happen within this three-day period, adjustments will be made to the next pay period.

If a payday falls during an employee's paid-time-off period, the employee's paycheck will be made available through his or her elected method of receiving compensation.

Employees may have pay directly deposited into their bank accounts if they provide advance written authorization to [**Practice Name Here**]. Employees will receive an itemized statement of wages when [**Practice Name Here**] makes direct deposits.

## Pay Deductions

The law requires that [**Practice Name Here**] make certain deductions from every employee's compensation; among these deductions are applicable federal, state, and local income taxes. [**Practice Name Here**] also must deduct Social

Security taxes on each employee's earnings up to a specified limit, which is called the Social Security "wage base." **[Practice Name Here]** matches the amount of Social Security taxes paid by each employee.

**[Practice Name Here]** has the right, absent state or federal law to the contrary, to deduct or withhold an employee's pay for the following circumstances:

- Employee is absent and has exhausted all accrued time off.
- Employee has not yet accrued sufficient time off.
- Full-day disciplinary suspensions are enacted for infractions of written policies and procedures.
- Amounts received as payment for jury and witness fees or military pay must be offset.

**[Practice Name Here]** offers programs and benefits beyond those required by law. Eligible employees may voluntarily authorize deductions from their paychecks to cover the costs of participation in these programs. If an employee has any questions concerning why deductions were made from his or her paycheck or how the deductions were calculated, management can assist in answering any questions.

Employee pay **will not** be reduced for any of the following reasons:

- Absences for jury duty, attendance as a witness, or military leave in any week in which an employee has performed any work
- Any other deductions prohibited by state and federal law

*Please note* that it is not an improper deduction to reduce an employee's accrued paid time-off bank for full- or partial-day absences for unforeseen/unplanned personal reasons (including tardiness and early release).

**Administrative Pay Corrections**

It is the practice and policy of **[Practice Name Here]** to accurately compensate employees and to do so in compliance with all applicable state and federal laws. Every effort is made to ensure that our employees are paid correctly.

Every employee must maintain a record of the total hours worked each day. In the unlikely event that an error occurs in the amount of pay, the employee should promptly bring the discrepancy to the attention of management so that corrections can be made as quickly as possible.

# Dress Code

**Personal Appearance and Dress Code**

Dress, grooming, and personal cleanliness standards contribute to the morale of all employees and affect the business image [**Practice Name Here**] presents to patients and visitors.

During business hours or when representing [**Practice Name Here**], you are expected to present a clean, neat, and tasteful appearance. You should dress and groom yourself according to the requirements of your position and accepted business standards. This is particularly true if your position involves dealing directly with patients, families, and visitors in person.

If management feels your personal appearance is inappropriate, you may be asked to leave the workplace until you can return properly dressed or groomed. Under such circumstances, you will not be compensated for the time away from work.

While we do not wish to unduly restrict individual tastes, employees should follow these personal appearance guidelines:

- Authorized scrubs **must** be clean and pressed.
- Shoes must provide safe, secure footing and offer protection against hazards.
- Canvas or athletic-type shoes are not appropriate professional attire unless they are worn with the authorized scrubs.
- Spaghetti strap–style tank tops or halter tops may not be worn under any circumstances.
- Facial hair must be clean, well trimmed, and neat.
- Hairstyles are expected to be in good professional taste.
- Unnaturally colored hair and extreme hairstyles, such as spiked hair, do not present an appropriate professional appearance.
- Offensive body odor and poor personal hygiene are not professionally acceptable.
- Perfume, cologne, and aftershave lotions should be used moderately or avoided altogether, as some individuals (employees and/or patients) may be sensitive to strong fragrances.
- Jewelry should not be functionally restrictive, dangerous to job performance, or excessive.
- Facial jewelry, such as eyebrow rings, nose rings, lip rings, and tongue studs, are not professionally appropriate and may not be worn during business hours.
- Torso body jewelry that can be seen through or under clothing must not be worn during business hours.
- Visible tattoos and similar body art must be covered during business hours.
- Graphic or white T-shirts are not permitted.
- Clothing with brand-name graphics is not permitted.
- Torn or frayed clothing is prohibited.
- Jogging suits, sweat suits, and sweatshirts are prohibited.
- Extremely baggy clothing or clothing that is too tight, including but not limited to Lycra and spandex, is prohibited.
- Undergarments are meant to be kept under your clothes; revealing attire or visibility of undergarments is prohibited.
- Flip-flops or flip-flop-style platform shoes are prohibited.
- Shorts and miniskirts are prohibited. Capri pants must be below the calf.
- Open-toe sandals are permitted for nonclinical staff. Toenails must be clean and manicured, and if polish is present, it must not be chipped.
- Chipped fingernail and/or toenail polish is prohibited.
- Hats and baseball caps are prohibited during business hours and/or while patients are present.

For clinical positions, clean, wrinkle-free, matching scrubs with close-toed protective footwear is required.

# Employment Benefits

## Employee Benefits

Eligible employees at [**Practice Name Here**] are provided with a wide range of benefits. Benefit eligibility is dependent upon a variety of factors, including employee's classifications.

The following benefit programs are available to eligible employees:

- Medical insurance
- COBRA (Consolidated Omnibus Budget Reconciliation Act)
- Life insurance
- Workers' compensation insurance
- Paid time off
- 401(k) savings plan with matching contribution
- Direct deposit
- Holiday pay

## Medical Insurance

All full-time employees—those who are not in a temporary status and who are regularly scheduled to work at [**Practice Name Here**] for a minimum of thirty hours per week—are eligible for medical insurance. Please discuss this benefit with management for current detailed information.

## Benefits Continuation (COBRA)

The federal Consolidated Omnibus Budget Reconciliation Act (COBRA) gives employees and their qualified beneficiaries the opportunity to continue health-insurance coverage under [**Practice Name Here's**] health plan when a "qualifying event" would normally result in the loss of eligibility. Some common qualifying events include resignation, termination of employment, death of an employee, reduction in an employee's hours, employee leave of absence, employee divorce or legal separation, and a dependent child no longer meeting eligibility requirements.

Under COBRA, the employee or beneficiary pays the full cost of coverage at [**Practice Name Here's**] group rate plus an administration fee. [**Practice Name Here**] provides each eligible employee with a written notice describing the rights granted under COBRA when the employee becomes eligible for coverage under [**Practice Name Here's**] health-insurance plan.

## Life Insurance

All full-time employees—those who are not in a temporary status and who are regularly scheduled to work at [**Practice Name Here**] for a minimum of thirty hours per week—are eligible for life insurance. Please discuss this benefit with management for current detailed information.

## 401(k)

All full-time employees of [**Practice Name Here**] who have been continuously employed for one full year are eligible for the 401(k). Please discuss this benefit with management for current detailed information.

**Time Off**

**Paid Time Off Benefits**

Paid time off (PTO) is available to eligible employees to provide opportunities for rest, relaxation, and personal pursuits. Full-time employees (minimum of thirty hours per workweek) will receive eleven days per calendar year of paid time off. Only full-time employees are eligible for paid time off. Paid time off will be acquired at a rate of **[fill in rate, e.g., 0.917]** days per month or **[fill in rate, e.g., 0.458]** days per biweekly pay period. After the completion of five years of continuous full-time employment, employees will receive an additional five days of paid time off per calendar year, for a total of twenty days per calendar year.

Paid time off can be used in minimum increments of one-half days. To take paid time off, employees should make written requests at least three weeks prior for advance approval. Four weeks' advance notice is encouraged when requested paid time off will be attached to a paid holiday. Requests will be reviewed and approved based on a number of factors, including business needs and staffing requirements.

Time off is paid at the employee's base pay rate at the time of usage for the amount of hours absent. Payment in lieu of accrued time off is not allowed. Maximum carryover of unused paid time off is forty hours per calendar year end. In the event that available paid time off is not used by the end of the calendar year, employees will forfeit the unused time they have acquired over forty hours. Employees are not entitled to and will not be paid for accrued, unused paid time off at the time an employee separates from employment.

**Holidays**

**[Practice Name Here]** will grant holiday paid time off to all full-time employees on the holidays listed below:

- New Year's Day (January 1)
- Memorial Day (last Monday in May)
- Independence Day (July 4)
- Labor Day (first Monday in September)
- Thanksgiving (fourth Thursday in November)
- Day after Thanksgiving
- Christmas Eve (December 24)
- Christmas Day (December 25)

Employees who have completed ninety calendar days of full-time service will be compensated. Holiday pay will be calculated based on the employee's straight-time pay rate (as of the date of the holiday) times the number of hours the employee would otherwise have worked on that day.

If a recognized holiday falls during an eligible employee's paid absence (such as during paid time off), holiday pay will be provided instead of the paid time off benefit that otherwise would have applied.

**Sick Time**

Employees who are unable to report to work due to illness or injury should notify the office manager **before** the scheduled start of their work day. If an employee is absent for illness or injury for more than two business days, a physician's statement must be provided verifying the disability and its beginning and expected ending dates. Any time off due to illness or injury will be deducted from earned paid time off.

**Bereavement Leave**

All employees who wish to take time off due to the death of a family member should notify management immediately. Bereavement leave will be provided to eligible full-time employees at the rates listed below:

- Immediate family: three days (spouse, child, mother, father, sibling)
- Extended family: one day (employee's grandparent, grandchild)

Bereavement pay is calculated based on the base pay rate at the time of the absence. Employees may, with management approval, use any available acquired paid time off for additional days off.

**Military Leave**

A military leave of absence will be granted to employees who are absent from work because of service in the US uniformed services in accordance with the Uniformed Services Employment and Reemployment Rights Act (USERRA). Advance notice of military service is required, unless military necessity prevents such notice, or it is otherwise impossible or unreasonable to do so.

Although the leave will be unpaid, employees may use any available paid time off during their absence.

Continuation of health-insurance benefits is available as required by The Uniformed Services Employment and Reemployment Rights Act of 1994 (USERRA) based on the length of the leave and subject to the terms, conditions, and limitations of the applicable plans for which the employee is otherwise eligible.

Benefit accruals, such as paid time off and holiday benefits, will be suspended during the leave and will resume upon the employee's return to active employment.

Employees returning from military leave will be placed in the position they would have attained had they remained continuously employed or a comparable one, depending on the length of military service and in accordance with USERRA. Such employees will be treated as though they had been continuously employed for the purposes of determining benefits based on length of service.

**Limitations on Leaves of Absence**

Should an employee who has not accrued sufficient PTO or has exhausted all of his or her PTO continue to require or request time off, that employee will be subject to leave without pay (for all or part of the leave) or termination from employment. [**Practice Name Here**] will consider the circumstances and exercise its discretion in addressing such situations. Any employee who is allowed leave without pay in such circumstances is subject to termination at any time, at the discretion of [**Practice Name Here**], and in no circumstances will an employee be permitted to take more than eight weeks of leave without pay. This policy is subject to any local, state, or federal law that requires otherwise.

# Safety

**Safety**
Effective: **[Insert date here]**

Safety and Loss Control / OSHA Compliance Officer: _____

**[Practice Name Here]** is dedicated to providing a safe and healthy environment for its employees, patients, and visitors. To assist in providing a safe and healthful environment, **[Practice Name Here]** has established a workplace safety program. This program is a top priority for **[Practice Name Here]**. The Safety and Loss / OSHA (Occupational Safety and Health Administration) Compliance Officer (henceforth "the Compliance Officer") is responsible for implementing, administering, monitoring, and evaluating the safety program. Its success depends on the alertness and personal commitment of all.

**[Practice Name Here]** provides information to employees about workplace safety and health issues through regular internal communication channels such as management-employee meetings, bulletin board postings, memos, or other written communications.

Some of the best safety improvement ideas come from the employees. Those with ideas, concerns, or suggestions for improved safety in the workplace are encouraged to bring them to the attention of the Compliance Officer. Reports and concerns about workplace safety issues may be made anonymously if the employee wishes. All reports can be made without fear of reprisal.

Each employee is expected to obey safety rules and to exercise caution during all work activities. Employees must comply with all occupational safety and health standards and regulations established by OSHA and state and local regulations. Employees must immediately report any unsafe conditions to the Compliance Officer and/or management. Employees who violate safety standards, who cause hazardous or dangerous situations, or who fail to report or remedy such situations, where appropriate, may be subject to disciplinary action, up to and including suspension and/or termination of employment.

If you believe that you are being exposed to a known or suspected hazard when working with toxic chemicals or substances, you have the right under the Hazardous Communications Law to know about such hazards though Material Safety Data Sheets (MSDSs). The Compliance Officer and management will review the MSDS with you. In addition, you will receive information about any hazardous substances you may come into contact with in the workplace. You will be protected against any disciplining or termination that results from exercising your employee rights under the law.

In the case of accidents that result in injury, regardless of how significant the injury may appear, employees should immediately notify the Compliance Officer or management. Such reports are necessary to comply with laws and to initiate insurance and workers' compensation benefits procedures.

**Smoking**

In keeping with **[Practice Name Here's]** intent to provide a safe and healthful work environment, smoking is prohibited throughout the workplace. This policy applies equally to all partners, employees, customers, and visitors.

**Visitors in the Workplace**

To provide the safety and security of employees and patients of **[Practice Name Here]**, only authorized visitors are allowed in the workplace. The restricting of unauthorized visitors helps to maintain safety standards, protects against theft, ensures equipment safety, protects confidentiality of information, safeguards employee welfare, and avoids potential distractions and disturbances.

All visitors must enter **[Practice Name Here]** through the main entrance. Authorized visitors will receive directions or be escorted to their destination. Employees are responsible for the conduct and safety of their visitors.

If an employee observes an unauthorized individual on **[Practice Name Here's]** premises, the employee should immediately notify the manager and direct the individual to the waiting area.

**Emergency Closing**

At times emergencies such as severe weather, fires, or power failures can disrupt company operations. In extreme cases, these circumstances may require the closing of a work facility.

When operations are officially closed due to emergency conditions, the time off from scheduled work will be paid.

In cases where an emergency closing is not authorized, employees who fail to report to work will not be paid for the time off. Employees may request to use accrued PTO during such times.

**Workplace Violence Prevention**

**[Practice Name Here]** is committed to preventing workplace violence and to maintaining a safe work environment. **[Practice Name Here]** has adopted the following guidelines to deal with intimidation, harassment, and/or other threats of (or actual) violence that may occur during business hours or on its premises.

All employees, including contract and temporary employees, should be treated with courtesy and respect at all times. Employees are expected to refrain from fighting, horseplay, or other conduct that may be dangerous to others. Firearms, weapons, and other dangerous or hazardous devices or substances are prohibited from the premises of **[Practice Name Here]**.

Conduct that threatens, intimidates, or coerces another employee, patient, customer, vendor, or other member of the public at any time, including during off-duty periods, will not be tolerated. This prohibition includes all acts of harassment, including harassment that is based on an individual's sex, race, age, or any other characteristic protected by federal, state, or local laws.

All threats of (or actual) violence, both direct and indirect, should be reported as soon as possible to a physician or manager. This includes threats by customers, vendors, solicitors, or other members of the public. When reporting a threat of violence, you must be as specific and detailed as possible.

All suspicious individuals or activities should also be reported as soon as possible to management. Do not place yourself in peril. If you see or hear a commotion or disturbance near or within your work area, do not try to intercede or see what is happening.

**[Practice Name Here]** will properly and thoroughly investigate all reports of, threats of, or actual violence and of any suspicious individuals or activities. The identity of the individual making a report will be protected as much as is practical. In order to maintain workplace safety and the integrity of an investigation, **[Practice Name Here]** may suspend employees, either with or without pay, pending investigation.

**Drug and Alcohol Use**

It is **[Practice Name Here's]** desire to provide a drug-free, healthful, and safe workplace. To promote this goal, employees are required to report to work in the appropriate mental and physical condition necessary to perform their jobs in a safe and satisfactory manner.

While on **[Practice Name Here's]** premises and while conducting business-related activities off **[Practice Name Here's]** premises, no employee may use, possess, distribute, sell, or be under the influence of alcohol or illegal drugs. The legal use of prescribed drugs is permitted on the job only if doing so does not impair an employee's ability to perform the essential functions of the job effectively and in a safe manner that will not endanger other individuals in the workplace.

If **[Practice Name Here]** has a Drug-Free Workplace Program or if you are in a position that requires drug testing under state or federal law, you will be subject to drug testing under certain circumstances according to applicable laws.

Violations of this policy may lead to disciplinary action, up to and including immediate termination of employment and/or required participation in a substance abuse rehabilitation or treatment program. Such violations may also have legal consequences.

**Sexual and Other Unlawful Harassment**

**[Practice Name Here]** is committed to providing a work environment that is free from all forms of discrimination and conduct that could be considered harassing, coercive, or disruptive, including sexual harassment. Actions, words, jokes, or comments based on an individual's sex, race, color, national origin, age, religion, disability, sexual orientation, or any other legally protected characteristic will not be tolerated.

Sexual harassment is defined as unwanted sexual advances or visual, verbal, or physical conduct of a sexual nature. This definition includes many forms of offensive behavior and includes gender-based harassment of a person of the same sex as the harasser. The following is a partial list of sexual harassment examples:

- Unwanted sexual advances
- Offering employment benefits in exchange for sexual favors
- Making or threatening reprisals after receiving a negative response to sexual advances
- Visual conduct that includes leering, making sexual gestures, or displaying sexually suggestive objects, pictures, cartoons, or posters
- Verbal conduct that includes making or using derogatory comments, epithets, slurs, or jokes
- Verbal sexual advances or propositions
- Verbal abuse of a sexual nature, graphic verbal commentaries about an individual's body, sexually degrading words used to describe an individual, or suggestive or obscene letters, notes, or invitations
- Physical conduct that includes touching, assaulting, or impeding or blocking movements, which may include the following:
    - Unwelcome sexual advances (either verbal or physical), requests for sexual favors, and/or other verbal or physical conduct of a sexual nature all constitute sexual harassment when submission to such conduct is made either explicitly or implicitly a term or condition of employment.
    - Any submission to or rejection of such conduct that is used as a basis for making employment decisions constitutes sexual harassment.
    - Conduct that has the purpose or effect of interfering with work performance or of creating an intimidating, hostile, or offensive environment constitutes sexual harassment.

If you experience harassment in the workplace, report it to your supervisor or the office manager immediately. If the supervisor or office manager is unavailable, or if you believe it would be inappropriate to contact either of those persons, then you should immediately contact the supervising physician. You can raise concerns or make reports without fear of reprisal or retaliation.

All allegations of sexual harassment and/or other unlawful harassment will be quickly and discreetly investigated. To the extent possible, your confidentiality and that of any witnesses and the alleged harasser will be protected against unnecessary disclosure. Communications will be made to others only on a limited, need-to-know basis.

# Discipline

**Employee Discipline**

This section is to help you understand what is expected of you with regard to proper behavior, performance, and personal conduct. The purpose of this policy is to state [**Practice Name Here's**] position on administering equitable and consistent discipline for unsatisfactory conduct in the workplace. By complying with these standards, you will help to maintain a positive, safe work environment for you and your colleagues.

To address those times when you have not lived up to the position's standards, we may provide you with counseling or written notification; we may terminate your employment if your conduct warrants it. We have the discretion to decide whether counseling, written notification, or immediate termination is appropriate. The best disciplinary measure is the one that does not have to be enforced and comes from good leadership and fair supervision at all employment levels.

[**Practice Name Here's**] own best interest lies in ensuring fair treatment of all employees and in making certain that all disciplinary action is taken to correct the problem, prevent recurrence, and prepare the employee for satisfactory service in the future.

Although employment with [**Practice Name Here**] is based on mutual consent, and both the employee and [**Practice Name Here**] have the right to terminate employment at will, with or without cause or advance notice, [**Practice Name Here**] may use progressive discipline at its discretion.

Disciplinary action may call for any of four steps—verbal warning, written warning, suspension with or without pay, or termination of employment—depending on the severity of the problem and the number of occurrences. There may be circumstances when one or more steps are bypassed, as determined at the discretion of [**Practice Name Here**].

[**Practice Name Here**] recognizes that certain types of employee problems are serious enough to justify either a suspension or termination of employment without going through the usual progressive disciplinary steps; in these cases, [**Practice Name Here**] reserves the right to unilaterally decide if some or all disciplinary steps should be bypassed. By using employee discipline, we hope that most employee problems can be corrected at an early stage, thus benefiting both the employee and [**Practice Name Here**].

**Resignation**

Resignation is a voluntary act initiated by the employee to terminate employment with [**Practice Name Here**]. Although advance notice is not required, [**Practice Name Here**] suggests at least two weeks' written resignation notice from all employees. Employees in direct provision of care may have longer resignation periods within their employment contracts.

**Return of Property**

Employees are responsible for any items issued to them by [**Practice Name Here**] or any items in their possession or control, such as the following:

- credit cards
- equipment
- identification badges
- keys
- manuals
- pagers
- written material
- software

All **[Practice Name Here]** property must be returned by employees on or before their last day of work. Where permitted by applicable laws, **[Practice Name Here]** may withhold from the employee's check or final paycheck the cost of any items that are not returned when required. **[Practice Name Here]** may also take all action deemed appropriate to cover or protect its property.

# Business Travel

**Business Travel Expenses**

[**Practice Name Here**] will reimburse employees for reasonable business travel expenses incurred while on assignments away from the normal work location. All business travel must be approved in advance by the management of [**Practice Name Here**].

Employees whose travel plans have been approved are responsible for making their own travel arrangements.

When approved, the actual costs of travel, meals, lodging, and other expenses directly related to accomplishing business travel objectives will be reimbursed by [**Practice Name Here**]. Employees are expected to limit expenses to reasonable amounts.

Expenses that generally will be reimbursed include the following:

- Airfare for travel in coach or economy class or the lowest available fare
- Car rental fees (only compact or midsize cars)
- Fares for shuttle or airport bus service, where available; costs of public transportation for other ground travel
- Taxi fares (only when no less expensive alternatives are available)
- Mileage costs for use with personal cars (only when less expensive transportation is not available)
- Cost of standard accommodations in midpriced hotels, motels, or similar lodgings
- Cost of meals, up to a maximum of fifty dollars per day
- Tips up to 15 percent of the total cost of a meal or 10 percent of a taxi fare
- Charges for telephone calls, faxes, and Internet service required for business purposes

*Note*: reimbursement will only be allowed when accompanied by the original receipt.

Employees who are involved in an accident while traveling on business must promptly report the incident to management.

With prior approval, employees on business travel may be accompanied by a family member or friend, when the presence of a companion will not interfere with successful completion of the business objectives. Generally, employees are also permitted to combine personal travel with business travel, as long as time away from work is approved. Additional expenses arising from such nonbusiness travel are the responsibility of the employee.

Once travel is completed, employees should submit completed travel expense reports within ten days. Reports should be accompanied by all receipts for all individual expenses.

Employees should correspond with management for guidance and assistance on procedures related to travel arrangements, expense reports, reimbursement for specific expenses, or any other business travel issues.

Abuse of the business travel expense policy, including falsifying expense reports to reflect costs not incurred by the employee, may be grounds for disciplinary action, up to and including termination of employment.

Included in the privilege of paid off-site training for any employee comes the responsibility that a presentation will be provided to the other members of the practice when the information directly affects their job performance.

# Miscellaneous

**Solicitation**

In an effort to ensure a productive and harmonious work environment, persons not employed by **[Practice Name Here]** may not solicit or distribute literature or material in the workplace for any purpose.

While **[Practice Name Here]** recognizes that employees may have interests in events and organizations outside the workplace, employees may not solicit or distribute literature or materials concerning these activities during working time. Working time does not include lunch/meal periods.

Examples of impermissible forms of solicitation include

- the collection of money, goods, or gifts on behalf of community groups, religious groups, or political groups;
- the circulation of petitions;
- the distribution of literature not approved by management; and
- the solicitation of memberships, fees, or dues.

In addition, the posting of written solicitation on company bulletin boards is prohibited. Bulletin boards are reserved for official organization communications on such items as postings required by law and internal memoranda.

**Suggestion Program**

As an employee of **[Practice Name Here]**, you have the opportunity to contribute to our future success and growth by submitting suggestions for practical work-improvement or cost-saving ideas. All employees are eligible to participate in the suggestion program.

A suggestion is an idea that will benefit **[Practice Name Here]** by solving a problem, reducing costs, improving operations or procedures, enhancing customer service, eliminating waste or spoilage, or making **[Practice Name Here]** a better and safer place to work.

All suggestions should be submitted in writing and should contain a description of the problem or condition to be improved as well as a detailed explanation of the solution or improvement. Submit any suggestions to management; after review, you will be notified of the adoption or rejection of your suggestion.

## Appendix 2

## Common Office Job Description Forms

### Receptionist
### Position Description

**Position:** Receptionist
**Fair Labor Standards Act (FLSA) status:** Nonexempt

### Job Description
Receptionists are the first-line employees whom patients and other customers entering the practice interact with. They are responsible for answering and routing calls, greeting and welcoming patients and visitors, handling inquiries from the public, and providing information related to the practice. They may also assist other administrative staff with performing general administrative duties pertaining to front-desk clerical functions. They must be friendly, professional, and helpful to the visitors and always represent the practice in a positive light.

### Organizational Reporting Relationship
This position reports directly to the office manager.

### Job Summary
A nonexempt, clerical position responsible for receiving incoming telephone calls in a prompt, courteous, efficient, and professional manner and for greeting/assisting visitors in the same manner.

### Specific Duties and Responsibilities
1. Promptly and professionally answers telephone calls; routes calls appropriately, offering voice mail, paging, or redirection of calls as needed
2. Greets visitors and assists them as appropriate; phones or pages employees to meet visitors, directs visitors to appropriate waiting areas, and appropriately and courteously screens solicitors for relevance to the organization's needs
3. Explains financial requirements to the patients or responsible parties and collects copays/coinsurance as required, and places sign-in strip for each encounter
4. Collects copays and deductibles and posts to patient accounts; balances cash drawer against day-sheet payment report; informs patients of any additional financial responsibilities due to additional services or changes in procedures; documents these conversations into patient accounts
5. Determines what records and labs are needed for patient appointments and ensures that they are made available for each patient's visit
6. Performs other duties as assigned

### Performance Requirements
Knowledge
1. Knowledge of medical terminology and the organization's services
2. Knowledge of individual responsibilities to accurately direct callers

Skills and Abilities
1. Ability to use multiline phone system, including transferring calls and paging
2. Adequate hearing ability for answering phones and speaking with patients
3. Ability to interact with outside physician offices and vendors
4. Ability to interact with doctors, nurses, sonographers, and other team members
5. Ability to multitask and the possession of effective organizational skills
6. Display of dependability and initiative in job performance by being prompt in completing tasks and helping others as needed or when called upon to do so
7. Display of a courteous and polite demeanor with patients and fellow employees

8. Must have strong communicative and interpersonal skills and be able to effectively handle stressful or difficult situations with patients
9. Elicits appropriate information in order to route calls to the appropriate person
10. Shows understanding of patient's situation and why she is being seen
11. Is friendly and treats patients the way the employee would expect to be treated

**Education**
High school diploma or GED equivalent

**Required Licenses/Certifications**
Certification in medical terminology preferred

**Experience**
1. Two-year receptionist experience, including CPT coding and ICD-10 coding experience preferred
2. **[Optional]** Prior electronic health records (EHR) experience preferred
3. Ability to type 40 wpm and to operate computers, general office equipment (copier, fax, scanner), and multiline telephones

**Physical Requirements**
Bending, lifting up to 25 lbs. Must have the capacity to use phones, computer keyboards, and monitors.

**Working Conditions**
Business office environment, days (M–F); evening and weekend work may be required.

**Risk of Exposure to Blood-Borne Pathogens**
Employees in this job description are never expected to have contact with blood-borne pathogens. Familiarization with the Federal Occupational Safety and Health Administration's Bloodborne Pathogen Standard is provided during orientation and then annually.

I have read and understand the position description for Receptionist.

_____          _____
Signature                                Date

Copy to: Personnel office
        Employee

## Administrative Assistant
## Position Description

**Position:** Administrative Assistant
**Fair Labor Standards Act (FLSA) status:** Nonexempt

### Job Description
An administrative assistant provides administrative support by overseeing and managing all office procedures and tasks. Support to the office is offered through the coordination of administrative activities and by retrieving, organizing, and disseminating information to staff and clients. Duties include clerical, reception, and project-based work. Duties may be in the form of planning and scheduling meetings or appointments, organizing hard-copy and electronic files, typing, conducting research, and managing projects. Administrative assistants may also be required to arrange staff and/or guest travel accommodations. The tools used by administrative assistants on a daily basis include the desk phone, Internet, mail, and e-mail. The equipment they use may include computers, fax machines, scanners, videoconferencing systems, and photocopiers. Administrative assistants project an organizational image through in-person and phone interactions.

### Organizational Reporting Relationship
Position reports directly to the practice administrator

### Job Summary
Nonexempt position responsible for providing administrative support to the practice administrator

### Specific Duties and Responsibilities
1. Assists and/or oversees all aspects of general office coordination
2. Maintains office calendar to coordinate workflow and meetings
3. Monitors the current status of employee work hours, pulls hours from time clock, makes necessary corrections, and notifies payroll department
4. Oversees and/or collects and maintains inventory of office equipment and supplies; approves office inventory and coordinates its repair and maintenance
5. May supervise volunteers and other support personnel
6. Interacts with vendors, clients, and visitors
7. Answers telephones and transfers to appropriate staff member
8. Accounts payable (AP): responsible for prompt payment on accounts, researches discrepancies, prepares invoices for payment, and mails payments after checks are processed; also maintains AP files
9. Supervises travel arrangements for physicians, managers, and staff
10. Performs general clerical duties to include, but not limited to, bookkeeping, copying, faxing, mailing, and filing
11. Prepares responses to correspondence containing routine inquiries
12. Files and retrieves clinic documents, records, and reports
13. Monitors and assists with maintenance of the clinic's website
14. Handles a variety of matters involving contact with various staff, board members, medical committees, government agencies, and the public
15. Composes correspondence and disseminates to appropriate individuals
16. Prepares various documents and maintains confidentiality in all aspects of patient, staff, and clinic information in accordance with clinic rules and procedures
17. Coordinates and directs office services such as records, budget preparation, personnel, and housekeeping
18. Creates and modifies documents such as invoices, reports, memos, letters, and financial statements using word processing, spreadsheet, database, and/or other presentation software such as Microsoft Office, QuickBooks, or other programs
19. May conduct research, compile data, and prepare papers for consideration and presentation to the executive director, staff, and board of directors
20. Prepares credentialing packets required by insurance companies and maintains credentialing files

21. Processes daily incoming correspondence including faxes and e-mail and distributes it to appropriate staff, departments, or physicians
22. Coordinates and maintains various records for staff, tracking logs, uniform logs, and TB and hepatitis B employee tracking logs; also performs weekly check of all hospitals for the physicians to make sure medical records are up to date to avoid suspension of hospital privileges
23. Sets up and coordinates meetings and conferences
24. Prepares agendas and makes arrangements for committee or other meetings
25. Attends meetings as requested and records minutes
26. Compiles, transcribes, and distributes meeting minutes
27. Assists in special events, such as community fairs and other annual events
28. Assists with overall maintenance of the clinic and its offices
29. Performs other duties as assigned

## Performance Requirements

Knowledge
1. Computer literate
2. Good writing, analytical, and problem-solving skills
3. Knowledge of principles and practices of organization as well as planning, records management, and general administration
4. Ability to communicate effectively
5. Ability to operate standard office equipment, including but not limited to computers, telephone systems, typewriters, calculators, copiers, and facsimile machines
6. Ability to follow oral and written instructions
7. Knowledge of organizational policies, procedures, and systems
8. Knowledge of office management techniques and practices
9. Knowledge of computer systems, programs, and applications
10. Knowledge of research methods and procedures sufficient to compile data and prepare reports
11. Knowledge of grammar, spelling, and punctuation
12. Knowledge of purchasing, budgeting, and inventory control
13. Knowledge of principles and practices of basic office management and organization
14. Knowledge of the basic principles and practices of bookkeeping
15. Ability to work well either alone or as part of a team

Skills and Abilities
1. Ability to interact with outside vendors
2. Ability to interact with physicians, nurses, sonographers, and other team members
3. Ability to multitask
4. Ability to use a courteous and polite demeanor with outside vendors and fellow employees
5. Ability to establish and maintain effective working relationships with other employees and the public
6. Ability to communicate, present information, and work under pressure
7. Ability to read, interpret, and apply clinic policies and procedures
8. Ability to identify problems, recommend solutions, and organize and analyze information
9. Ability to establish priorities and coordinate work activities

## Education
1. High school graduate or completed GED
2. Completion of secretarial science program and/or medical assistant program required; degree preferred but not required
3. Computer literacy required

## Required Licenses/Certifications
Certification: Administrative Assistant

## Experience
At least three (3) years of experience in general office responsibilities and procedures

**Physical Requirements**
Bending, lifting up to 25 lbs. Must have the capacity for frequent use of phones, computer keyboards, and monitors.

**Working Conditions**
Exposure to normal office hazards; frequent standing, walking, sitting, reaching, filing, typing, and photocopying; occasional stooping, kneeling, and crouching; constant talking and listening. Business office environment, days (M–F)

**Risk of Exposure to Blood-Borne Pathogens**
Employees in this job description are never expected to have contact with blood-borne pathogens. Familiarization with the Federal Occupational Safety and Health Administration's Bloodborne Pathogen Standard is provided during orientation and then annually.

I have read and understand the position description for Administrative Assistant.

_____          _____
Signature                                                Date

Copy to: Personnel office
          Employee

# Appointment Scheduler
## Position Description

**Position:** Appointment Scheduler
**Fair Labor Standards Act (FLSA) status:** Nonexempt

## Job Description
An appointment scheduler is a person who arranges appointments for a physician in an office or hospital. Although scheduling appointments is the main focus, other duties are involved to help operate the practice.

## Organizational Reporting Relationship
This position reports directly to **[Insert to whom this position reports]**.

## Job Summary
Nonexempt clerical position responsible for providing professional customer service by obtaining and verifying necessary demographic and insurance information. Responsible for making and scheduling future patient appointments. Responsible for assisting and supporting physicians by performing clerical, reception, and communication activities supportive of the practice.

## Specific Duties and Responsibilities
1. Utilizes professional customer service skills to promptly and professionally answer telephone calls
2. Follows opening and closing procedures according to office guidelines
3. Effectively utilizes available scheduling software to appropriately schedule patients' appointments as they either phone in or arrive in person at checkout and end of office visit
4. Utilizes the computerized system to accurately match physician/clinician availability with patient preferences in terms of date and time; ensures that appropriate notes are entered as needed and/or coding of the appointment is done based on the purpose of the visit
5. Maintains and updates (e.g., cancellations or additions) daily current information on physician schedules or master schedule to ensure that patients are scheduled properly
6. Assists front desk as needed
7. Maintains scheduling system so records are accurate and complete and can be used to analyze patient/staffing patterns
8. Distributes daily physicians' schedule sheets to physicians/clinicians or medical/technical assistants for the following day. Additional copies distributed to other staff such as receptionists or registration staff as needed
9. Maintains strictest confidentiality and adheres to all HIPAA (Health Insurance Portability and Accountability Act) guidelines/regulations
10. Collaborates with other staff such as triage nurses or genetic counselors to accommodate scheduling requests
11. Communicates as needed with physicians/clinicians and other staff about any patient concerns/issues related to scheduling. Consults with officer manager about any system problems
12. Uses customer service principles and techniques to deal with patients calmly and pleasantly
13. Obtains insurance information; may require verification by contacting insurance companies
14. Collects all copays and balances as required by office policies. Understands and can apply payments to balances
15. Reviews all forms for accuracy and completion according to office policies prior to accepting
16. Applies billing codes accurately at checkout
17. Proves out at closing to show the day's total receipts; matches the day's transactions and completes deposit slips
18. Effectively communicates with referring physician offices, ensuring that requests are directed to the appropriate physician or team member
19. Performs other duties as assigned

## Performance Requirements
Knowledge
1. Knowledge of medical terminology and organization services

2. Knowledge of individual responsibilities to accurately direct callers
3. Knowledge of customer service concepts and techniques
4. Knowledge of grammar, spelling, and punctuation to type patient information into appropriate records or computer system

Skills and Abilities
1. Medical terminology and computer literacy required
2. Ability to interact with patients in stressful situations and changing work environments related to changing patient needs
3. Ability to perform work accurately and to pay attention to details, often changing from one task to another without loss of efficiency or composure
4. Ability to work cooperatively and to effectively interact with health system, patients, family members, and multidisciplinary team members (e.g., physicians, sonographers, vendors, and other staff)
5. Ability to utilize effective time management skills to set priorities, multitask, perform job-related responsibilities, and respond quickly to emergency situations
6. Ability to demonstrate effective organizational, critical thinking, and analytical skills
7. Expertise in the use of computers and related computer software
8. Ability to use multiline phone system, including transferring calls and paging
9. Adequate hearing ability for answering phones and speaking with patients
10. Demonstration of dependability and initiative in job performance by being prompt in completing tasks and helping others as needed or when called upon to do so
11. Ability to demonstrate effective customer service skills with patients and families, fellow employees, physicians, and other clients
12. Strong communicative and interpersonal skills and ability to effectively handle stressful or difficult situations with patients
13. Ability to elicit appropriate information to route calls to the appropriate person
14. Demonstrated effectiveness of skills in communicating with empathy toward patients as the need arises

**Education**
High school diploma or GED equivalent

**Required Licenses/Certifications**
Certificate of completion from a recognized medical training program

**Experience**
1. Minimum two years of receptionist experience, including CPT coding, ICD-10 coding, and medical terminology experience
2. Ability to type 40 wpm and operate computers, general office equipment (copier, fax, scanner), and multiline telephones
3. **[Optional]** Prior electronic health records (EHR) experience preferred

**Physical Requirements**
Assists with lifting, pushing, or pulling of up to 25 lbs. Must have the capacity to use phones, computer keyboards, and monitors.

**Working Conditions**
Business office environment, days (M–F). Evening and weekend work may be required. Exposure to normal office hazards. Position requires frequent standing, walking, sitting, reaching, filing, typing, and photocopying; occasional stooping, kneeling, and crouching; and constant talking and listening.

**Risk of Exposure to Blood-Borne Pathogens**
Employees in this job description are never expected to have contact with blood-borne pathogens. Familiarization with the Federal Occupational Safety and Health Administration's Bloodborne Pathogen Standard provided during orientation and as needed.

I have read and understand the position description for Appointment Scheduler.

_____                                _____
Signature                                                                                          Date

Copy to: Personnel office
                Employee

## Prior Authorization Department
## Position Description

**Position: Prior Authorization**
**Fair Labor Standards Act (FLSA) status: Nonexempt**

### Job Description
Nonexempt clerical position responsible for obtaining authorization for services performed in the office for outgoing referrals by contacting patients' insurance via fax, web submittal, or by phone to ensure appropriate payment of claims.

### Organizational Reporting Relationship
This position reports directly to the office manager.

### Specific Duties and Responsibilities
1. Enters appropriate CPT codes in the appointment block within EMR for new patients, as well as for follow-up appointments based on physician diagnoses
2. Prints encounters daily for the following date of service and writes the corresponding CPTs on the encounter
3. Submits authorization requests two weeks prior to scheduled patient appointment to ensure that authorizations are approved prior to the patient's office visit
4. Creates referral within EMR to keep track of authorizations
5. Submits retro-authorization requests, appeals, and authorization requests for outgoing referrals and genetic testing
6. Exercises ability to reschedule patients due to pending authorization
7. Communicates with data entry, billing, benefits, nurses, front office, and other staff members to ensure CPTs are being performed and distributed properly per insurance guidelines as well as per medical necessity guidelines
8. Communicates with patients and physicians when insurance denies authorization
9. Demonstrates comprehensive knowledge of medical terminology, CPT codes, and ICD-10 codes in order to provide medical criteria for authorization requests
10. Performs other duties as assigned

### Performance Requirements
Knowledge
1. Knowledge of medical terminology and organization services
2. Knowledge of individual responsibilities to accurately direct callers

Skills and Abilities
1. Ability to use multiline phone system, including transferring calls and paging
2. Adequate hearing ability for answering phones and speaking with patients
3. Ability to interact with outside physician offices and vendors
4. Ability to interact with doctors, nurses, sonographers, and other team members
5. Ability to multitask
6. Demonstration of dependability and initiative in job performance by being prompt in completing tasks and helping others as needed or when called upon to do so
7. Demonstration of a courteous and polite demeanor with patients and fellow employees
8. Must have strong communicative and interpersonal skills and be able to effectively handle stressful or difficult situations with patients
9. Elicits appropriate information to route calls to the appropriate person
10. Shows understanding of patients' situations and why they are being seen
11. Is friendly and treats patients the way the employee would expect to be treated

**Education**
High school diploma or GED equivalent

**Experience**
1. Minimum two-year prior authorization experience including CPT coding and ICD-10 coding experience
2. Ability to type 40 wpm and operate computers, general office equipment (copier, fax, scanner), and multiline telephones
3. Prior electronic health records (EHR) experience preferred

**Physical Requirements**
Bending, lifting up to 25 lbs. Must have the capacity to use phones, computers, Internet, keyboards, and monitors. Must establish usernames and passwords with the various insurances we use to obtain authorization via the Internet.

**Working Conditions**
Business office environment, days (M–F). Evening and weekend work may be required.

**Risk of Exposure to Blood-Borne Pathogens**
Employees in this job description are never expected to have contact with blood-borne pathogens. Familiarization with the Federal Occupational Safety and Health Administration's Bloodborne Pathogen Standard is provided during orientation and then annually.


I have read and understand the position description for Prior Authorization.

_____                                    _____
Signature                                                          Date

Copy to: Personnel office
         Employee

Office Manager
Position Description

**Position: Office Manager**
**Fair Labor Standards Act (FLSA) status: Exempt**

## Job Description
Office managers supervise administrative support workers such as receptionists, secretaries, and administrative assistants as well as coordinate administrative support activities. Office managers may head the entire office, especially in a large practice or in administrative support operations in a small practice. In either case, the office manager is responsible for directing clerical staff and seeing that their jobs are done efficiently as well as providing the necessary training where needed.

## Organizational Reporting Relationship
This position reports directly to **[Insert to whom this position reports]**.

## Job Summary
Exempt management position responsible for managing the daily operations of the office

## Specific Duties and Responsibilities
1. Oversees daily office operations and delegates authority to assigned supervisors
2. Assists supervisors in developing and implementing short- and long-term work plans and objectives for clerical functions
3. Assists supervisors in understanding/implementing clinic policies and procedures
4. Develops guidelines for prioritizing work activities, evaluating effectiveness, and modifying activities as necessary; ensures that office is staffed appropriately
5. Assists in the recruiting, hiring, orientation, development, and evaluation of clerical staff
6. Establishes and maintains an efficient and responsive patient-flow system
7. Oversees and approves office supply inventory, ensures that mail is opened and processed and that offices are opened and closed according to procedures
8. Supports and upholds established policies, procedures, objectives, quality improvement, safety, environmental and infection control, and codes and requirements of accreditation and regulatory agencies
9. Assists development, implementation, and monitoring of customer satisfaction initiatives
10. Assists development, implementation, and monitoring of performance improvement initiatives pertaining to access-related issues, patient flow, wait time, and other customer service or patient care issues
11. Assists in promoting teamwork among all office staff
12. Exemplifies effective customer service skills
13. Performs other duties as assigned

## Performance Requirements
Knowledge
1. Knowledge of medical practices, terminology, and reimbursement policies
2. Knowledge of electronic medical records (EMR) system, with ability to use it
3. Knowledge of business management and basic accounting principles to direct the business office
4. Sufficient knowledge of policies and procedures to accurately answer questions from internal and external customers
5. Knowledge of customer service standards
6. Knowledge of performance improvement principles

Skills and Abilities
1. Proficient in software applications including Microsoft Word, Excel, and PowerPoint or graphics software
2. Good organizational skills

3. Proficient in planning, delegating, and supervising employees
4. Excellent use of discretion in confidential matters
5. Ability to communicate effectively (orally and in writing)
6. Ability to effectively interact with customers to meet their needs
7. Ability to work independently with minimal direct supervision
8. Ability to work cooperatively within a team environment
9. Ability to handle frequent interruptions and adapt to changes in workload and work schedule
10. Ability to set priorities, make effective decisions, and respond quickly to customers' needs
11. Ability to recognize and deal with problematic situations and to prioritize
12. Ability to recognize and implement systems for continuous improvement of patient satisfaction, workflow, and overall office functions
13. Ability to interact with patients in stressful situations and changing work environments related to changing patient needs
14. Ability to read, interpret, and apply policies and procedures
15. Ability to recognize, evaluate, and solve problems and to correct errors
16. Ability to set priorities among multiple requests
17. Ability to interact effectively with patients, medical and administrative staff, and the public

## Education
Bachelor's degree, preferably with coursework in health-care administration

## Required Licenses/Certifications
[As determined by the organization.]

## Experience
1. Minimum of three years of supervisory experience desired
2. Ability to type 40 wpm and operate computers and general office equipment
3. Knowledge of various software, including the Microsoft Office suite (Excel, Word, PowerPoint, and Outlook)
4. EMR experience preferred

## Physical Requirements
Bending, lifting up to 25 lbs.; intermittent walking and sitting. This employee must have the capacity to use phones, computer keyboards, and monitors plus have the ability to multitask and use excellent communication skills.

## Working Conditions
Business office environment, days (M–F). Evening and weekend work may be required. Exposure to normal office hazards. Assists with lifting, pushing, or pulling of up to 25 lbs. Position requires frequent standing, walking, sitting, reaching, filing, typing, and photocopying; occasional stooping, kneeling, and crouching; and constant talking and listening.

## Risk of Exposure to Blood-Borne Pathogens
Employees in this job description are never expected to have contact with blood-borne pathogens. Familiarization with the Federal Occupational Safety and Health Administration's Bloodborne Pathogen Standard is provided during orientation and then annually.

I have read and understand the position description for Office Manager.

_____          _____
Signature                                Date


Copy to: Personnel office
        Employee

# Practice Liaison
# Position Description

**Position:** Practice Liaison
**Fair Labor Standards Act (FLSA) status:** Exempt

## Job Description

The practice liaison is responsible for developing and maintaining strong relationships between the practice and the physician community throughout the practice's service area. The position works closely with the members of the organizational senior leadership team and the practice physicians. The practice liaison focuses on sales and customer relations with physicians and physician office/practice staff for the development of practice referral relationships and growth of targeted services.

## Organizational Reporting Relationship

This position reports to the practice manager.

## Job Summary

Exempt professional position responsible for establishing and maintaining referral relationships, developing contact lists of new referral sources, and acting as a liaison between referring physicians and the group practice.

## Specific Duties and Responsibilities
1. Establishes and maintains referral relationships
2. Maintains a database of physician contacts and referrals, tracking results and trends
3. Collaborates with the managing physician partner, physician team, and practice administrator to develop new marketing strategies and new business
4. Works with the managing partner and practice administrator to develop new marketing materials
5. Schedules periodic in-services with referring ob-gyns (OBs) to discuss new tests or procedures; involves the genetic counselors to update OBs in the area of genetic testing
6. Performs other duties as assigned

## Performance Requirements

Knowledge
1. Knowledge of computer database applications
2. Knowledge of marketing/sales strategies

Skills and Abilities
1. Skill in sales and in attracting new customers
2. Skill in effective oral and written communication
3. Ability to develop and maintain effective relationships
4. Ability to organize and analyze data
5. Ability to utilize basic medical terminology, primarily obstetric and gynecological terms

## Education

Bachelor's degree in marketing, communications, or business administration

## Experience
1. Minimum three years of experience in sales/service, preferably in the health-care industry
2. Ability to type 45 wpm and to operate computers and general office equipment
3. Customer service training a plus

## Physical Requirements

Bending, lifting up to 25 lbs. Must have the ability to use phones, computer keyboards, monitors, and cell phone.

## Working Conditions

This position works out of the office approximately 80 percent of the time, thus requiring the ability to use a cell phone to return calls and e-mails. Must have reliable transportation that is licensed and insured in the appropriate state.

## Risk of Exposure to Blood-Borne Pathogens

Employees in this job description are never expected to have contact with blood-borne pathogens. Familiarization with the Federal Occupational Safety and Health Administration's Bloodborne Pathogen Standard is provided during orientation and then annually.

I have read and understand the position description for Practice Liaison.

_____          _____
Signature                                Date


Copy to: Personnel office
         Employee

## Medical Records / Health Information Technician
## Position Description

**Position: Medical Records / Health Information Technician**
**Fair Labor Standards Act (FLSA) status: Nonexempt**

**Job Summary**
Nonexempt position responsible for uploading/scanning information into patients' electronic medical record (EMR) system in an accurate and complete manner.

**Organizational Reporting Relationship**
This position reports directly to the office manager.

**Specific Duties and Responsibilities**
1. Assembles patients' health information, including patient symptoms and medical history, exam results, X-ray reports, lab tests, diagnoses, and treatment plans. Checks to ensure that all forms are completed, properly identified, and signed and that all necessary information is then scanned into the patient's electronic file in the preferred manner and proper category
2. Communicates as needed with physicians and other health-care professionals to clarify diagnoses or to obtain additional information
3. Submits files/documentation to physicians and other clinicians (as requested) for review, quality assurance checks, and other purposes
4. Provides charts/documents requested for use in legal actions, following patient consent/confidentiality protocols
5. Forwards consultation notes to referring provider in a timely manner
6. Uses computer programs (if requested) to tabulate and analyze data in order to improve patient care, control costs, respond to surveys, or use in research studies
7. Performs other duties as assigned

**Performance Requirements**
Knowledge
1. Knowledge of medical terminology and the organization's services
2. Knowledge of individual responsibilities to efficiently use EMR system
3. Knowledge of customer service concepts and techniques
4. Knowledge of grammar, spelling, and punctuation to type patient information into EMR system

Skills and Abilities
1. Ability to use multiline phone system, including transferring calls and paging
2. Adequate hearing ability for answering phones and speaking with patients
3. Ability to interact with outside physician offices and vendors
4. Ability to interact with doctors, nurses, sonographers, and other team members
5. Ability to multitask
6. Demonstration of dependability and initiative in job performance by being prompt in completing tasks and helping others as needed or when called upon to do so
7. Demonstration of courteous and polite demeanor with patients and fellow employees
8. Demonstration of strong communicative and interpersonal skills and ability to effectively handle stressful or difficult situations with patients
9. Shows understanding of patients' situations and why they are being seen
10. Must be friendly and treat patients the way the employee would expect to be treated

**Education**
1. High school diploma or GED equivalent

2. Registered health information technician (RHIT) designation preferred (but not required), offered by the American Health Information Management Association; designation awarded after successful completion of written exam

**Experience**
1. Minimum two years of medical records clerk / health information technician experience in a medical practice setting
2. Ability to type 45 wpm and to operate computers and general office equipment

**Physical Requirements**
Bending, lifting up to 25 lbs. Must have the capacity to use phones, computer keyboards, and monitors.

**Working Conditions**
Business office environment, days (M–F). Evening and weekend work may be required.

**Risk of Exposure to Blood-Borne Pathogens**
Employees in this job description are never expected to have contact with blood-borne pathogens. Familiarization with the Federal Occupational Safety and Health Administration's Bloodborne Pathogen Standard is provided during orientation and then annually.

I have read and understand the position description for Medical Records / Health Information Technician.

_____        _____
Signature                         Date

Copy to: Personnel office
         Employee

Benefits Coordinator
Position Description

---

**Position: Benefits Coordinator**
**Fair Labor Standards Act (FLSA) status: Nonexempt**

---

**Job Summary**
Nonexempt clerical position responsible for obtaining patients' eligibility and benefits, annotating the same in the patients' electronic health records (EHR) system, and calling and confirming patients' appointment dates and services to be provided. Responsible for scanning various information/paperwork into our EHR system.

**Organizational Reporting Relationship**
This position reports directly to the office manager.

**Specific Duties and Responsibilities**
1. Obtains patients' eligibility and benefits for services being provided and adds billing comments into patients' EHR
2. Checks daily schedule for add-ons and obtains eligibility and benefits prior to scheduled appointment times
3. Calls patients to confirm next appointment dates/times and to explain financial responsibilities for services being rendered
4. Enters patient demographics and copay/coinsurance requirements within our EHR system
5. Uses customer service principles and techniques to deal with patients in a calm and pleasant manner
6. Obtains Medicaid benefits three to five business days prior to the next month, adding comments as needed
7. Performs other duties as assigned

**Performance Requirements**
Knowledge
1. Knowledge of medical terminology and of the organization's services
2. Knowledge of individual responsibilities to accurately direct callers
3. Knowledge of customer service concepts and techniques
4. Knowledge of grammar, spelling, and punctuation to type patient information into our EHR system

Skills and Abilities
1. Ability to use multiline phone system, including transferring calls and paging
2. Adequate hearing ability for answering phones and speaking with patients
3. Ability to interact with outside physician offices and vendors
4. Ability to interact with doctors, nurses, sonographers, and other team members
5. Ability to multitask
6. Demonstration of dependability and initiative in job performance by being prompt in completing tasks and helping others as needed or when called upon to do so
7. Demonstration of a courteous and polite demeanor with patients and fellow employees
8. Demonstration of strong communicative and interpersonal skills and ability to effectively handle stressful or difficult situations with patients
9. Ability to elicit appropriate information to route calls to the appropriate person
10. Shows understanding of patients' situations and why they are being seen
11. Is friendly and treats patients the way the employee would expect to be treated

**Education**
High school diploma or GED equivalent

**Experience**
1. Minimum two years of medical office experience, including CPT coding and ICD-10 coding experience

2. Ability to type 40 wpm and operate computers, general office equipment (copier, fax, scanner), and multiline telephones
3. Prior EHR experience preferred

**Physical Requirements**

Bending, lifting up to 25 lbs. Must have the capacity to use phones, computers, Internet, keyboards, and monitors. Must establish usernames and passwords with the various insurances we use as well as obtain authorization via the Internet.

**Working Conditions**

Business office environment, days (M–F). Evening and weekend work may be required.

**Risk of Exposure to Blood-Borne Pathogens**

Employees in this job description are never expected to have contact with blood-borne pathogens. Familiarization with the Federal Occupational Safety and Health Administration's Bloodborne Pathogen Standard is provided during orientation and then annually.


I have read and understand the position description for Benefits Coordinator.


_____          _____
Signature                                Date


Copy to: Personnel office
         Employee

**Billing and Collection Specialist**
**Position Description**

---

**Position: Billing and Collection Specialist**
**Fair Labor Standards Act (FLSA) status: Nonexempt**

---

### Job Description
Billing and collection specialists are responsible for obtaining any payments due to the practice. They attempt to reach patients who have not paid, either by phone or mail (and occasionally both). They often keep track of accounts with a computer, making notations or taking credit card payments once they establish contact with a customer.

### Organizational Reporting Relationship
This position reports directly to the practice administrator.

### Job Summary
Verifies and posts charges and payments to patient and insurance company accounts. Audits patients and insurance accounts for accuracy in billing and performs functions for the collection of accounts receivable.

### Specific Duties and Responsibilities
1. Analyzes accounts for billing; contacts insurance companies for status of outstanding claims
2. Analyzes patient accounts for collections, bad debt, and uncollectible accounts
3. Analyzes patient accounts for billing cycle
4. Posts entries into accounts as necessary
5. Audits and files electronic claims; responsible for auditing and transmitting electronics claims
6. Generates HCFAs, claims, and patient statements; responsible for mailing HCFAs and patient statements
7. Continuously follows up on accounts in collection module
8. Posts entries for billing cycles, accounts receivable (A/R), bankruptcies, and write-offs
9. Pulls bulk explanation of benefits (EOBs) for accuracy of posting and for filing of secondary claims
10. Reviews and works daily incoming lock-box mail/checks
11. Accurately posts payments, reviewing accounts for any payment errors and then rebilling claims and filing appeals if necessary
12. Takes incoming calls and answers patients' questions regarding their account balances, covered benefits, and copay/coinsurance
13. Responds to insurance company inquires
14. Reviews payer rejection reports
15. Performs other duties as assigned

### Performance Requirements
1. Demonstrates a courteous and polite demeanor with patients and fellow employees
2. Displays dependability and initiative in job performance by being prompt in completing tasks and helping others as needed or when called upon to do so
3. Must have strong communicative and interpersonal skills and be able to effectively handle stressful or difficult situations with patients

### Education
High school diploma or GED equivalent

### Experience
1. Minimum two years of payment posting or billing experience, including CPT coding and ICD-10 coding experience
2. Ability to type 40 wpm and operate computers and general office equipment

**Physical Requirements**
Bending, lifting up to 25 lbs. Must have the capacity to use phones, computer keyboards, and monitors.

**Working Conditions**
Business office environment, days (M–F). Some evening and weekend work may be required.

**Risk of Exposure to Blood-Borne Pathogens**
Employees in this job description are never expected to have contact with blood-borne pathogens. Familiarization with the Federal Occupational Safety and Health Administration's Bloodborne Pathogen Standard is provided during orientation and then annually.

I have read and understand the position description of Billing and Collection Specialist.


Signature:_____    Date:_____


Copy to: Personnel office
         Employee

# Medical Biller
# Position Description

**Position: Medical Biller**
**Fair Labor Standards Act (FLSA) status: Nonexempt**

### Job Description
Medical billers compile and track the outstanding balances owed to the practice. They maintain the payment records of all patients, make payment arrangements, and collect on past-due accounts.

### Job Summary
Verifies patient accounts for accuracy in billing patients and insurance companies.

### Organizational Reporting Relationship
This position reports directly to the practice administrator and the director of accounts receivable (A/R).

### Specific Duties and Responsibilities
1. Reviews and corrects HCFAs
2. Assists front office in insurance contract interpretation
3. Answers patients' questions regarding their account balances, covered benefits, and copays
4. Serves as liaison between posting office and front office; assists checkout when necessary
5. Assists posting department and center administrator in identifying deficiencies of front-office operations
6. Performs A/R follow-up
7. Assists physicals department with billing
8. Relays information to the A/R director
9. Responds to insurance company requests
10. Performs other duties as assigned

### Performance Requirements
1. Demonstrates a courteous and polite demeanor with patients and fellow employees
2. Displays dependability and initiative in job performance by being prompt in completing tasks and helping others as needed or when called upon to do so
3. Must have strong communicative and interpersonal skills and be able to effectively handle stressful or difficult situations with patients

### Education
High school diploma or GED equivalent

### Experience
1. Minimum of two years of medical front office, billing, or collections experience
2. Ability to type 40 wpm and operate computers and general office equipment

### Physical Requirements
Bending, lifting up to 25 lbs. Must have the capacity to use phones, computer keyboards, and monitors.

### Working Conditions
Office and medical center environment. Evening and weekend work may be required.

### Risk of Exposure to Blood-Borne Pathogens
Employees in this job description are never expected to have contact with blood-borne pathogens. Familiarization with the Federal Occupational Safety and Health Administration's Bloodborne Pathogen Standard is provided during orientation and then annually.

I have read and understand the position description for Medical Biller.

_____              _____
Signature                                     Date

Copy to: Personnel office
         Employee

# Accounts Receivable (A/R) Supervisor
# Position Description

**Position:** Accounts Receivable (A/R) Supervisor
**Fair Labor Standards Act (FLSA) status:** Nonexempt

## Job Description
The accounts receivable (A/R) supervisor oversees activities in the A/R function. The A/R supervisor is responsible for collection activities such as sending follow-up inquiries, negotiating with past-due accounts, maintaining cash receipts, and referring accounts to collection agencies. Maintaining accurate records and ensuring that the day-to-day accounting operations of the practice are completed are important functions of this role.

## Job Summary
Directs and coordinates functions of accounts receivable.

## Organizational Reporting Relationship
This position reports directly to the director of accounts receivable or the billing supervisor.

## Specific Duties and Responsibilities
1. Directs and performs audits and analyses of patient accounts for collections, bad debt, and uncollectible accounts
2. Ensures that accounts are processed for collection and are followed up on continuously
3. Coordinates and directs a systematic and continuous follow-up of accounts receivable
4. Coordinates posting for billing cycles, A/R, bankruptcies, and write-offs
5. Ensures that staffing is adequate and cost effective, assisting in all personnel-related duties including hiring, time and attendance, disciplinary actions, and evaluations
6. Instructs and trains personnel in collection, billing, and A/R functions
7. Furnishes director of A/R with monthly reports as specified
8. Performs all other duties as assigned

## Performance Requirements
1. Displays an excellent understanding of medical center computer billing systems
2. Displays knowledge of billing and collection procedures for all medical insurance programs including HMOs, PPOs, Medicare, workers' compensation group billing, per diem, and private pay
3. Displays skill in exercising initiative, judgment, problem-solving, and objective decision-making
4. Displays dependability and initiative in job performance by being prompt in completing tasks and organizing workload, prioritizing duties to meet fluctuating daily schedules so that duties are accomplished in an organized and effective manner, even under pressure
5. Must have strong communicative and interpersonal skills and be able to effectively communicate with executives, peers, and subordinates
6. Must demonstrate evidence of physical and emotional well-being

## Education
1. High school diploma or GED equivalent
2. Certification as a Professional Coder

## Experience
1. Minimum five to eight years of medical billing experience
2. Minimum three to five years of supervisory experience
3. Excellent computer skills

**Physical Requirements**
Requires hand-eye coordination and manual dexterity sufficient to handle general administrative and clerical functions.

**Working Conditions**
Administrative office environment (usually M–F). Evening and weekend work may be required.

**Risk of Exposure to Blood-Borne Pathogens**
Employees in this job description are never expected to have contact with blood-borne pathogens. Familiarization with the Federal Occupational Safety and Health Administration's Bloodborne Pathogen Standard is provided during orientation and then annually.


I have read and understand the position description for Accounts Receivable (A/R) Supervisor.


_____                    _____
Signature                                                                          Date


Copy to: Personnel office
            Employee

**Medical Assistant**
**Position Description**

---

**Position:** Medical Assistant
**Fair Labor Standards Act (FLSA) status:** Nonexempt

---

### Job Description
The medical assistant is a multiskilled health professional who works interdependently with other health-care professionals to provide quality health care to the patient. The medical assistant is educated and trained to perform both administrative and clinical skills in the medical care environment.

### Job Summary
Nonexempt position responsible for performing a variety of medical duties in both the clinical and administrative areas, including assisting physicians with patient care as well as handling clerical, environmental, and organizational tasks.

### Organizational Reporting Relationship
This position reports directly to the office manager.

### Specific Duties and Responsibilities
1. Fulfills patient care responsibilities as assigned, which may include checking schedules and organizing patient flow; accompanying patients to exam/procedure room; assisting patients as needed with walking transfers, dressing, collecting specimens, performing vital signs, preparing for exams, and so on; collecting patient history; performing screenings per provider guidelines; assisting physicians/nurses with various procedures; charting; relaying instructions to patients/families; answering calls and providing pertinent information
2. Fulfills clerical responsibilities as assigned, which may include sending/receiving patient medical records; obtaining lab/X-ray reports, hospital notes, referral information, and so on; completing forms/requisitions as needed; scheduling appointments; verifying insurance coverage and patient demographics; managing and updating charts to ensure that information is complete and filed appropriately
3. Fulfills environmental responsibilities as assigned, which may include setting up instruments and equipment according to department protocols; cleaning exam/procedure rooms, instruments, and equipment between patient visits to maintain infection control; cleaning sterilizer according to scheduled maintenance program and keeping appropriate records; ordering, sorting, storing supplies; restocking exam/procedure rooms
4. Fulfills organizational responsibilities as assigned, including respecting/promoting patient rights; responding appropriately to emergency codes; sharing problems relating to patients and/or staff with immediate supervisor
5. Fulfills clinical medical assisting responsibilities, which vary according to state law; these may include medical/surgical asepsis, sterilization, and instrument wrapping and autoclaving; checking vital signs or menstruations; physical examination preparations; clinical pharmacology; drug administration through various routes including injections; prescription verifications with physician's orders; minor surgery assists, including surgical tray setup pre/postsurgical care, applying dressings, and suture removal; biohazard waste disposal and monitoring; laboratory procedures, including Occupational Safety and Health Administration (OSHA) guidelines; quality control methods; Clinical Laboratory Improvement Amendment (CLIA)-waived testing; specimen handling such as urine, vaginal, emergency triage, and first aid. Medical assistants must adhere to the MA scope of practice in the laboratory.
6. Performs other duties as assigned

### Performance Requirements
Knowledge
1. Knowledge of health-care field and medical office protocols/procedures
2. Knowledge of specific assisting tasks related to particular medical practice
3. Knowledge of information that must be conveyed to patients and families

Skills and Abilities
1. Skill in performing medical assistance tasks appropriately
2. Skill in tact and diplomacy in interpersonal interactions
3. Skill in understanding patient education needs by effectively sharing information with patients and families
4. Ability to learn and retain information regarding patient care procedures
5. Ability to project a pleasant and professional image
6. Ability to plan, prioritize, and complete delegated tasks
7. Ability to demonstrate compassion and caring in dealing with others

**Education**
1. High school diploma or GED, medical assistant diploma from an accredited vocational institution, or community college course in medical assisting
2. Current documentation of a national certification for registered medical assistants (RMAs) through the American Medical Technologists (AMT) or for certified assistants through the American Association of Medical Assistants (AAMA)
3. Current CPR certification

**Experience**
1. Minimum one year of recent experience working in a medical facility as a medical assistant
2. Ability to type 40 wpm and operate computers and general office equipment

**Physical Requirements**
Bending, lifting up to 25 lbs. Must have the capacity to use phones, computer keyboards, and monitors.

**Working Conditions**
Business office environment, days (M–F). Evening and weekend work may be required.

**Risk of Exposure to Blood-Borne Pathogens**
Employees in this job description are expected to have contact with blood-borne pathogens, and as such they are required to be oriented and annually trained under the Federal Occupational Safety and Health Administration's Bloodborne Pathogen Standard.

I have read and understand the position description of Medical Assistant.

_____       _____

Signature                                                                          Date

Copy to: Personnel office
           Employee

# Genetic Counselor
# Position Description

**Position:** Genetic Counselor
**Fair Labor Standards Act (FLSA) status:** Exempt

## Job Description
Genetic counselors work with families and couples to understand their family history, counsel those who may be at risk for inherited conditions, and help them adapt to birth defects or genetic disorders. They spend a great deal of time evaluating the family history and what the history means from a genetic point of view. This is a very in-depth process in order to fully understand the history of each family member. Genetic counselors must have patience while they thoroughly record the medical history of each patient and spend time evaluating the medical data. They work in a scientific-based role in which they take the information gathered and apply it to their evaluation of what the family history means for each individual.

## Organizational Reporting Relationship
This position reports directly to **[Insert to whom this position reports]**.

## Job Summary
Exempt position for a health professional with a specialized graduate degree and experience in the area of medical genetics and counseling. The genetic counselor works as a member of the health-care team, providing information and support to families who have a member with birth defects or genetic disorders as well as to families who may be at risk for a variety of inherited conditions.

## Specific Duties and Responsibilities
A. Patient Information Gathering and Evaluation
   1. Verifies patient identification and that genetic counseling service has been requested
   2. Explains the nature of genetics evaluation to families; utilizes interviewing techniques to obtain and review relevant information from the family using standard pedigree nomenclature

B. Patient Education, Communication, Support, and Care Management
   1. Evaluates data supplied and determines appropriate diagnosis and plan of treatment
   2. Provides comprehensive counseling to families about a wide range of prenatal and preconception indications
   3. Explains to families (verbally and/or in writing) medical information regarding the diagnosis and/or potential occurrence of a genetic condition or birth defect
   4. Discusses and provides education regarding available options and delineates risks, benefits, and limitations of appropriate tests and clinical assessments
   5. Orders tests under physician supervision and performs assessments in accordance with local, state, and federal regulations
   6. Provides ongoing emotional support to families throughout the counseling process and during extensive genetic tests (including invasive procedures); assists them with difficult aspects of findings
   7. Identifies and facilitates access to local, regional, and national resources such as support groups and ancillary services; discusses the availability of such resources with families and provides referrals as necessary
   8. Documents case information clearly and concisely in the medical records and in correspondence to the referring provider; discusses case information with other members of the health-care team as necessary

C. Performance Improvement, Quality of Care, and Customer Service Excellence
   1. Maintains up-to-date knowledge in the field and participates in clinical research programs as appropriate or when applicable; shares knowledge and expertise with colleagues and other members of the health-care team
   2. Participates in performance improvement processes for continuous improvement of patient care quality
   3. Works in partnership with other members of the health-care team to provide quality patient care; promotes a positive and collaborative work environment with all members of the patient care team

4. Adheres to the accepted professional ethical standards and exercises effective customer service skills related to services, excellence, respect, values, and ethics
5. Performs other duties as assigned

**Performance Requirements**

Knowledge
1. Knowledge of medical practices, terminology, and reimbursement policies
2. Knowledge of and ability to use electronic medical record (EMR) system
3. Sufficient knowledge of policies and procedures to accurately answer questions from internal and external customers

Skills
1. Skill in planning and organizing
2. Skill in evaluating the effectiveness of existing methods and procedures
3. Skill in critical thinking problem-solving
4. Must have strong communicative and interpersonal skills and be able to effectively handle stressful or difficult situations with patients
5. Must display dependability and initiative in job performance by being prompt in completing tasks and helping others as needed or when called upon to do so
6. Must demonstrate a courteous and polite demeanor with patients and fellow employees
7. Skill in working effectively as a member of a team
8. Skill in decision-making

Abilities
1. Ability to read, interpret, and apply policies and procedures
2. Ability to recognize, evaluate, and solve problems and correct errors
3. Ability to set priorities among multiple requests
4. Ability to interact effectively with patients, medical and administrative staff, and the public
5. Ability to interact with a diverse population and different age groups

**Education**
1. Baccalaureate degree (the majority of genetic counselors have a background in biology, genetics, psychology, nursing, social work, or public health)
2. Master's degree from an accredited genetic counseling program

**Required Licenses/Certifications**
1. Certification is provided through the American Board of Genetic Counseling (ABGC).
2. Certification is provided to those genetic counselors who demonstrate that they meet established standards for professional practice through documentation of specialized training and clinical experience as well as the successful completion of the ABGC certification exam.
3. Recertification must be completed every five years.

**Experience**
1. Minimum two (2) years of experience in a genetic counseling role preferred
2. Ability to type 40 wpm and operate computers and general office equipment
3. **[Optional]** Prior EMR experience preferred

**Physical Requirements**
Bending, lifting up to 25 lbs. Must have the capacity to use phones, computer keyboards, monitors, and Microsoft software. Must have the ability to multitask and have effective communication and customer service skills. Must comply with all appropriate regulatory requirements.

**Working Conditions**
Normal business office/hospital environment, days (M–F). Evening and weekend work may be required.

**Risk of Exposure to Blood-Borne Pathogens**
Employees in this job description may have some contact with blood-borne pathogens, and as such they are required to be oriented and annually trained under the Federal Occupational Safety and Health Administration's Bloodborne Pathogen Standard.

I have read and understand the position description for Genetic Counselor.

_____                    _____
Signature                                                                                  Date

Copy to: Personnel office
             Employee

## Registered Nurse
## Position Description

**Position: Registered Nurse**
**Fair Labor Standards Act (FLSA) status: Exempt**

### Job Description
Registered nurses (RNs) work to promote good health and to prevent illness. They treat and educate patients and the public about various medical conditions, and they also provide advice and emotional support to patients' family members. RNs record patients' medical histories and symptoms, help perform diagnostic tests and analyze results, operate medical machinery, administer treatment and medications, and help with patient follow-up and rehabilitation. RNs teach patients and their families how to manage their illnesses or injuries, explaining post-treatment home-care needs; diet, nutrition, and exercise programs; and self-administration of medication and physical therapy. Some RNs may work to promote general health by educating the public on warning signs and symptoms of disease. RNs also might run general health screening or immunization clinics, blood drives, and public seminars on various conditions. When caring for patients, RNs establish a care plan or contribute to an existing plan. Plans may include numerous activities, such as administering medications, including careful checking of dosages and avoiding interactions; administering therapies and treatments; observing the patient and recording those observations; and consulting with physicians and other health-care clinicians. Some RNs provide direction to licensed practical nurses and nursing aides regarding patient care.

### Organizational Reporting Relationship
This position reports directly to the practice manager.

### Job Summary
This is an exempt position responsible for providing primary care to patients, including assessment, treatment, care planning, and medical care evaluation.

### Specific Duties and Responsibilities
A. Patient Information Gathering and Evaluation
1. Verifies patient identification and that the requested services correspond with the patient's clinical history and presentation
2. Obtains patient history, chief complaints, and vital signs and gathers relevant information from the patient or patient's representative and the patient's medical records regarding the patient's health status and medical history
3. Effectively uses the nursing process to develop, implement, and evaluate the patient's plan of care

B. Patient Care, Education and Communication, Support and Management
1. Identifies, recognizes, and implements appropriate educational content and methodologies required to meet the patient's and/or family member's specific needs
2. Educates patients and families about health status, health maintenance, and management of acute and chronic conditions
3. In collaboration with maternal-fetal medicine (MFM) subspecialists and genetic counselors, identifies and facilitates access to local, regional, and national resources such as support groups and ancillary services; discusses the availability of such resources with families and provide referrals as necessary
4. Effectively collaborates with the entire team in the practice to develop and prioritize the patient's care
5. Responds appropriately to changing workloads and crisis and/or emergency situations within the practice in a professional, caring, and expedient manner
6. Executes prescribed treatments and medical interventions, administers prescribed medications, and monitors and documents treatment progress and patient response
7. Delegates as allowed under the Nurse Practice Act; refers to/consults with physicians, other health providers, and community resources to prevent/resolve problems or concerns

8. Documents patient assessment and intervention data using established medical record forms and automated systems and documentation practices
9. Obtains prior authorization as applicable

C. Performance Improvement, Quality of Care, and Customer Service Excellence
1. Participates in multidisciplinary teams in implementing performance improvement processes and outcomes; tracks quality assurance data and monitors for acute and chronic care management
2. Assists in maintaining a clean, organized, and safe working environment at all times
3. Pursues personal growth and development
4. Delegates and communicates patient-specific tasks and activities to the appropriate staff members and follows through with team members to ascertain if outcomes were achieved within predetermined time frames
5. Participates in the mentoring and professional development of personnel such as new nurses and licensed practical (vocational) nurses
6. Performs other duties as required or assigned

**Performance Requirements**

Knowledge
1. Knowledge of nursing processes, community resources, and health-care systems, structures, and functions; understanding of health-care technology, equipment, and supplies; familiarity with state laws on nursing care, nurse practice guidelines, and clinic policies and procedures
2. Knowledge of wellness/illness, growth and development, human behavior, psychosocial factors, and alternative health-care treatments
3. Knowledge of chart/medical record documentation requirements and federal/state laws related to release of health-care information

Skills
1. Effective oral and written communication skills, including speech clarity, understanding the information relayed, and deductive and inductive reasoning skills (the ability to apply general rules to specific problems to produce answers that make sense and the ability to combine pieces of information to/from general rules or conclusion, respectively)
2. Detail oriented and skilled in time management, problem-solving, multitasking, prioritizing, and medical care coordination
3. Skill in initiating appropriate crisis interventions and emergency response
4. Skill in patient triage in person and on the phone
5. Demonstration of a courteous and polite demeanor with patients and fellow employees

Abilities
1. Ability to analyze options and then counsel patients and families about choices and make referrals to other providers and resources
2. Ability to engage clients and families in the development and implementation of care plans
3. Ability to read and interpret physicians' orders and notes from other providers
4. Ability to calculate and administer drug dosages and injections and measure results
5. Ability to work cooperatively within health system and with multidisciplinary team members

**Education**
Completion of an RN program from an accredited program with a bachelor's of science degree in nursing (BSN), an associate degree in nursing (ADN), or a diploma. BSN preferred.

**Required Licenses/Certifications**
1. Current state-registered nurse license
2. Current BLS/CPR certificate
3. Up-to-date training in fetal monitoring
4. **[Optional]** Current knowledge in diabetic education

**Experience**
1. Minimum of five years of professional nursing experience in labor and delivery; physician practice office experience also preferred
2. **[Optional]** Prior electronic medical records (EMR) experience preferred
3. Ability to type 40 wpm and operate computers and general office equipment

**Physical Requirements**
Bending, lifting up to 25 lbs. Must have the capacity to use phones, computer keyboards, and monitors. Involves standing, walking, bending, grasping, manipulating, and squatting. Occasional need to lift patients during transfer/turn process with or without assistance.

**Working Conditions**
Business office environment, days (M–F). Evening, weekend, and holiday work may be required. Medical exam/treatment rooms and medical offices. Controlled lighting, acoustics, air quality, and temperature settings. Environmental hazards may be unpredictable, including exposure to communicable diseases and biohazards.

**Risk of Exposure to Blood-Borne Pathogens**
Employees in this job description are expected to have contact with blood-borne pathogens, and as such they are required to be oriented and annually trained under the Federal Occupational Safety and Health Administration's Bloodborne Pathogen Standard.

I have read and understand the position description for Registered Nurse.

_____                              _____
Signature                                                    Date

Copy to: Personnel office
         Employee

# Sonographer
# Position Description

**Position: Sonographer**
**Fair Labor Standards Act (FLSA) status: Nonexempt**

## Job Description
A sonographer is a diagnostic ultrasound professional who is qualified by professional credentialing and academic and clinical experience to provide diagnostic patient care services using ultrasound and related diagnostic procedures. The scope of practice of the diagnostic medical sonographer includes those procedures, acts, and processes permitted by law for which the individual has received education and clinical experience, has demonstrated competency, and has completed the appropriate American Registry for Diagnostic Medical Sonography (ARDMS) certification(s), which is the standard of practice in ultrasound.

## Organizational Reporting Relationship
This position reports directly to the practice manager.

## Job Summary
Responsible for the independent operation of diagnostic medical equipment to diagnose various ob-gyn conditions and for performing and communicating results of diagnostic examinations using sonography. Sonography, or ultrasonography, is the use of sound waves to generate an image for assessment and diagnosis. This position will specialize in perinatal sonography. Ultrasound examinations include a variety of conditions ranging from routine ob-gyn to high-risk obstetrical scans and include (but are not limited to) nuchal translucency, fetal anatomy survey, Doppler studies, biophysical profile, and endovaginal scans. Experience also includes ability to perform guidance for amniocentesis, chronic villus sampling, and other invasive procedures commonly performed in a maternal-fetal medicine (MFM) program. Must be able to work independently and have thorough knowledge of high-risk situations. The sonographer is responsible for the daily operations of the sonographic laboratory, patient schedule, equipment maintenance, the report of equipment failures, and quality assessment (QA).

## Specific Duties and Responsibilities
A. Patient Information Gathering and Evaluation
1. Verifies patient identification and that the requested procedure correlates with the patient's clinical history and presentation. In the event that the requested procedure does not correlate, either the interpreting physician or the referring physician will be notified.
2. Uses interviewing techniques to gather relevant information from the patient or patient's representative and the patient's medical records regarding the patient's health status and medical history
3. Assesses the patient's ability to tolerate procedures
4. Evaluates any contraindications to the procedure, such as medications, insufficient patient preparation, or the patient's inability or unwillingness to tolerate the procedure

B. Patient Education and Communication, Support, and Management
1. Communicates with the patient in a manner appropriate to the patient's ability to understand; presents explanations and instructions in a manner that can be easily understood by the patient and other healthcare providers
2. Explains the examination procedure to the patient and responds to patient questions and concerns
3. Refers specific diagnostic, treatment, or prognosis questions to the patient's physicians

C. Analysis and Determination of Procedure Plan for Conducting the Diagnostic Examination
1. Analyzes the previously gathered information and develops a procedure plan for the diagnostic procedure; each procedure plan is based on age-appropriate and gender-appropriate considerations and actions
2. Uses independent professional judgment to adapt the procedure plan to optimize examination results; performs the ultrasound procedure under general or direct supervision, as defined by the procedure

3. Consults appropriate medical personnel, when necessary, in order to optimize examination results
4. Confers with the interpreting physician, when appropriate, to determine if contrast media administration will enhance image quality and provide additional diagnostic information
5. Determines the need for accessory equipment and uses it when appropriate
6. Determines the need for additional personnel to assist in the examination if applicable

D. Implementation of the Procedure Plan
1. Implements a procedure plan that falls within established protocols
2. Elicits the cooperation of the patient in order to carry out the procedure plan
3. Modifies the procedure plan according to the patient's disease process or condition
4. Modifies the procedure plan, as required, according to the physical circumstances under which the procedure must be performed (ultrasound room, patient's bedside [if inpatient], etc.)
5. Assesses and monitors the patient's physical and mental status during the examination
6. Modifies the procedure plan according to changes in the patient's clinical status during the procedure
7. Initiates first aid in emergency situations, as required by employer policy
8. Performs basic patient care tasks, as needed
9. Requests the assistance of additional personnel, when warranted
10. Recognizes sonographic characteristics of normal and abnormal tissues, structures, and blood flow; adjusts scanning technique to optimize image quality and spectral waveform characteristics
11. Analyzes sonography findings throughout the course of the examination so that a comprehensive exam is completed and sufficient data is provided to the physician in order to direct patient management and render a final diagnosis
12. Performs measurements and calculations according to laboratory protocols
13. Strives to minimize patient exposure to acoustic energy without compromising examination quality or completeness

E. Evaluation of Diagnostic Examination Results
1. Establishes that the examination, as performed, complies with applicable protocols and guidelines
2. Identifies any exceptions to the expected outcome
3. Documents any exceptions clearly, concisely, and completely; when necessary, develops a revised procedure plan in order to achieve the intended outcome
4. Initiates additional scanning techniques as indicated by the examination
5. Notifies an appropriate health provider when immediate medical attention is necessary, based on procedural findings and patient conditions
6. Evaluates the patient's physical and mental status prior to discharge from the ultrasound room
7. Upon assessment of the examination findings, recognizes the need for an urgent rather than routine report and takes appropriate action
8. Provides a written or oral summary of preliminary findings to the physician

F. Production of Clear and Precise Documentation Necessary for Continuity of Care, Accuracy of Care, and Quality Improvement
1. Documents diagnostic and patient data in the appropriate record, according to established policies and procedures
2. Records diagnostic images and data for use by the interpreting physician in rendering a diagnosis and for archival purposes
3. Provides an oral or written summary of preliminary findings to the interpreting physician

G. Participates in the Quality Improvement Process and Is Proactive in Fostering the Team Process throughout the Organization
1. Strives to maintain a safe workplace environment
2. Performs equipment quality assurance procedures, as required, to determine that equipment operates at an acceptable performance level
3. Seeks to ensure that the work site has in place policy manuals that address environmental safety, equipment maintenance standards, and equipment operation standards and that these policy manuals are reviewed and revised on a regular basis; knows, understands, and implements the policies set forth

4. Strives to become knowledgeable about the theory and practice of improvement process as they are applied in the clinical environment; works with all concerned parties to implement such methods and procedures, with the objective of continuously improving the quality of MFM ultrasound diagnostic services
5. Utilizes performance improvement outcome data to assist in developing written procedure protocols that meet or exceed established guidelines
6. Adheres to established policy and procedural guidelines

H. Performance Improvement, Quality of Care, and Customer Service
1. Works in partnership with the other health-care professionals to provide the best care possible for all patients, maintaining an attitude of service and excellence at all times
2. Maintains knowledge in own field of expertise
3. Participates in continuing education activities through professional societies and organizations to enhance knowledge, skills, and performance
4. Promotes a positive and collaborative atmosphere with all members of the health-care team
5. Effectively communicates with all members of the health-care team regarding the welfare of the patient
6. Shares knowledge and expertise with colleagues, patients, students, and all members of the health-care team
7. Adheres to accepted professional ethical standards and exercises appropriate customer service skills related to service, excellence, respect, value, and ethics
8. Is accountable for professional judgments and decisions

**Performance Requirements**

Knowledge
1. Knowledge of medical practices, terminology, and reimbursement policies
2. Knowledge of and ability to use electronic medical record (EMR) system
3. Sufficient knowledge of policies and procedures to accurately answer questions from internal and external customers

Skills
1. Skill in planning and organizing
2. Skill in evaluating the effectiveness of existing methods and procedures
3. Skill in problem-solving
4. Strong communicative and interpersonal skills and ability to effectively handle stressful or difficult situations with patients
5. Demonstration of dependability and initiative in job performance by being prompt in completing tasks and helping others as needed or when called upon to do so
6. Demonstration of a courteous and polite demeanor with patients and fellow employees

Abilities
1. Ability to read, interpret, and apply policies and procedures
2. Ability to recognize, evaluate, and solve problems and correct errors
3. Ability to set priorities among multiple requests
4. Ability to interact effectively with patients, medical and administrative staff, and the public

**Education**
1. Associate's or bachelor's degree in sonography from accredited school. Training may be available in hospitals, vocational-technical institutions, and the US armed forces.
2. American Registry for Diagnostic Medical Sonography (ARDMS) registration in obstetrics

**Required Licenses/Certifications**
1. Current certification with the ARDMS required
2. Nuchal translucency and nasal bone certification within one year of hire

**Experience**

1. Minimum one or more years of experience and/or training with graduate sonographer; new graduates have one year upon hiring to obtain licensure
2. Ability to type 40 wpm and operate computers and general office equipment
3. Prior EMR experience preferred

**Physical Requirements**
Standing for extended periods of time; frequent walking, sitting, carrying, lifting, balancing, bending, stooping, squatting, crouching, twisting, reaching, handling, kneeling, and the need for wrist and digital dexterity. May include patient lifting, ambulating, and the transfer of patients in wheelchairs, gurneys, and beds and/or use of mechanical lifts; speaking, hearing, and visual acuity for performing tests on patients and receiving and interpreting instructions. Ability to use phones and computer keyboards.

**Working Conditions**
In a business office or hospital, using ultrasound equipment. The ultrasound examination room lighting may be dimmed for visualization of image pictures. Employment full-time at 32 hours or more per week.

**Risk of Exposure to Blood-Borne Pathogens**
Possible exposure to potentially dangerous substances, needles, and blood. This position may have exposure to blood-borne pathogens and as such is required to be trained under the Federal Occupational Safety and Health Administration's Bloodborne Pathogen Standard.

I have read and understand the position description for Sonographer.

_____        _____
Signature                             Date


Copy to: Personnel office
         Employee

# Appendix 3

## Patient Office Forms

**[Insert Practice Name here]**

---

<u>Please print very clearly.</u>

■ Patient Information

Name (Last, First, Middle)_____

Birthdate _____ Soc. Sec. # _____

Home Phone _____ Cell Phone _____Work Phone_____

Address _____

City _____ State _____Zip_____

Sex: ☐ M ☐ F          Marital Status: ☐ Single ☐ Married ☐ Divorced
                                     ☐ Widowed ☐ Legally Separated

E-mail address _____

Employer _____

Ethnicity: ☐ Hispanic ☐ Non-Hispanic

Primary Language Spoken: ☐ English ☐ Spanish ☐ Other _____

Race: ☐ White ☐ Hispanic ☐ African American ☐ Indian ☐ Asian ☐ Pacific Islander
☐ Other_____

Referring Physician _____

Phone_____

■ Spouse / Legal Guardian

Name (Last, First, Middle) _____

Home Phone _____Cell Phone _____

Birthdate _____ Soc. Sec. # _____

Address _____

Employer _____

City _____ State _____ Zip _____ Sex: ☐ M ☐ F

■ Emergency Contact

Name (Last, First) _____Phone Number _____

Relationship _____

■ Primary Insurance

Insurance Company_____

Insurance ID #_____Group #_____

*Please enter the policyholder's information below.*

*If you are the policyholder yourself, check this box ☐ and skip to the next section.*

Policyholder's Name (Last, First, Middle)_____

Relationship to Patient_____ Soc. Sec. # _____

Birthdate _____

Address_____

Home Phone _____

Employer _____

Work Phone _____

■ Secondary Insurance *(If not applicable, please cross out section. If you have tertiary insurance, please ask the receptionist for another page.)*

Insurance Company _____

Insurance ID # _____

Group # _____

*Please enter the policyholder's information below. If you are the policyholder yourself, check this box ☐ and skip to the next section.*

Policyholder's Name (Last, First, Middle) _____

Relationship to Patient_____Soc. Sec. # _____

Birthdate _____

Address_____

Home Phone _____

Employer _____

Work Phone _____

■ Assignment and Release

**I hereby authorize payment directly to [Insert Practice Name Here] of all insurance benefits otherwise payable to me for services rendered. I understand that I am financially responsible for all charges, whether or not paid by insurance, and for all services rendered for me or for my dependents. I authorize the doctors and/or any provider or supplier of services in this office to release the information required to secure the payment of benefits. I authorize the use of my signature on all insurance submissions. I authorize a copy of this document to be used in place of the original. I have read and agreed to the above.**

**Signature:** _____

**Date:** _____

**If the patient is a minor (under 18 years of age), the responsible parent or guardian must sign above and fill in the information below.**

**Parent/Guardian Name (print):** _____

**Relationship to Patient:** _____

Patient Name:_____    Date:_____

## ■ Medical Information

Please state the reason(s) for your visit today:_____

Primary Care Physician's Name_____    Phone_____

Preferred Pharmacy Name_____    City & State_____
Pharmacy Telephone Number_____    Pharmacy Fax_____

                                                   **Yes No**

1. Are you currently under medical treatment: ☐ ☐
   Please describe:_____
   _____

                                                                                                          **Yes No**

2. Have you ever had any serious illnesses
   or operations:................................☐ ☐         Aspirin................................☐ ☐
   Please describe:_____       Other..................................☐ ☐
   _____      Please describe:_____
                                                                                                      _____

3. Are you taking any medications: ...........☐ ☐   9. Women Only:
   Please list:_____          Do you have regular periods? ..........☐ ☐
   _____       Are you using birth control pills /
4. Do you smoke? .........................................☐ ☐     patch / injection?..............................☐ ☐
5. Do you drink alcohol? .............................☐ ☐     Are you pregnant now? ....................☐ ☐
6. Do you use cocaine or other drugs? ..........☐ ☐    Have you ever been pregnant? .........☐ ☐
7. Do you have religious beliefs that could          Number of Pregnancies:_____
   impact your decision to accept
   blood products? .........................................☐ ☐
8. Have you had any allergic reactions to
   the following:
       Local Anesthetics (eg. Novacaine) ....☐ ☐
       Penicillin or other Antibiotics ..............☐ ☐
       Sulfa Drugs ........................................☐ ☐
       Barbiturates (sleeping pills) ...............☐ ☐
       Other Sedatives .................................☐ ☐
       Iodine .................................................☐ ☐

**Please indicate which of the following conditions/illnesses you have or have not had:**

|  | Yes | No |  | Yes | No |
|---|---|---|---|---|---|
| Anemia (low blood count) | ☐ | ☐ | Measles | ☐ | ☐ |
| Anorexia (no appetite) | ☐ | ☐ | Migraine | ☐ | ☐ |
| Arthritis | ☐ | ☐ | | Yes | No |
| Asthma | ☐ | ☐ | Headaches | ☐ | ☐ |
| Back Problems | ☐ | ☐ | Mitral Valve Prolapse | ☐ | ☐ |
| Bleeding Tendency | ☐ | ☐ | Mumps | ☐ | ☐ |
| Blood Disease | ☐ | ☐ | Multiple Sclerosis | ☐ | ☐ |
| Cancer | ☐ | ☐ | Pacemaker | ☐ | ☐ |
| Chemical Dependency (drug addiction) ☐ | | | Pneumonia | ☐ | ☐ |
| | ☐ | | Polio | ☐ | ☐ |
| Chemotherapy | ☐ | ☐ | Prostate Problem | ☐ | ☐ |
| Chicken Pox | ☐ | ☐ | Psychiatric Care | ☐ | ☐ |
| Chronic Fatigue Syndrome | ☐ | ☐ | Respiratory Disease | ☐ | ☐ |
| Circulatory Problems | ☐ | ☐ | Rheumatic Fever | ☐ | ☐ |
| Congenital Heart Lesions | ☐ | ☐ | Scarlet Fever | ☐ | ☐ |
| Cough – persistent or bloody | ☐ | ☐ | Shortness of Breath | ☐ | ☐ |
| Diabetes | ☐ | ☐ | Sinus Trouble | ☐ | ☐ |
| Emphysema | ☐ | ☐ | Skin Rash | ☐ | ☐ |
| Epilepsy | ☐ | ☐ | Stroke | ☐ | ☐ |
| Glaucoma | ☐ | ☐ | Thyroid Problems | ☐ | ☐ |
| Heart Murmur | ☐ | ☐ | Tonsillitis | ☐ | ☐ |
| Heart Disease | ☐ | ☐ | Tuberculosis | ☐ | ☐ |
| Hepatitis – Type ____ | ☐ | ☐ | Ulcer | ☐ | ☐ |
| Hernia | ☐ | ☐ | Venereal Disease | ☐ | ☐ |
| Herpes | ☐ | ☐ | Any Other Condition | ☐ | ☐ |
| High Blood Pressure | ☐ | ☐ | Please Describe: _____ | | |
| HIV / AIDS | ☐ | ☐ | _____ | | |
| Jaundice | ☐ | ☐ | | | |
| Kidney Disease | ☐ | ☐ | | | |
| Latex Sensitivity | ☐ | ☐ | | | |
| Liver Disease | ☐ | ☐ | | | |
| Low Blood Pressure | ☐ | ☐ | | | |

[Insert Practice Name here]

## Billing and Collection Policies

**Our goal is to provide you with high-quality and efficient care.** There are many details involved in the process of payment for the services that you receive. In order for this process to flow smoothly, it is essential that you understand what information we must share with one another and with health-insurance companies, and what both parties' responsibilities are.

**Upon scheduling and registration,** we require you to provide your medical insurance card (if you have coverage), photo identification, address, date of birth, and phone number. If you receive health benefits through a spouse, partner, or parent, we require you to provide that person's address, date of birth, and phone number as well. Our billing process works more smoothly if you provide Social Security numbers as well.

**Health-insurance cards:** Upon scheduling each appointment, our team will ask to verify your insurance information, and they will ask to see your insurance card upon check-in at each appointment. Please bring your card to every appointment and notify the office at your first appointment after that if there are changes. Intentionally failing to notify us of changes to your insurance coverage may constitute fraud, and we may be obliged to report such behavior to the authorities. We will not engage in any fraudulent practices under any circumstances.

**Keeping appointments:** In the event that you do not arrive for a scheduled appointment, unless that appointment has been cancelled at least one full business day in advance, you may be charged **[$50.00]** for each no-show occurrence. Should this occur more than twice within a twelve-month period, you may be dismissed from the practice. By signing below, you accept these policies.

**Health-insurance plans:** It is your responsibility to understand the provisions of your health-insurance plan and coverage. As helpful as we pride ourselves on being, our team cannot be expected to know the details of your particular plan, as we see hundreds of different plans every week. We recommend contacting your carrier prior to receiving services in order to verify your coverage levels and responsibilities.

**Authorizations:** You are responsible for obtaining all necessary referrals or other required documentation prior to your appointment. If our office determines that your plan requires a referral, and you do not provide such referral, you may be required to sign a waiver in order to receive services. Additionally, even should our team fail to request such a waiver, you will nonetheless be responsible for all charges that are not paid by your insurance carrier due to lack of authorization. By signing below, you accept these policies.

**Copayments:** It is our responsibility, as detailed by the terms of our contracts with health-insurance companies, to collect any copayment amounts at the time of your appointment. It is your responsibility, as detailed by the terms of your health-insurance coverage, to pay any copayment amounts at the time of your appointment. Please have your payment ready upon check-in. By signing below, you accept these policies.

**Previous balances and/or deductibles:** It is our responsibility, as detailed by the terms of our contracts with the health-insurance companies we participate with, to bill you for any portion of your treatment that your health-insurance carrier assigns to your responsibility. It is your responsibility, as detailed by the terms of your health-insurance coverage, to pay any such portion. If you do not remit full payment on any such bills within a reasonable period and with reasonable notice, your account will be sent to collections (and subject to an additional collection fee) and/or legal action will be pursued. You may be dismissed as a patient by our practice for failure to meet your financial obligations. By signing below, you accept these policies.

**Health-insurance nonpayment:** Services that have not been paid by your health-insurance carrier within sixty days of claim submission will become your responsibility to pay in full. Should your health-insurance carrier later pay us for those services you have paid for, you will be reimbursed. By signing below, you accept these policies.

**Self-pay patients:** If you do not have health insurance, have coverage through a carrier with which we do not participate, or are receiving a known noncovered service, it is our policy that you must pay for your service in full before leaving the office. By signing below, you accept these policies.

**I have read, fully understand, accept, and agree to comply with all the above policies. I consent to the assignment of authorized health-insurance benefits by my health insurer to** [Insert Practice Name here] **for any services furnished to me or my dependents.**

Signature of Patient: _____

Date: _____

If the patient is a minor (under 18 years of age), the responsible parent or guardian must sign above and indicate the relationship to the patient.

## Privacy Practices Acknowledgment and Consent Form

♦ I have received your Notice of Privacy Practices and/or I have been provided an opportunity to review it.

♦ I agree that telephone messages regarding my appointments, prescription renewals, lab results, and all other Protected Health Information* (PHI) may be left for me on voice-mail systems and answering machines at the following telephone numbers, in addition to any other numbers provided to you by me:

(\_\_ \_\_ \_\_) \_\_ \_\_ \_\_ - \_\_ \_\_ \_\_ \_\_Home / Office / Cell / Other: _____
_____

(\_\_ \_\_ \_\_) \_\_ \_\_ \_\_ - \_\_ \_\_ \_\_ \_\_Home / Office / Cell / Other: _____
_____

(\_\_ \_\_ \_\_) \_\_ \_\_ \_\_ - \_\_ \_\_ \_\_ \_\_Home / Office / Cell / Other: _____
_____

*[If we need to contact you with lab results, please place a check mark next to the preferred contact number, if any.]*

♦ I agree that my PHI may be shared with my spouse.
_____

♦ I agree that my PHI may be shared with the following other people:

_____    _____
_____    _____
_____    _____
_____    _____

♦ I understand that I can change any of the foregoing agreements, at any time, by providing written notice to **[Insert Practice Name here]**.

*\* As defined in the Health Insurance Portability and Accountability Act (HIPAA) of 1996 and its regulations, as may be amended from time to time.*

**Patient Name (print):**_____

Signature: _____

Date: _____
If the patient is a minor (under 18 years of age), the responsible parent or guardian must sign above and fill in the information below.
Parent/Guardian Name (print):   _____

Relationship to Patient: _____

Insert Logo Here

## Patient Intake Form

Date: _____  Appointment Date: _____
Patient Name: _____  Appointment Time: _____
Date of Birth: _____ **New patients please arrive ½ hour prior to appt**
Home Phone: _____ Social Security #: _____
Cell Phone: _____ Acct: _____
Initials of Preparer: _____

| Primary Insurance: | Secondary Insurance: |
|---|---|
| Subscriber: | Subscriber: |
| ID #: | ID #: |
| Group #: | Group #: |
| Employer: | Employer: |
| Phone #: | Phone #: |

**Must check one box:**
☐ Consultation and indicated diagnostic services (ultrasound, antepartum testing, amnio, cvs, invasive procedure)
☐ Diagnostic services (ultrasound, antepartum testing, amnio, cvs, invasive procedure) and indicated consultation
**Reason for referral:**
_____
_____
_____

LMP:_____ EDC: _____ by LMP / sono / exam / IVF

Weeks Pregnant: ____ Height: _____ Weight:_____

Singleton:____ Twins:____ Other:__

Gravida: ____ Fullterm:____ Preterm: ____ SAB: ____ TAB: ____ Living:_____

    **Screenings completed by referring provider:**

    ____CONF VIAB U/S ___FTS/NT ____NIPT (Cell Free/MaterniT21) ____CF ____SMA ____FragileX
    ____Quad/Penta/MSAFP

    Lab Used: _____Quest _____LabCorp Records Attached: Y / N

Referring Provider:_____ Office Phone:_____
Spoke With: _____

Please make sure previous ultrasound reports are attached along with all patient records!
Visit us on the web @ www.webadress.com
Phone: xxx-xxx-xxxx

**[Insert Practice Name/Logo here]**

## Ultrasound Consent Form

Your physician has ordered an ultrasound on you and your unborn child. There are many reasons that this diagnostic test may have been ordered. Some of these include evaluation of your baby for birth defects, growth patterns, amniotic fluid level, Doppler flow indices, abnormal blood test results, or as adjuncts to diagnostic therapeutic testing or procedures. The quality of an ultrasound examination is extremely dependent on the equipment utilized, the sonographer doing the ultrasound, the position of your baby within your womb, your body size, previous abdominal surgery, and the physician who interprets your exam.

Ultrasound examinations have never been shown to damage you or your baby. This is not an X-ray. Ultrasound uses sound waves. The ultrasound produces a small burst of high-frequency sound and then listens for the "echo" of the sound in your body. A computer then integrates this information to make the picture that you see on the screen. Many things can be seen about your baby, such as birth defects and growth abnormalities. Ultrasound is also used to see where the baby is in relation to the needle when certain invasive procedures are done, such as amniocentesis.

Failure to have this ultrasound done may make it difficult, if not impossible, to care for you and your pregnancy in the best way possible. There may be abnormalities of your reproductive system that may benefit from diagnosis and treatment. You may not be able to take advantage of many options afforded to you by law. The birth of your baby may be compromised by not being able to have the appropriate specialists present during your pregnancy and at the time of your delivery whom your baby may need. Without ultrasound, therapeutic measures would also not be possible, and this may result in a damaged baby or even the loss of the life of your baby.

The utmost care and concern is given to you and your unborn child. Even so, ultrasound is not a perfect science and things may not be seen. Factors that may limit the accuracy of the ultrasound include the gestational age of your baby, your body composition, any previous abdominal surgery, and the position of your baby within the womb. Some abnormalities are never seen with ultrasound.

*I understand that ultrasound cannot see all things in my unborn child or me but that it may be a very helpful tool to help manage my pregnancy and to plan the delivery.*

**I have read this consent, fully understand the above information, and have had all my questions answered to my satisfaction.**

☐ I wish to have an ultrasound performed on me.

☐ I decline to have an ultrasound performed on me.

Signed:_____ Date: _____

Witness:_____ Date: _____

# List of Contributors

**Brian K. Iriye, MD**
Managing partner
High Risk Pregnancy Center, Las Vegas, Nevada
Past chair, Association for Maternal Fetal Medicine Management
President-elect, Society for Maternal-Fetal Medicine
Editor; author, "Introduction" and chapters 10, 11, 19, and 23

**Anthony C. Sciscione, DO**
Director
Division of Maternal Fetal Medicine
Delaware Center for Maternal Fetal Medicine of Christiana Care, Newark, Delaware
Co-editor; author, chapter 9

**Daniel F. O'Keeffe, MD**
Executive vice president
Society for Maternal-Fetal Medicine
Co-editor; author, chapters 2, 5, and 6

**David C. Lagrew Jr., MD**
Executive medical director, women's services
Providence St. Joseph Health System—Southern California Region
Professor of clinical medicine, University of California, Irvine
Department of Obstetrics and Gynecology, Division of Maternal Fetal Medicine
Coauthor, chapter 1

**James Keller, MD, MHSA**
Vice president of medical management
Advocate Trinity Hospital, Chicago, Illinois
Division director of maternal-fetal medicine, Advocate Children's Hospital
Chair, Practice Management Division, Society for Maternal-Fetal Medicine
Author, chapter 3

**Donna D. Johnson, MD**
Professor and chair, Lawrence L. Hester Endowed Chair
Department of Obstetrics and Gynecology
Medical University of South Carolina
Author, chapter 4

**Michael R. Foley, MD**
Professor and chair
Department of Obstetrics and Gynecology
University of Arizona College of Medicine—Phoenix
Author, chapter 5

**Idahlynn Karre, PhD**
Chief executive officer
Council on Healthcare Leadership
Author, chapter 5

**Nubia Sandhu, BS**
Supervising office manager
High Risk Pregnancy Center, Las Vegas, Nevada
Author, chapter 7

**Dina Costanzo, CMOM (Certified Medical Office Manager)**
Assistant practice manager
Delaware Center for Maternal and Fetal Medicine of Christiana Care, Newark, Delaware
Author, chapter 8

**Vanita D. Jain, MD**
Director, Perinatal Special Care Unit & Antenatal Step-Down
Director, High Risk Clinics
Delaware Center for Maternal Fetal Medicine of Christiana Care, Newark, Delaware
Author, chapter 9

**Elizabeth Williams, RDMS**
Practice manager
Delaware Center for Maternal and Fetal Medicine of Christiana Care, Newark, Delaware
Author, chapter 10

**Daniel Thibodeau, MHP, PA-C, DFAAPA**
Associate Professor
Director, Clinical Education, Recruitment, and Support
Eastern Virginia Medical School, Norfolk, Virginia
Coauthor, chapter 12

**Erin McCartney, MPAS, PA-C**
Division of Maternal Fetal Medicine
Eastern Virginia Medical School, Norfolk, Virginia
Coauthor, chapter 12

**Aleece Fosnight, MPAS, PA-C**
Past president
Association of Physician Assistants in Obstetrics and Gynecology
Brevard, North Carolina
Coauthor, chapter 12

**Alfred Abuhamad, MD**
Professor and chair
Eastern Virginia Medical School Obstetrics and Gynecology, Norfolk, Virginia
Vice dean for clinical affairs, Eastern Virginia Medical School
Mason C. Andrews Chair in Obstetrics and Gynecology
Coauthor, chapter 12

**Thomas Lee, MD, MBA**
Managing Partner, Northwest Perinatal Center / Women's Healthcare Associates LLC, Portland, Oregon
Author, chapter 13

**C. Andrew Combs, MD, PhD**
Director of quality
Obstetrix Medical Group, San Jose, California
Associate director of research for Obstetrix, Division of Clinical Services, Mednax National Medical Group, Sunrise, Florida
Coauthor, chapter 14

**Alan Fishman, MD**
Medical director
Obstetrix Medical Group, San Jose, California
Director of Clinical Operations for Obstetrix, Mednax National Medical Group, Sunrise, Florida
Coauthor, chapter 14

**Stewart Gandolf, MBA**
CEO
Healthcare Success, Medical marketing and healthcare advertising agency
www.healthcaresuccess.com
Author, chapter 15

**Arnold W. Cohen, MD**
Chairman emeritus
Department of Ob-Gyn, Einstein Healthcare Network
Professor of obstetrics and gynecology
Sydney Kimmel Medical College, Philadelphia
Author, chapter 16

**Dirk Feinblatt, BS**
Practice Manager
High Risk Pregnancy Center, Las Vegas, NV
Author, chapter 17

**Fadi Bsat, MD**
Immediate Past Chair, Society for Maternal-Fetal Medicine (SMFM) Coding Committee
Associate professor
Tufts University School of Medicine
Coauthor, chapter 18

**Pamela K. Kostantenaco, LPN, CPC (Certified Practice Consultant), CMC (Certified Medical Coder)**
President
PKK Consulting Inc.
Coauthor, chapter 18

**Wilbert Fortson Jr., MD**
Staff perinatologist
Kaiser Permanente, Fontana, California
Author, chapter 20

**Frank Ciafone, MBA**
Principal consultant
Affina Healthcare Consulting, Phoenix, Arizona
Author, chapter 21

**Greg Ferrante, MCSE (Microsoft Certified Systems Engineer), CCNA (Cisco Certified Network Administrator)**
Co-executive principal
Blue Water Networks, Las Vegas, Nevada
Coauthor, chapter 22

**Megan Ferrante, BS**
Co-executive principal
Blue Water Networks, Las Vegas, Nevada
Coauthor, chapter 22

Made in the USA
Columbia, SC
24 April 2018